Reflectance Confocal Microscopy of Cutaneous Tumors

Reflectance Confocal Microscopy of Cutaneous Tumors
An Atlas with Clinical, Dermoscopic and Histological Correlations

Edited by

Salvador González MD PhD

Dermatology Service, Department of Medicine,
Memorial Sloan-Kettering Cancer Center
New York, NY
USA

Melissa Gill MD

Department of Pathology, Memorial Sloan-Kettering Cancer Center
New York, NY
USA

Allan C Halpern MD

Dermatology Service, Department of Medicine,
Memorial Sloan-Kettering Cancer Center
New York, NY
USA

informa
healthcare

First published in the United Kingdom in 2008 by Informa Healthcare, Telephone House, 69-77 Paul Street, London EC2A 4LQ. Informa Healthcare is a trading division of Informa UK Ltd. Registered Office: 37/41 Mortimer Street, London W1T 3JH. Registered in England and Wales number 1072954.

Tel: +44 (0)20 7017 5000
Fax: +44 (0)20 7017 6699
Website: www.informahealthcare.com

A CIP record for this book is available from the British Library.
Library of Congress Cataloging-in-Publication Data

Data available on application

ISBN-10: 0 415 45104 3
ISBN-13: 978 0 415 45104 8

Distributed in North and South America by
Taylor & Francis
6000 Broken Sound Parkway, NW, (Suite 300)
Boca Raton, FL 33487, USA

Within Continental USA
Tel: 1 (800) 272 7737; Fax: 1 (800) 374 3401
Outside Continental USA
Tel: (561) 994 0555; Fax: (561) 361 6018
Email: orders@crcpress.com

Distributed in the rest of the world by
Thomson Publishing Services
Cheriton House
North Way
Andover, Hampshire SP10 5BE, UK
Tel: +44 (0)1264 332424
Email: tps.tandfsalesorder@thomson.com

Composition by Exeter Premedia Services Private Ltd., Chennai, India
Printed and bound in India by Nutech Photolithographers

Contents

Contributors

Anna Liza C Agero MD
Dermatology Service, Department of Medicine
Memorial Sloan-Kettering Cancer Center
New York, NY
USA

Marco Ardigo MD
San Gallicano Dermatological Institute, IRCCS
Rome
Italy

Susanne Astner MD
Department of Dermatology
Skin Cancer Charité
University Hospital of Berlin
Berlin
Germany

Lorea Bagazgoitia MD
Department of Dermatology
Ramon y Cajal Hospital
Alcala de Henares University
Madrid
Spain

Sara Bassoli MD
Department of Dermatology
University of Modena and Reggio Emilia
Modena
Italy

Cristiane Benvenuto-Andrade MD
Dermatology Service, Department of Medicine
Memorial Sloan-Kettering Cancer Center
New York, NY
USA

Klaus J Busam MD
Department of Pathology
Memorial Sloan-Kettering Cancer Center
New York, NY
USA

Jesus Cuevas MD
Department of Pathology
University Hospital of Guadalajara
Alcala de Henares University
Guadalajara
Spain

Ruby Delgado MD
Department of Pathology
Memorial Sloan-Kettering Cancer Center
New York, NY
USA

Daniel S Gareau PhD
Dermatology Service, Department of Medicine
Memorial Sloan-Kettering Cancer Center
New York, NY
USA

Melissa Gill MD
Department of Pathology
Memorial Sloan-Kettering Cancer Center
New York, NY
USA

Salvador González MD PhD
Dermatology Service, Department of Medicine
Memorial Sloan-Kettering Cancer Center
New York, NY
USA

Allan C Halpern MD MS
Dermatology Service, Department of Medicine
Memorial Sloan-Kettering Cancer Center
New York, NY
USA

Pedro Jaen MD
Dermatology Service
Ramon y Cajal Hospital
Alcala de Henares University
Madrid
Spain

Jocelyn A Lieb MD
Dermatology Service, Department of Medicine
Memorial Sloan-Kettering Cancer Center
New York, NY
USA

Caterina Longo MD
Dermatology of Department
University of Modena and Reggio Emilia
Modena
Italy

Josep Malvehy MD
Dermatology Department (Melanoma Unit)
Hospital Clinic, Barcelona
Villaroel, Barcelona
Spain

Sanjay K Mandal MD
Dermatology Service, Department of Medicine
Memorial Sloan-Kettering Cancer Center
New York, NY
USA

Ashfaq A Marghoob MD
Dermatology Service, Department of Medicine
Memorial Sloan-Kettering Cancer Center
New York, NY
USA

Patricia Myskowski MD
Dermatology Service, Department of Medicine
Memorial Sloan-Kettering Cancer Center
New York, NY
USA

Kishwer S Nehal MD
Dermatology Service, Department of Medicine
Memorial Sloan-Kettering Cancer Center
New York, NY
USA

Yogesh G Patel MS
Dermatology Service, Department of Medicine
Memorial Sloan-Kettering Cancer Center
New York, NY
USA

Giovanni Pellacani MD
Department of Dermatology
University of Modena and Reggio Emilia
Modena
Italy

Susana Puig MD
Dermatology Department (Melanoma Unit)
Hospital Clinic, Barcelona
Villaroel, Barcelona
Spain

Milind Rajadhyaksha PhD
Dermatology Service, Department of Medicine
Memorial Sloan-Kettering Cancer Center
New York, NY
USA

Juan Luis Santiago Sánchez-Mateos MD
Department of Dermatology
Ramon y Cajal Hospital
Alcala de Henares University
Madrid
Spain

Alon Scope MD
Dermatology Service, Department of Medicine
Memorial Sloan-Kettering Cancer Center
New York, NY
USA

Stefania Seidenari MD
Department of Dermatology
University of Modena and Reggio Emilia
Modena
Italy

Martina Ulrich MD
Department of Dermatology
Skin Cancer Charité
University Hospital of Berlin
Berlin
Germany

Preface

Since the dawn of recorded medical history, the skin has been recognized as a window to the diagnosis and evaluation of disease. Ironically, the skin has been largely ignored and bypassed in the recent evolution of non-invasive diagnostic imaging technologies due to the readiness of visual inspection of the skin and ease of invasive skin biopsy. At the same time, a growing reliance on skin biopsy, blood tests, and radiologic assessments has diminished the morphologic dermatologic acumen of most clinicians including dermatologists. Fortunately, this situation has recently begun to change for the better. The growing popularity of dermoscopy has revived and expanded the attention of dermatologists to surface and subsurface morphologic details. At the same time, a host of exciting non-invasive technologies are being developed and investigated as adjuncts to the clinical examination. Examples of these technologies include high-frequency ultrasound, optical coherence tomography, spectroscopy, surface magnetic resonance imaging, and reflectance confocal microscopy (RCM).

Among these exciting new skin imaging technologies, RCM has especially caught the attention of the dermatology community. This probably reflects the strong reliance on skin biopsy and dermatopathology in clinical practice as well as the emphasis of dermatopathology in the training of dermatologists. Among all of the non-invasive imaging techniques, only RCM provides morphologic imaging with sufficient resolution to permit recognition of individual cells, resulting in quasi-histologic images.

Large expensive bench-top transmission confocal microscopes are widely used in the laboratory for high-resolution imaging of thin samples of living tissues. Smaller reflectance confocal microscopes have been developed for superficial subsurface imaging of intact skin. The technique permits real-time imaging of the epidermis and superficial dermis with sufficient resolution to resolve individual cells. The process is completely safe and painless, allowing repetitive application of the technique and observation of dynamic changes in situ over time.

This is the first atlas of RCM of the skin. It focuses on cutaneous tumor. In this atlas, we present RCM images of the most common skin neoplasms with their associated clinical, dermoscopic, and histologic appearance. Whereas we have gone to great lengths to provide good-quality RCM images, the individual frame still images included in the atlas fail to capture the wealth of information that can be gleaned during a real-time imaging session. At the bedside, images can be acquired at multiple depths within the skin, permitting one to focus up and down on individual elements within an area of interest and thus provide a three-dimensional context. Furthermore, dynamic processes such as blood flow can be observed in real time.

In the atlas, we cover various applications of confocal microscopy to the diagnosis, evaluation, and surgical management of cutaneous neoplasms. In this very young field, there are a limited number of centers studying RCM of skin tumors. This atlas represents a highly collaborative effort among many of the leaders in the field. It is a first step in what promises to be a very exciting and productive process of bringing this new technology into clinical practice. This process will require the development of a new lexicon for the description and interpretation of RCM images. A glossary provided at the end of the text (Appendix 1) will help the reader begin to become familiar with the current usage of RCM terminology.

We hope that you will share our enthusiasm for this technology and enjoy the outstanding contributions of our collaborators and colleagues.

Salvador González
Melissa Gill
Allan C Halpern

CHAPTER 1

Basic principles of reflectance confocal microscopy

Daniel S Gareau, Yogesh G Patel, and Milind Rajadhyaksha

HISTORY

The confocal microscope was invented by Marvin Minsky in 1957.[1,2] Minsky's initial instrument scanned the sample with respect to the microscope to form an image. Subsequently, the confocal microscope was adapted to image human skin in vivo, using a white light source and a spinning disk of pinholes.[3–6] Further developments included the use of a laser light source and spinning polygon mirror.[7–9] Both confocal scanning technologies have been commercialized: the spinning disc by Noran Inc. (Madison, Wisconsin, USA) and the spinning polygon by Lucid Inc. (Rochester, New York, USA).

In 1992, Noran Instruments (Madison, Wisconsin, USA) developed the tandem scanning microscope (TSM): a confocal system based on a spinning Nipkow disk using broadband illumination and providing video-rate image acquisition in reflectance mode with a 40× objective lens. This instrument was later adapted to perform in-vivo skin imaging, taking advantage of its acquisition speed. Later, a fast laser scanning confocal microscope was developed based on acousto-optic scanning technology that was also adapted and commercialized as an in-vivo skin imager that provided simultaneous reflectance and fluorescence images of the human skin.[10]

The spinning polygon design was commercialized in 1997 when Lucid Inc. produced the VivaScope 1000, which featured image acquisition over a 1.5 mm square area by sequential acquisition and mosaicing of adjacent images. Each individual image displayed a field-of-view of 500 μm. A second version produced in 2000, called the VivaScope 1500, featured the ability to mosaic over a 4 mm square area. A third version, the VivaScope 2500, is for use on ex-vivo samples and offers mosaicing of up to 20 mm square area. The latest version, introduced in 2006, is the VivaScope 3000, which is a handheld confocal microscope for in-vivo skin imaging.

OPTICAL PRINCIPLES

The common wide-field microscope illuminates and images a large volume of tissue such that ultrastructural detail is not resolved or seen. Thus, thin sections must be first prepared, as in histology, to enable observation of nuclear, cellular, and ultrastructural detail.

By comparison, the confocal microscope illuminates a small volume (voxel) from which reflected light is collected to produce a pixel. Scanning the voxel in two dimensions creates an illuminated plane that produces an image pixel by pixel. A confocal microscope images thin optical sections within whole-tissue samples such as skin in-vivo. Confocal microscopy offers clinicians a noninvasive in-vivo high-resolution real-time view of the skin.

A confocal microscope consists of a point source of light, condenser and objective lenses, and a point detector (Figure 1.1). Point illumination (i.e. of a voxel) is achieved by focusing a point or small source of light into the sample. Point detection (i.e. of a pixel) is achieved by placing a pinhole in front of the photodetector. The pinhole collects light emanating only from the focus (solid lines in Figure 1.1) and blocks light from elsewhere (dashed lines in Figure 1.1). The point source of light, the voxel within the sample and the pinhole lie in optically conjugate focal planes, leading to the name confocal. This arrangement is sensitive only to the illuminated voxel in the focus and insensitive to out-of-focus light from all other locations. Scanning the voxel in the focal plane of the objective lens enables optical sectioning: noninvasive imaging of a thin (<5 μm) section within a thick sample. This optical sectioning capability of confocal microscopy is thus an attractive adjunct to physical sectioning that is routinely performed for histology.

The mechanism of bright contrast in reflectance confocal microscopy is backscattering of light. In gray-scale confocal images, structures that appear bright (white) have components with high refractive index compared with their surroundings and/or are similar in size to the wavelength of light. Backscattering of light is primarily governed by the structures' refractive index (n) compared to the surrounding medium. Highly reflective skin components include melanin ($n = 1.72$),[11] hydrated collagen ($n = 1.43$),[12] and keratin ($n = 1.51$).[13] These components appear bright when surrounded by epidermis ($n = 1.34$) and dermis ($n = 1.41$).[13] A secondary mechanism that determines reflectivity is the size of the tissue component: tissue components that are similar in size to the wavelength of light appear bright in the image. Predictions of reflectivity based on size and refractive index can be made using Mie theory.[14]

Typical parameters of reflectance confocal microscopy are compared to those of histology in Table 1.1.

OPERATING METHODS

The commercially available confocal reflectance microscope (Figures 1.2–1.4) uses a laser with wavelength of 830 nm and a 30× water immersion objective lens with numerical aperture of 0.9. The laser power is typically 5–10 mW on the skin and causes no tissue damage. A metal ring with either a polymer or glass window is attached to the skin with medical-grade adhesive. The ring (with the attached skin) is then magnetically connected to the objective lens housing to stabilize the site of imaging (Figure 1.3D). A small drop of immersion oil is applied to the skin lesion because oil's refractive index (typically 1.50) is sufficiently close to that of the stratum corneum (1.55) and that of the polymer or glass window (1.52).

Table 1.1 Typical parameters of confocal microscopy compared to routine histology

Parameter	*Confocal*	*Histology*
Wavelength	Selectable, 400–1064 nm	Broadband white light, 400–700 nm
Maximum imaging depth	50–100 μm at 488 nm	–
	150–250 μm at 830 nm	
	300–400 μm at 1064 nm	
Section thickness	1–5 μm	5 μm
	Noninvasive, optical	Physical
Lateral resolution	0.1–1 μm	0.1–4 μm
Numerical aperture	0.7–1.4	0.1–1.4
Immersion media	Water or oil immersion	Air or oil immersion
Magnification	40–100×	1–100×
Field of view	0.5–0.2 mm	20–0.2 mm
Pinhole size	50–500 μm	–
Contrast mechanism	Endogenous reflective microstructures	Exogenous absorbing dyes
Contrast agents/stains	Melanin	Hematoxylin and eosin
	Keratin	Methylene blue
	Collagen	Toluidine blue

The immersion oil optically couples the window to the sample. The water immersion lens requires the use of water (1.33) or water-based gels such as ultrasound gel (1.35) or hair gel (1.34) placed between the window and objective lens. The water-based immersion mediums have a refractive index close to that of the epidermis (1.34), thus allowing sufficient imaging through the epidermis and into the dermis.

The objective lens may be translated parallel to the skin surface and a two-dimensional sequence of images captured and stitched in software to create a mosaic. A mosaic, called a Vivablock, displays a larger field of view (Figure 1.6). For example, the VivaScope 1500 creates a mosaic of 8 × 8 images to display a 4 × 4 mm field-of-view. Each image displays a field-of-view of 500 μm with 30× magnification; thus the mosaic displays a field-of-view of 4 mm that is equivalent to about 4× magnification. Similarly, a sequence of images may be captured in depth to display a z-stack, called a VivaStack (Figure 1.7). Furthermore, a sequence of mosaics may be captured in depth to display a cube-shaped volume of skin, called a 'Vivasuite.' Video at 15–25 frames per second (adjustable) can also be captured to document dynamic events such as leukocyte trafficking and blood flow.

REFERENCES

1. Minsky M. Microscopy Apparatus. US Patent #3013467, 1961.
2. Minsky M. Memoir on inventing the confocal scanning microscope. Scanning 1988; 10:123–8.
3. Corcuff P, Bertrand C, Leveque JL. Morphometry of human epidermis in vivo by real-time confocal microscopy. Archiv Dermatol Res 1993; 285(8):475–81.
4. Corcuff P, Leveque JL. In vivo vision of the human skin with the tandem scanning microscope. Dermatology 1993; 186(1):50–4.
5. Bertrand C, Corcuff P. In vivo spatio-temporal visualization of the human skin by real-time confocal microscopy. Scanning 1994; 16(3):150–4.
6. New K, Petroll W, Boyde A et al. In vivo imaging of human teeth and skin using real-time confocal microscopy. Scanning 1991; 13:369–72.
7. Rajadhyaksha M, Anderson RR, Webb RH. Video-rate confocal scanning laser microscope for imaging human tissues in vivo. Appl Opt 1999; 38: 2105–15.
8. Rajadhyaksha M, Gonzalez S, Zavislan JM, Anderson RR, Webb RH. In vivo confocal scanning laser microscopy of human skin II: advances in instrumentation and comparison with histology. J Invest Dermatol 1999; 113(3):293–303.
9. Rajadhyaksha M, Grossman M, Esterowitz D, Webb RH, Anderson RR. In vivo confocal scanning laser microscopy of human skin: melanin provides strong contrast. J Invest Dermatol 1995; 104(6):946–52.
10. Corcuff P, Gonnord G, Pierard GE, Leveque JL. In vivo confocal microscopy of human skin: a new design for cosmetology and dermatology. Scanning 1996; 18(5):351–5.
11. Vitkin IA, Woolsey J, Wilson BC, Anderson RR. Optical and thermal characterization of natural *(Sepia officinalis)* melanin. Photochem Photobiol 1994; 59(4): 455–62.
12. Wang X, Milner T, Chang M, Nelson J. Group refractive index measurement of dry and hydrated type I collagen films using optical low-coherence reflectometry. J Biomed Opt 1996; 1:212–16.
13. Tearney G, Brezinski M, Southern JF et al. Determination of the refractive index of highly scattering human tissue by optical coherence tomography. Opt Lett 1995; 20(21):2258–60.
14. Rajadhyaksha M, Gonzalez S, Zavislan JM. Detectability of contrast agents for confocal reflectance imaging of skin and microcirculation. J Biomed Opt 2004; 9(2):323–31.

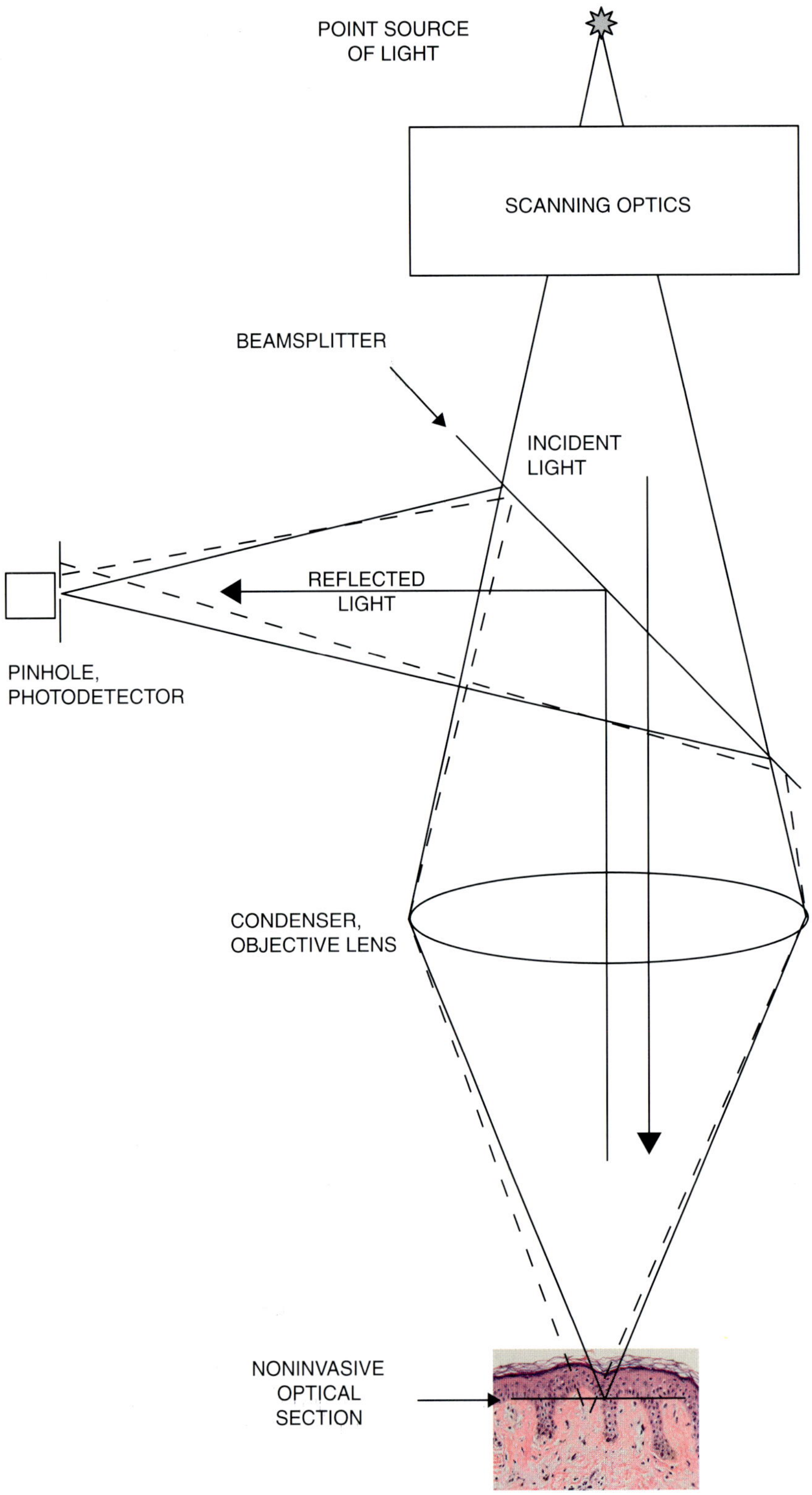

▲ **Figure 1.1** The schematic of a confocal microscope illustrating point illumination and detection. Light from out-of-focus regions (dashed line) is blocked from detection by the pinhole. The scanning optics scan the illumination point (voxel) and detection point (pixel) laterally in an en-face plane such that a thin optical section is imaged.

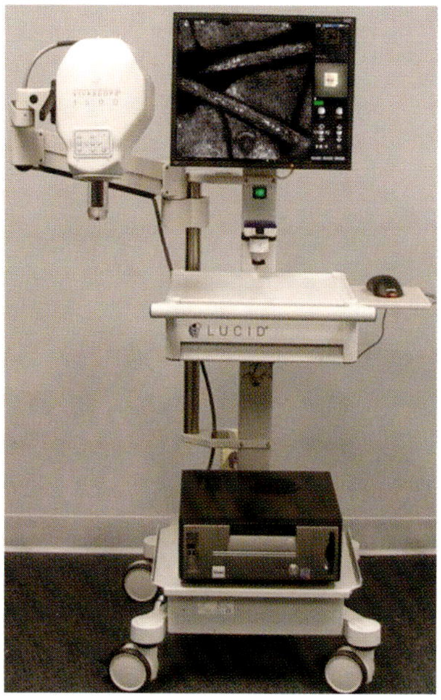

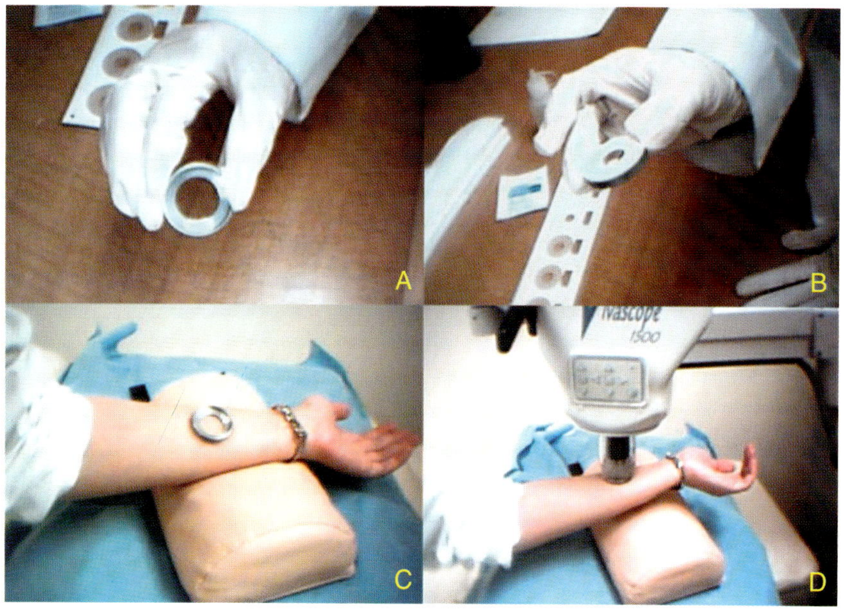

▲ **Figures 1.2, 1.3** The VivaScope 1500. An oil-based immersion medium is placed on the surface of the skin lesion. (A) Metal ring for placement on skin lesion. (B) Application of medical-grade adhesive onto metallic ring for secure attachment on skin lesion. (C) The placement of the metallic ring with medical adhesive onto skin lesion creates a well for holding a water-based immersion medium through which the objective lens images. (D) Magnetic attachment of VivaScope objective lens housing onto skin lesion to secure and stabilize site of imaging.

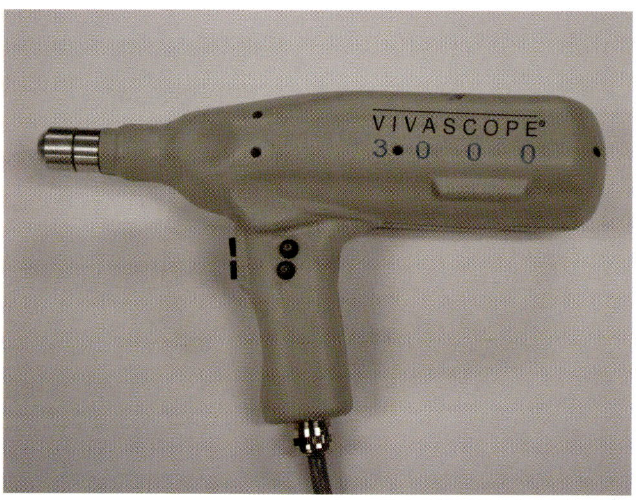

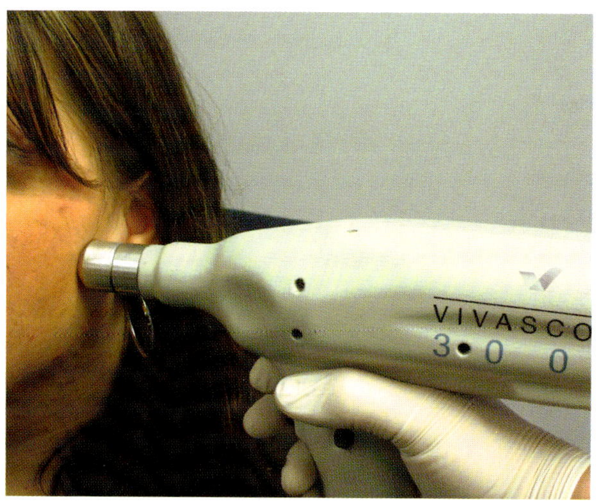

▲ **Figures 1.4, 1.5** The VivaScope 3000 handheld design connects to the computer like the articulating head of the VivaScope 1500. Application to the patient requires only immersion medium and no adhesive metallic ring.

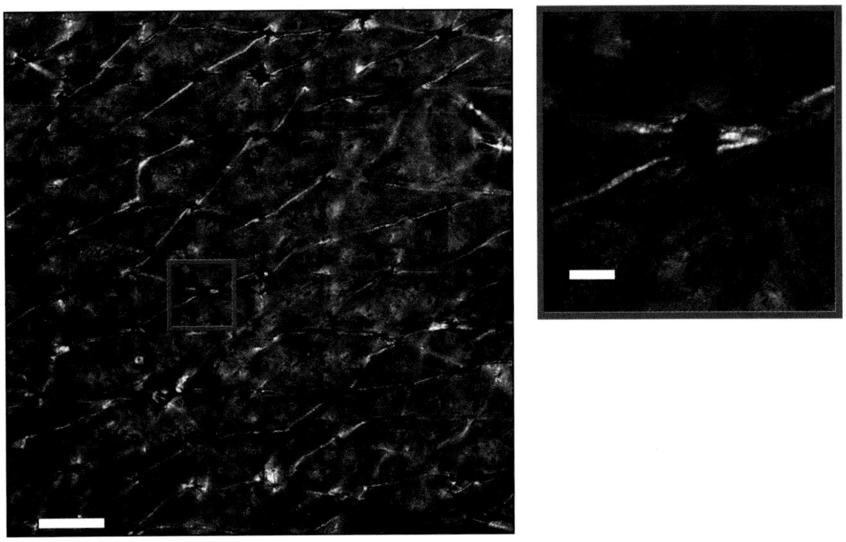

Figure 1.6

The VivaBlock from the VivaScope 1500 is a two-dimensional composite mosaic of images stitched together to create a larger field-of-view. Mosaics may be created to display 4 mm × 4 mm, 3 mm × 3 mm, or 2 mm × 2 mm field-of-view. Scale bar 500 µm. Each image (blue box) displays a 500 µm field-of-view. Scale bar 100 µm.

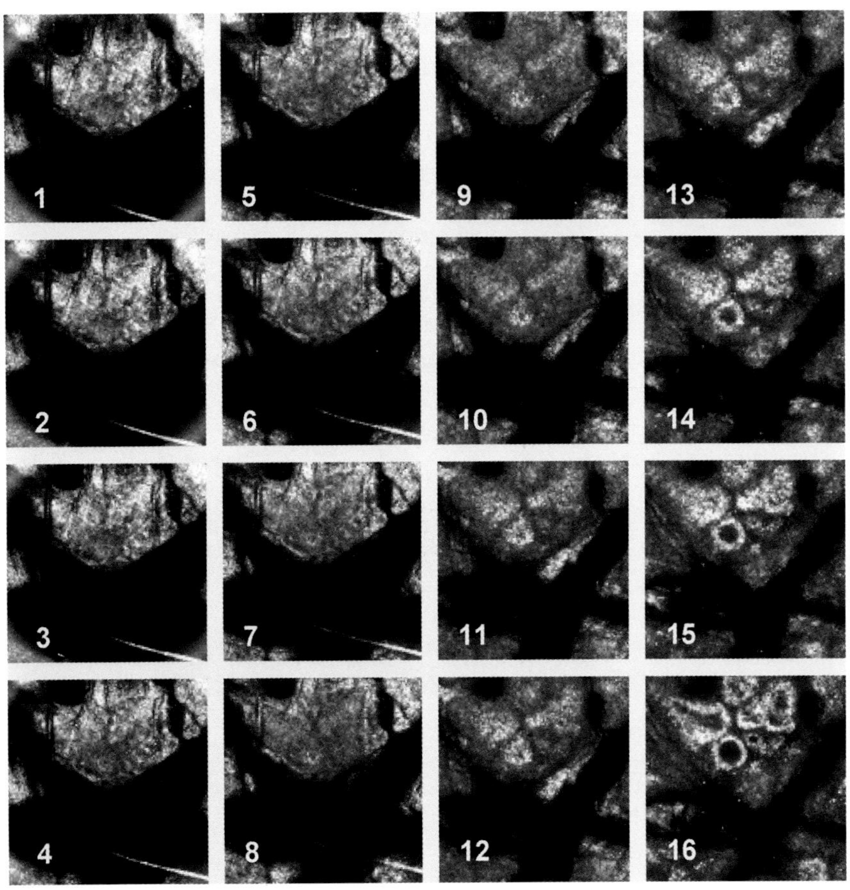

Figure 1.7

A VivaStack from the VivaScope 1500 is a z-stack of images, each image displaying a 500 µm field-of-view. The z-depth between captured images may be varied, with the typical being 3 µm. This VivaStack begins at the stratum corneum (1) and images through the dermal–epidermal junction into the papillary dermis (16).

CHAPTER 2

Normal skin

Jocelyn A Lieb, Melissa Gill, Yogesh G Patel, Milind Rajadhyaksha, and Salvador González

To appreciate features of pathologic processes as seen with reflectance confocal microscopy (RCM), a basic understanding of the attributes of normal skin is essential.

Conventional histology of excised human skin generally produces 5-μm thick sections oriented perpendicular to the skin surface, or vertical sections (Figure 2.1). In-vivo RCM produces real-time optical sections less than 5 μm in thickness, with a lateral resolution of 0.5–1.0 μm, oriented parallel to the skin surface (Figure 2.2).[1] Real-time confocal images, therefore, correspond best with histology performed in the horizontal plane (Figures 2.2, 2.3). For optimal imaging results, slight circumferential traction should be applied to the skin to create a taut surface before ring placement. Ex-vivo RCM allows for optical sectioning in any plane and from any tissue edge (surface, lateral, or deep).

The maximum in-vivo imaging depth of RCM is approximately 150–350 μm (dependent on tissue) and generally allows for imaging from the surface of the skin to the papillary dermis or upper reticular dermis in areas characterized by thin epidermis, such as the inner forearm.[1] However, in areas characterized by thick epidermis, such as palmoplantar skin, only the very superficial papillary dermis can be imaged. A technique called 'tape stripping' may be employed to remove layers of the stratum corneum, enabling deeper imaging of hyperkeratotic skin.

The epidermis is composed primarily of keratinocytes, with minority populations of dendritic cells (melanocytes and Langerhans cells). The dermis consists of blood vessels, nerves, inflammatory cells, and fibroblasts enveloped in a network of collagen and elastic fibers. The papillary dermis forms upward finger-like projections into the epidermis, called dermal papillae. The dermis and epidermis meet at the undulating dermal–epidermal junction (DEJ), which is architecturally similar to the topographical surface of an egg carton; the papillary dermis forms the egg carton and the epidermis is a mold poured over the egg carton.

In the epidermis, keratinocytes differentiate to constitute the four epidermal layers. Using RCM, it is possible to distinguish the epidermal layers based on architectural and cytologic features as well as location/depth. Table 2.1 shows the depth levels of normal skin structures on RCM.[2] Table 2.2 shows the refractive (contrast) intensity of various structures on RCM.

EPIDERMAL LEVELS

Stratum corneum

The stratum corneum (corneal layer) is the most superficial layer of the epidermis and is composed of flattened anucleated keratinocytes (Figure 2.6). This layer varies in thickness depending on topographic site and sun exposure, being thickest on the palms and soles. The stratum corneum is found at an approximate depth of 0–15 μm from the skin surface. By RCM, this layer appears as a variably refractile surface with visible skin folds and large polygonal-shaped anucleated keratinocytes, each with an approximate dimension of 25–50 μm (Figures 2.4, 2.5).[1,2] Skin folds (dermatoglyphs)

Table 2.1 Depth of normal skin structures on RCM

Structure	*Depth*	*Mean keratinocyte width*
Stratum corneum	0–15 μm	25–50 μm
Stratum granulosum	10–20 μm	25–35 μm
Stratum spinosum	20–100 μm	15–25 μm
Stratum basalis	40–130 μm	7–12 μm
Papillary dermis	50–150 μm	–
Reticular dermis	>150 μm	–

appear as non-refractile or dark, linear valleys between groups of keratinocytes. The depth of the skin fold, which may extend as deep as the spinous layer, depends on factors such as skin phototype, topographic area, and sun exposure. The amount of traction applied to the skin prior to ring placement may also influence the appearance and depth of skin folds.

Stratum granulosum

The stratum granulosum (granular layer) is composed of somewhat flattened keratinocytes containing cytoplasmic keratohyaline granules and large, oval nuclei (Figure 2.9). This layer varies from 1 to 3 cells in thickness to 10 cells in thickness in hypercornified sites such as the palms and soles.[3] The stratum granulosum is found at an approximate depth of 10–20 μm from the skin surface, depending on topographic site.[1,2] By RCM, a granular keratinocyte has an approximate dimension of 25–35 μm and contains a round to oval dark central area, corresponding to its nucleus, with a surrounding rim of bright grainy cytoplasm. Commonly seen within the dark nucleus of granular keratinocytes is the nucleolus, which appears as a central white dot. The cytoplasm appears bright due to the presence of numerous, refractile 0.1–1.0 μm structures, which correspond to organelles and keratohyaline granules.[2] The keratinocytes have clearly demarcated cell borders and are arranged in a honeycomb pattern (Figures 2.7, 2.8).

Stratum spinosum

The stratum spinosum (spinous layer) is composed of polygonal-shaped keratinocytes, which progressively flatten towards the surface (Figure 2.11). The spinous layer usually varies from 5 to 10 cells in thickness and is found at an approximate depth of 20–100 μm below the skin surface.[1–3] By RCM, a spinous keratinocyte has an approximate dimension of 15–25 μm, is polygonal in shape, contains an oval to round dark central area, corresponding to its nucleus, and a bright rim of cytoplasm.[2] The keratinocytes have clearly demarcated cell borders and are arranged in a honeycomb pattern (Figure 2.10).

Stratum basalis

The stratum basalis (basal layer) is a single layer of columnar keratinocytes with randomly dispersed melanocytes, located just above the basement membrane. Histologically, these actively proliferating keratinocytes often contain supranuclear melanin (Figures 2.14, 2.17). Melanocytes appear as small round to stellate cells dispersed among the basal keratinocytes at an average rate of 1 per every 10 basal keratinocytes.[3] The basal layer is found at an approximate depth of 40–130 μm below the skin surface.[2] Melanin is a major source of contrast for RCM of the epidermis.[4] These keratinocytes generally appear brighter than spinous keratinocytes, are uniform in size and shape, and each measures approximately 7–12 μm in dimension[4] (Figures 2.12, 2.13, 2.15, 2.16). In skin phototype I, the basal keratinocytes have low refractility (contrast) and are difficult to elucidate (Figure 2.21). In skin phototypes II–VI, confocal sections through the upper aspect of the basal layer reveal a cobblestone pattern created by clusters of relatively bright round cells, corresponding to supranuclear melanin caps (Figures 2.12, 2.13, 2.18). Upon deeper imaging through these cells, the dark nucleus is seen with a moderately bright rim of cytoplasm. In anatomic sites with rete ridges, these cells are arranged in a circular pattern surrounding a dark dermal papilla, termed a dermal papillary ring (Figures 2.15, 2.16, 2.18). However, in areas with flattened rete ridges this circular arrangement is not seen (Figure 2.31C, D). Interspersed melanocytes may appear as bright stellate cells.[5]

Dermal–epidermal junction

The dermis and epidermis meet at the undulating DEJ, where, as discussed above, the dermis forms upward finger-like projections into the epidermis called dermal papillae. By RCM, the dermal papillae appear as dark areas with microcirculation through capillary loops and minimal refractile collagen, surrounded by a ring of basal keratinocytes (Figures 2.15, 2.16, 2.18E,F). In light-skinned individuals dermal papillary rings may not be visualized, whereas in darker-skinned individuals dermal papillary rings are very noticeable, appearing as bright, well-demarcated keratinocytes arranged in rings surrounding dermal papillae (Figures 2.21, 2.22, 2.35–2.37).

Other cell types

Langerhans cells are normally inconspicuous on both histology and RCM. When activated, Langerhans cells appear as highly refractile dendritic cells, which are difficult to distinguish from dendritic melanocytes, reactive or neoplastic, by RCM (Figures 2.19, 2.20).[6]

DERMAL LEVELS

Below the dermal–epidermal junction is the dermis, which varies in overall thickness from 0.3 mm on the eyelid to 3.0 mm on the back and can be subdivided into two anatomic subunits, papillary dermis and reticular dermis.[7]

Papillary dermis

The papillary dermis includes the dermal papillae and the thin layer of dermis between the base of the rete ridges and the superficial vascular plexus. It is composed of a finely woven network of collagen and elastin, fibroblasts, blood vessels, lymphatics, nerve endings, and scattered inflammatory cells (Figure 2.24). The papillary dermis is found at an approximate depth of 50–150 μm beneath the skin surface.[1,2] By RCM, the papillary dermis is usually darker than the epidermis, lacks visible nuclei, and contains varying amounts of refractile collagen (Figures 2.21, 2.22). When rete ridges are preserved, the papillary dermis appears dark with gray collagen fibers and is surrounded by a ring of bright basal keratinocytes. Collagen fibers may appear as a reticulated meshwork or as bright bundles (see 'Collagen' section). During real-time imaging or on video capture, capillary loops with circulating blood cells can be seen (see 'Blood Vessels' section).

Reticular dermis

The reticular dermis extends from the base of the superficial vascular plexus to the subcutis and is composed of thickened collagen bundles, elastic fibers, fibroblasts, inflammatory cells, a network of blood vessels, lymphatics, and nerves, and contains site-specific adnexal structures (Figure 2.24). The reticular dermis is found at an approximate depth of >150 μm beneath the skin surface.[1,2] Only the upper reticular dermis can be visualized by in-vivo RCM, and it is often difficult to assess through intact skin due to backscatter of light from the overlying structures. When assessable by in-vivo RCM, the reticular dermis reveals gray, thick, slightly hyper-refractile bundles of collagen arranged in a fascicular pattern with interspersed dark lumina, corresponding to blood vessels, and a few small, refractile cells, corresponding to inflammatory cells (Figure 2.23).

Collagen

Collagen appears as low to moderately refractile fibrillar structures arranged in a reticulated or web-like pattern or as bundles gathered into large fascicles.[2] The reticulated pattern is typically seen in the papillary dermis (Figures 2.21, 2.22), while the fasciculated pattern is more commonly seen in the reticular dermis (Figure 2.23). Fibrillar collagen has a diameter of 1–5 μm and bundled collagen has a diameter of 5–25 μm.[2]

Blood vessels

Blood vessels walls are weakly refractile and serum appears dark/black. Erythrocytes measure 6–9 μm in diameter and are weakly refractile.[1] Leukocytes vary from 6 to 30 μm in diameter and range from weakly refractile (most lymphocytes) to bright and granular (granulocytes).[1] Platelets measure 2–5 μm in diameter and are moderately bright and granular.[1] Blood vessels therefore appear as dark tubular or canalicular structures containing a mixture of weakly refractile and brightly refractile cells (Figure 2.25). Blood vessels are best visualized during real-time imaging, where they can be identified by the movement of bloods cells through their lumina. Typically, leukocytes can be seen rolling slowly along the vessel wall, whereas erythrocytes move quickly through the vessel lumen.[1]

ADNEXAL STRUCTURES

Due to the restricted imaging depth of RCM, in-vivo imaging of intact skin only visualizes the upper portion of adnexal structures, whereas deeper aspects can be seen using ex-vivo imaging.

Follicle

The infundibular portion of the hair follicle is the only segment of the follicle visualized by in-vivo RCM. The follicle appears as an ostium lined by central rough, refractile keratin debris, often containing a central hair shaft (see 'Hair shaft' section) (Figures 2.26, 2.27). Beneath the keratin are cells of different sizes in an ordered pattern, reflecting the various layers of the infundibular epithelium similar to surface epidermis. The cells vary from small, ovoid, or polygonal basal cells to larger, flatter surface cells. Occasionally, well-defined, weakly refractile structures, probably representing *Demodex* mites, are seen within the follicle (Figures 2.28, 2.29).

Hair shaft

The hair shaft appears as a long cylindrical acellular structure with a highly refractile surface and a somewhat less refractile central core. It is typically seen emanating from a round, non-refractile hair follicle lumen (see 'Follicle' section) (Figure 2.30A–D).

Eccrine duct/gland

The intraepidermal eccrine duct, or the acrosyringium, and the superficial intradermal eccrine duct are the only portions of the eccrine sweat apparatus visualized with in-vivo RCM. The acrosyringium is 3–4 cell-thick, keratinizing epithelium, which spirals through the epidermis and opens onto the skin surface (Figure 2.31F). By RCM, the acrosyringium appears as an ostium lined by highly refractile debris, which spirals through the epidermis (Figure 2.31A–D). It is reminiscent of a hair follicle, but typically has a smaller diameter, is less straight, and does not contain a central hair shaft. The intradermal eccrine duct is a bilayer composed of a luminal, cuboidal layer and an outer, flattened basal layer. By RCM, the intradermal eccrine duct appears as an often grouped, round, weakly refractile donut-shaped structure with a darker outer ring, an internal weakly refractile donut shape, and a central, small dark lumen (Figure 2.31E).

Apocrine duct/gland

Apocrine ducts are generally not seen, as they usually insert into the follicular infundibulum just above the insertion point of the sebaceous duct. Occasionally, the apocrine duct may not insert into the follicle, but rather independently passes through the epidermis directly opening onto the skin surface. These intraepidermal apocrine ducts may be visualized by in-vivo RCM; they are usually located adjacent to a follicle, are straight not coiled, resembling a follicle without a hair shaft rather than an acrosyringium, and they are only found in specialized sites such as groin and axilla.

Sebaceous duct/gland

Sebaceous glands are found in highest concentration on the face, where the epidermis is relatively thin. As a result, occasionally the surface of a sebaceous gland can be visualized, especially in the context of sebaceous hyperplasia. The lipid droplets contained within the sebaceous acinar cells are highly refractile on RCM, giving the glands a bright morular appearance. Each individual sebocyte contains a central, round, dark area, corresponding to its nucleus and a well-defined rim of bright speckled cytoplasm (Figures 2.32, 2.33).

ANATOMIC/TOPOGRAPHIC SITE VARIATION

Face

The skin of the face differs greatly from that of the torso and extremities. On the face, the rete ridges

Table 2.2 Refractile structures in decreasing brightness

High refractility	Bright
Melanin-containing cells	
Melanocyte cytoplasm	
Melanophage cytoplasm	
Pigmented keratinocyte cytoplasm	
Keratin-containing structures	
Stratum corneum	
Infundibular epithelium	
Hair shaft	
Acrosyringium	
Activated Langerhans cell cytoplasm	
Granulocyte (WBC) cytoplasm	
Medium refractility	
Spinous keratinocyte cytoplasm	
Sebocyte cytoplasm	
Keratohyaline granules	
Nucleoli	
Collagen	
Low refractility	
Red blood cells	
Lymphocytes	
Skin folds (very low)	
Nuclei (very low)	
No refractility	
Air	
Serum	Dark

are flattened with increased density of pilosebaceous units.[2] In fair-skinned individuals lacking brightly refractile basal cell melanin caps, the transition from epidermis to dermis is very subtle, and, on the face, because of the increased numeric density of pilosebaceous units, it can be difficult to detect (Figure 2.34A–B).

Palmoplantar

The epidermis of the palms and soles is thicker than that of the rest of the body and therefore appears different on RCM. The stratum corneum is thicker, as are the stratum granulosum and stratum spinosum.[2] Additionally, the palms and soles show a much higher concentration of eccrine ducts/glands relative to other sites and a total absence of hair follicles (Figure 2.34C, D). Because of the increased thickness of the stratum corneum, imaging of the lower epidermal layers and the dermis is more challenging than on other anatomic sites.

Back/extremities

Normal skin of the back is associated with a decreased en-face density of granular keratinocytes, an increased en-face density of spinous keratinocytes, and a decreased number of basal keratinocytes per millimeter of DEJ as compared to the cheek, forehead, inner forearm, outer forearm, and leg (Figure 2.34E, F). Normal skin of the leg is associated with a thinner stratum corneum and a thicker stratum granulosum as compared to the cheek, forehead, inner forearm, outer forearm, and back. Normal skin of the inner forearm has a thinner stratum corneum, a thicker stratum granulosum, a decreased en-face density of granular keratinocytes, and an increased en-face density of spinous keratinocytes as compared to the outer forearm.[2]

SKIN PHOTOTYPES

The cytoplasm of keratinocytes in darkly pigmented skin is markedly more refractile than that of lightly pigmented skin because melanin provides strong cytoplasmic contrast.[4] This increased contrast aids in the proper identification of the epidermal layers and, more specifically, the basal layer.[4] In skin phototype I, it may be difficult to distinguish the basal layer from the spinous layer, and, consequently, the transition to papillary dermis (Figures 2.21, 2.35). Due to the relative lack of epidermal contrast as compared to other phototypes, dermal collagen bundles often appear relatively more refractile than the epidermis (Figure 2.21). In skin phototypes II–VI, with increasing phototype, basal keratinocytes are progressively more refractile due to changing quality and quantity of intracellular melanin (Figures 2.36, 2.37).[4] In progressively higher phototypes, refractile melanin is also seen in suprabasal keratinocytes, which can result in increased refractility of the overlying epidermal layers and contribute to the increased brightness of the stratum corneum seen in darker-skinned individuals.[2,4]

SUN-PROTECTED, SUN-EXPOSED, AND SUN-DAMAGED SKIN

Sun-protected sites

In sun-protected sites, the stratum corneum is thinner, while the stratum granulosum is thicker. There is a decreased en-face density of granular keratinocytes and an increased en-face density of spinous keratinocytes. Dermal papillae appear evenly distributed and are round to ellipse in shape. They occur less frequently, but are significantly larger in diameter than dermal papillae in areas with chronic sun exposure. Papillary dermal capillaries are fewer in number, larger in diameter, and arranged in isolated loops. Collagen fibers are well defined, elongated, and fibrillar, forming delicate networks in the papillary dermis.[2] With increasing age, there is progressive flattening of the epidermis, decreased pigmentation, fewer melanocytes and Langerhans cells, thinner and fewer elastic fibers, coarser and somewhat haphazard collagen fibers, and fine, temporary wrinkles, or wrinkles that reduce with stretching.[8]

Sun-exposed and sun-damaged sites

In sun-exposed sites, the stratum corneum appears brighter and is thicker, while the stratum granulosum is thinner. The en-face density of keratinocytes in the stratum granulosum is increased, while the en-face density of keratinocytes in the stratum spinosum is decreased. In the stratum spinosum, intercellular demarcations can be increased in thickness and, in frankly sun-damaged skin, random keratinocytic atypia is often encountered. Dermal papillae appear randomly distributed and are irregular in shape. They occur with higher frequency, but have smaller and more varied diameters than dermal papillae in sun-protected sites. Papillary dermal capillaries are greater in number, smaller in diameter, and arranged in small clusters. In the superficial dermis of sun-exposed and sun-damaged skin, a network of thicker, refractile collagen bundles are intermixed with varying amounts of slightly less refractile, fragmented, fuzzy, lacy or spiral structures, corresponding to solar elastosis (Figures 2.38–2.40).[2] Additional features of frankly sun-damaged skin which can be appreciated on RCM include epidermal atrophy or mild epidermal acanthosis, rete ridge effacement, increased pigmentation, extensive solar elastosis, decreased amount of dermal collagen, and permanent deep coarse wrinkles, which do not reduce with stretching.[8]

Key RCM features of normal skin

- Stratum corneum: highly refractile and granular
- Stratum granulosum: regular honeycomb pattern formed by polygonal cells with moderately refractile granular cytoplasm and dark central nuclei
- Stratum spinosum: regular honeycomb pattern formed by smaller polygonal cells with moderately refractile cytoplasm and dark central nuclei
- Stratum basalis (skin phototypes II–VI): bright supranuclear melanin caps form a regular cobblestone pattern
- Stratum basalis (skin phototype I): poorly pigmented basal cells are difficult to distinguish from surrounding cells
- Dermal–epidermal junction (skin phototypes II–VI): bright basal cells with dark basal nuclei form rings around dark central dermal papillae or bright dermal papillary rings
- Dermal–epidermal junction (skin phototype I): weakly refractile basal cells form rings around relatively brighter central dermal papillae or dark dermal papillary rings
- Dermis: moderately refractile collagen bundles and blood vessels with dark lumina containing bright granulocytes and weakly refractile erythrocytes

REFERENCES

1. Rajadhyaksha M, Gonzalez S, Zavislan JM, Anderson RR, Webb RH. In vivo confocal scanning laser microscopy of human skin II: advances in instrumentation and comparison with histology. J Invest Dermatol 1999; 113(3):293–303.
2. Huzaira M, Rius F, Rajadhyaksha M, Anderson RR, Gonzalez S. Topographic variations in normal skin, as viewed by in vivo reflectance confocal microscopy. J Invest Dermatol 2001; 116(6):846–52.
3. Murphy G. Histology of the skin. In: Elder DE, Elenitsas R, Johnson BL Jr, Murphy GF, eds. Lever's Histopathology of the Skin, 9th edn. Philadelphia: Lippincott Williams & Wilkins; 2005: 9–58.
4. Rajadhyaksha M, Grossman M, Esterowitz D, Webb RH, Anderson RR. In vivo confocal scanning laser microscopy of human skin: melanin provides strong contrast. J Invest Dermatol 1995; 104(6):946–52.

5. Busam KJ, Charles C, Lee G, Halpern AC. Morphologic features of melanocytes, pigmented keratinocytes, and melanophages by in vivo confocal scanning laser microscopy. Mod Pathol 2001; 14(9):862–8.

6. Busam KJ, Marghoob AA, Halpern A. Melanoma diagnosis by confocal microscopy: promise and pitfalls. J Invest Dermatol 2005; 125(3):vii.

7. Habif T. A Color Guide to Diagnosis and Therapy. In: Clinical Dermatology, 4th edn. Philadelphia: Mosby; 2004.

8. McKee PH, Calonje E, Granter SR. Diseases of collagen and elastic tissue: cutaneous effects of chronic sun damage and chronological aging. In: McKee PH, Calonje E, Granter SR, eds. Pathology of the Skin with Clinical Correlations, Vol. 2, 3rd edn. Philadelphia: Elsevier Mosby; 2005: 1053–4.

NORMAL SKIN

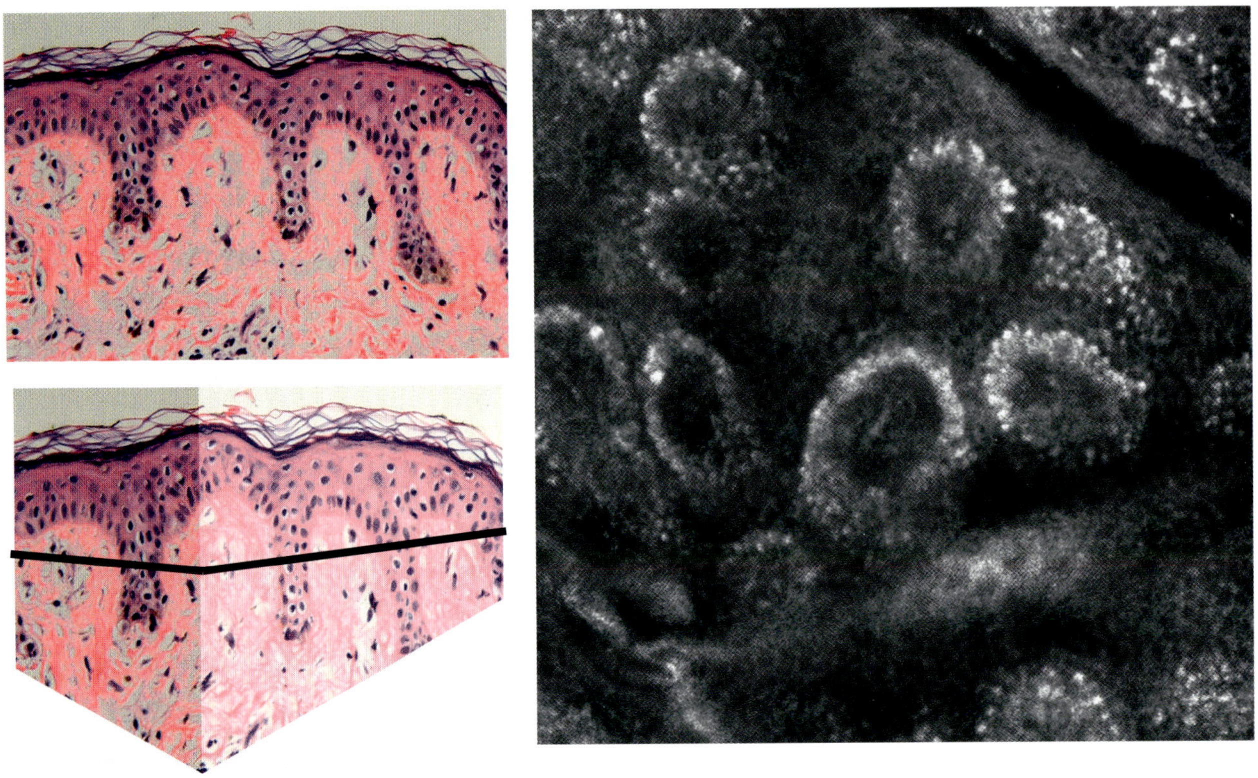

▲ **Figures 2.1–2.3** Upper left: vertical histologic section of the skin. Lower left: schematic demonstrating the horizontal axis of the RCM image (black line). Right panel: the corresponding horizontal (en-face) plane of the RCM image (0.5 mm × 0.5 mm).

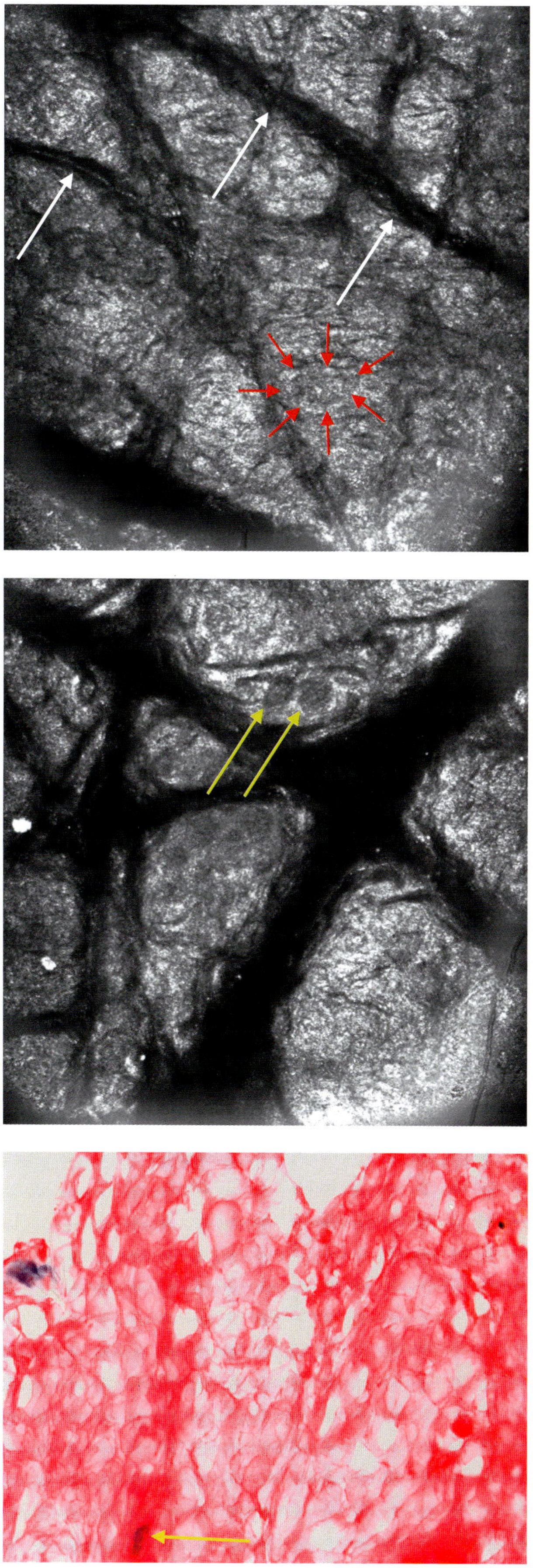

◂ **Figures 2.4–2.6**

These en-face RCM images (0.5 mm × 0.5 mm) show the stratum corneum with its highly refractile surface and prominent skin folds (white arrows). The centre image is from a slightly deeper level and shows a few nucleated cells which are transitioning from granular keratinocytes to anucleated corneocytes (yellow arrows). The fully differentiated anucleated corneocytes have poorly demarcated cell borders and blend together (red arrows). Horizontal frozen section histology (40×) shows the en-face appearance of large anucleated keratinocytes of the stratum corneum and a single transitioning granular keratinocyte (yellow arrow).

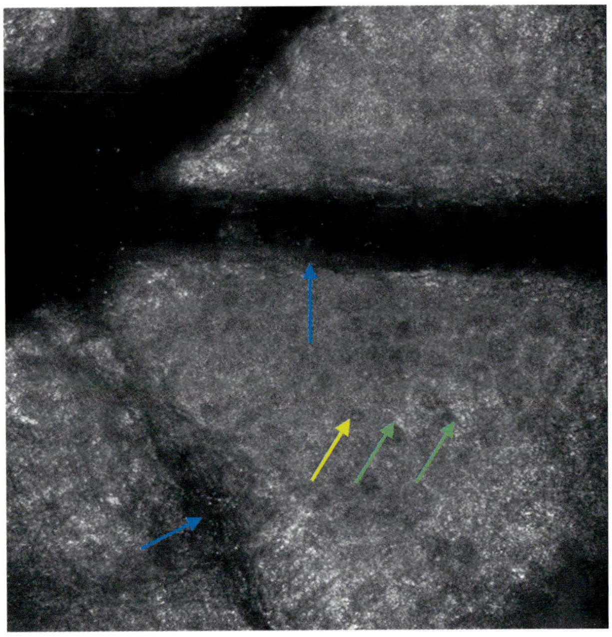

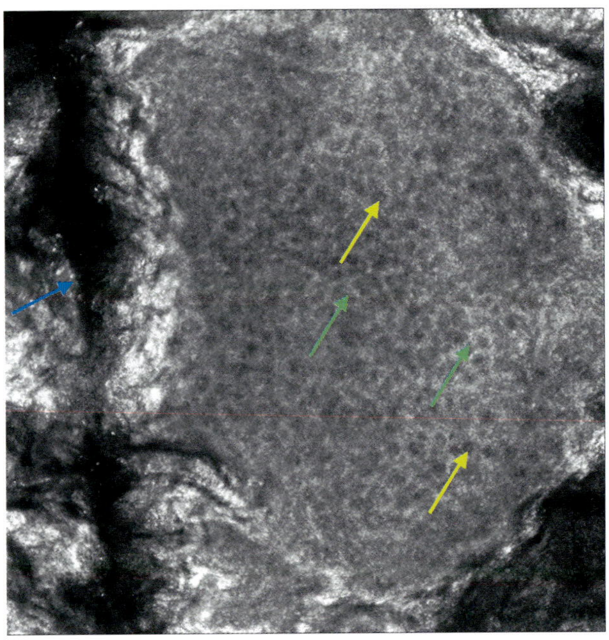

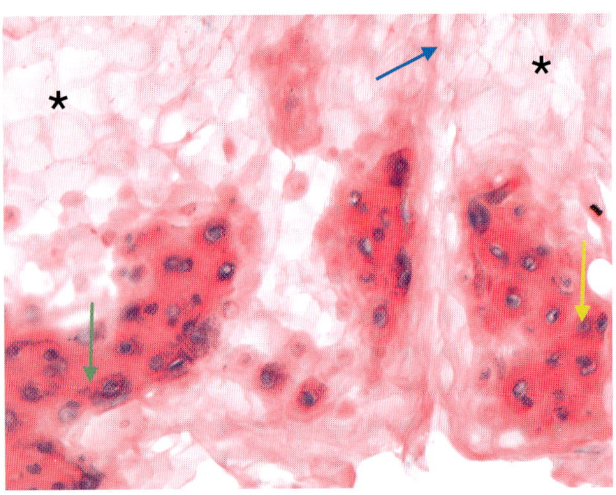

◀ **Figures 2.7–2.9**

These en-face RCM images (0.5 mm × 0.5 mm) of the stratum granulosum show polygonal keratinocytes with grainy cytoplasms (green arrows) and dark central nuclei containing nucleoli (yellow arrows) arranged in a honeycomb pattern, surrounded by skin folds (blue arrows). Horizontal frozen section histology (40×) shows the en-face appearance of the stratum corneum (asterisks) and stratum granulosum.

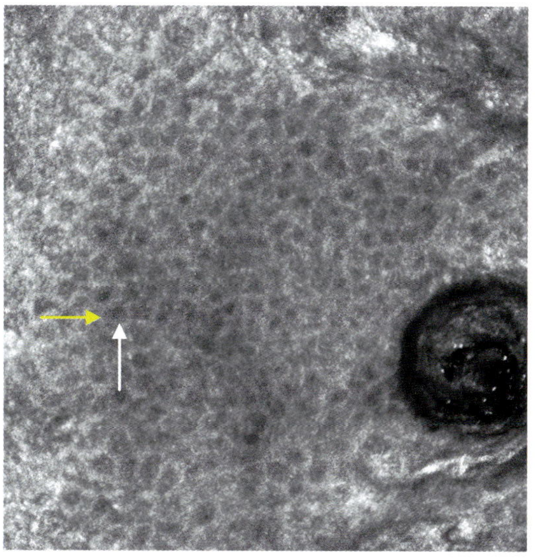

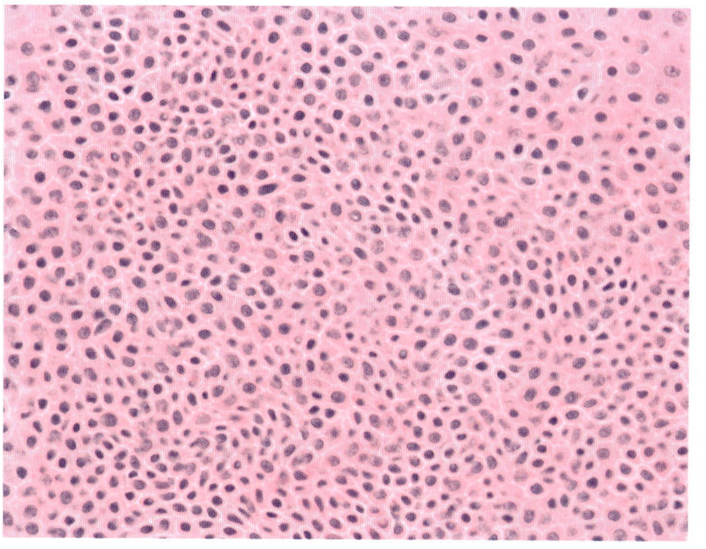

▲ **Figures 2.10, 2.11** This en-face RCM image (0.5 mm × 0.5 mm) of the stratum spinosum shows polygonal keratinocytes with dark central nuclei (white arrow) surrounded by a rim of bright cytoplasm (yellow arrow) arranged in a honeycomb pattern. Horizontal frozen section histology (40×) shows the en-face appearance of the stratum spinosum.

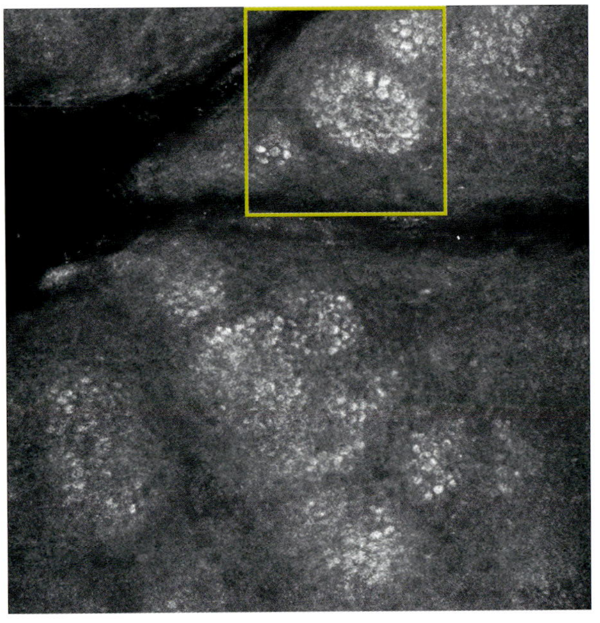

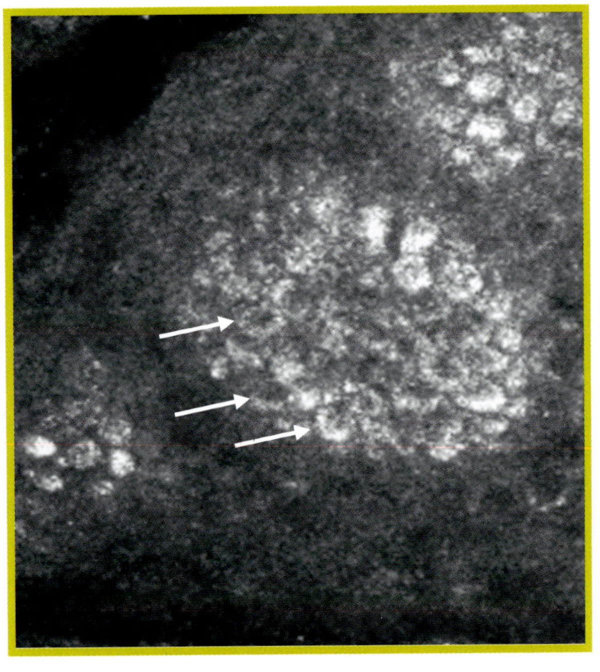

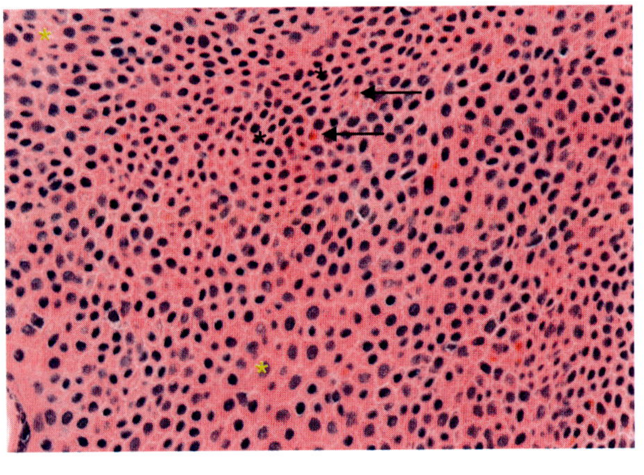

◀ **Figures 2.12–2.14**

En-face RCM (0.5 mm × 0.5 mm, upper) of the superficial stratum basalis shows a cobblestone pattern formed by clusters of bright, round cells, which correspond to supranuclear melanin caps. A subimage (yellow square, upper and 0.2 mm × 0.2 mm, lower) reveals some cells with central dark areas (arrows), or nuclei, indicating that these cells are in a slightly higher plane and thus have been transected at a slightly deeper level. Horizontal frozen section histology (40×) shows the en-face appearance of larger poorly pigmented deep spinous keratinocytes (yellow asterisks), and smaller, pigmented basal cells transected through the supranuclear melanin cap (arrows) or the nucleus (black asterisks).

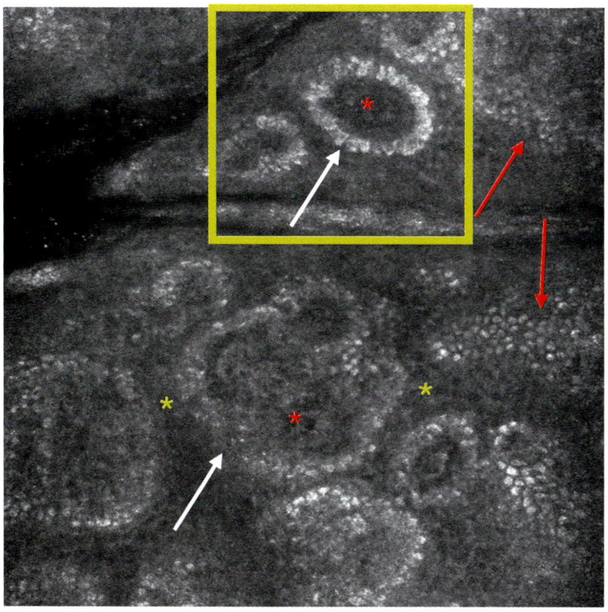

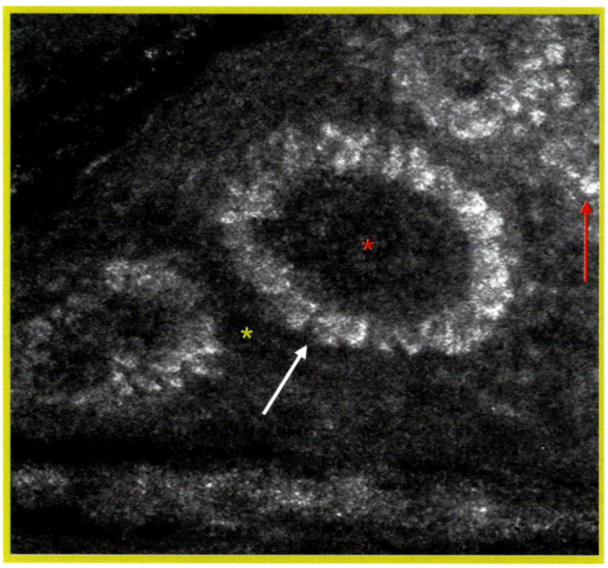

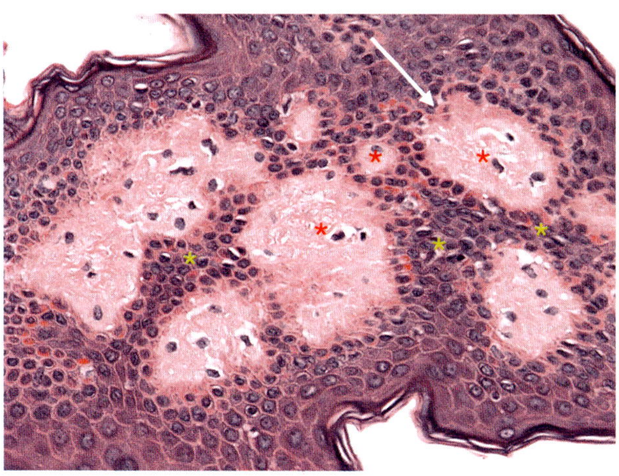

◀ **Figures 2.15–2.17**

The en-face RCM image and subimage (0.5 mm × 0.5 mm, upper ; and 0.3 mm × 0.27 mm, lower) at the level of the superficial DEJ of a patient with skin phototype III demonstrate dermal papillary rings (white arrows) surrounding dermal papillae (red asterisks). Some dermal papillae are smaller in diameter, indicating they have been imaged more superficially or that the suprapapillary plate slightly thicker. In other areas, a cobblestone patttern is seen (red arrows), indicating transection through the supranuclear melanin caps of the stratum basalis. Between the dermal papillary rings are downward extensions of epidermis forming a meshwork of rete ridges, which show a honeycomb pattern (yellow asterisks). Horizontal frozen section histology (40×) from a less-pigmented individual shows the en-face appearance of the superficial DEJ.

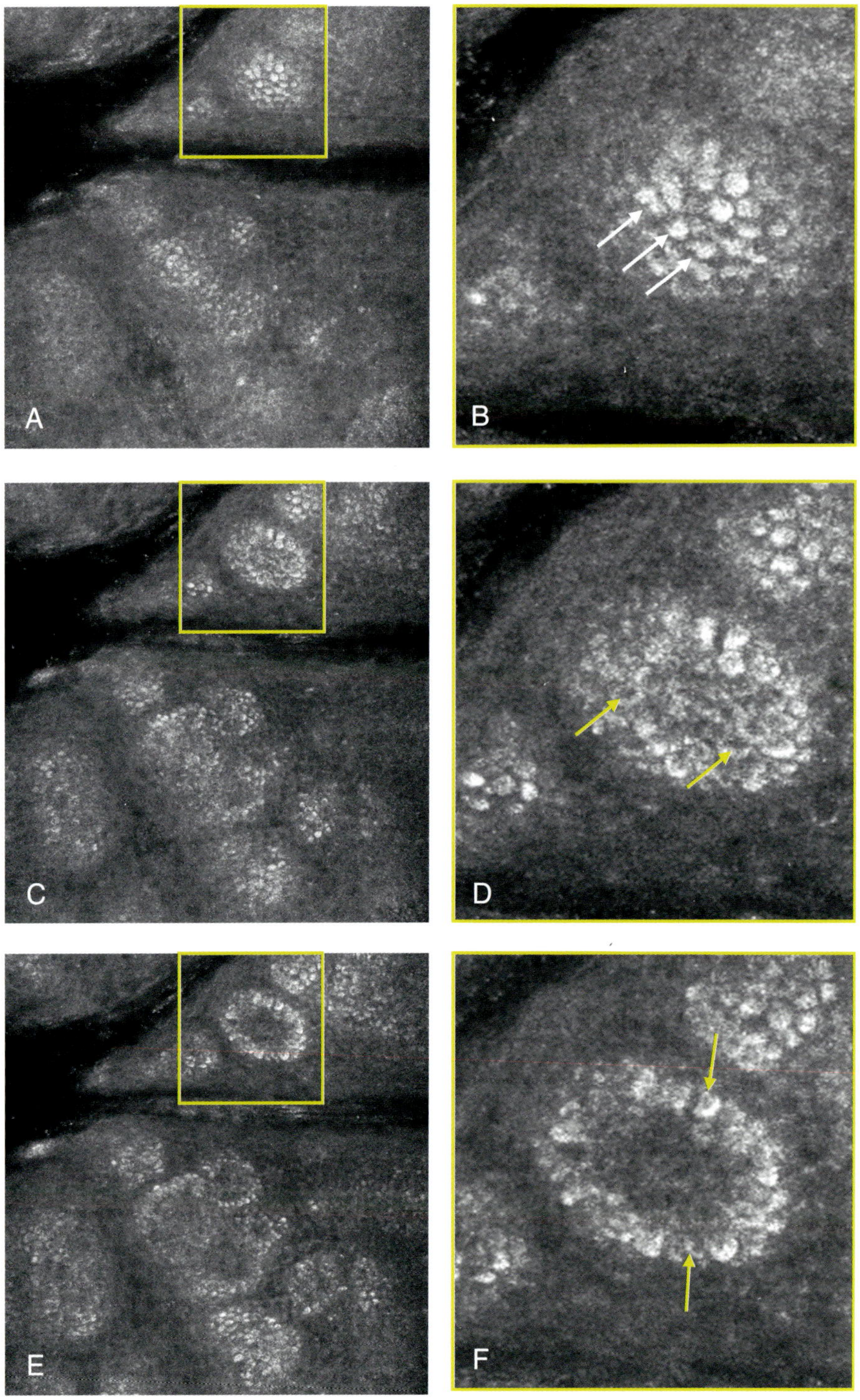

▲ **Figure 2.18A–F** This series of en-face RCM images with associated subimages demonstrates the appearance of the stratum basalis at the level of the supranuclear melanin caps of the suprapapillary plate (**A**, 0.5 mm × 0.5 mm; **B**, 0.2 mm × 0.2 mm), basal cell nuclei of the suprapapillary plate (**C**, 0.5 mm × 0.5 mm; **D**, 0.2 mm × 0.2 mm), and the superficial DEJ (**E**, 0.5 mm × 0.5 mm; **F**, 0.2 mm × 0.2 mm) sequentially revealing a cobblestone pattern (white arrows), a peripheral cobblestone pattern with central nucleated bright basal cells (yellow arrows), and dermal papillary rings, composed of nucleated bright cells (yellow arrows).

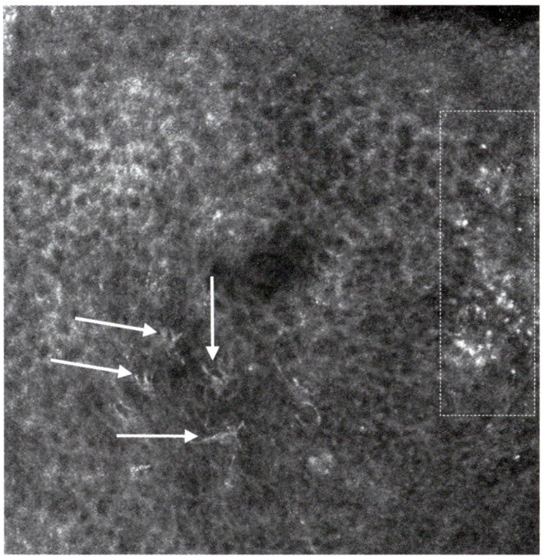

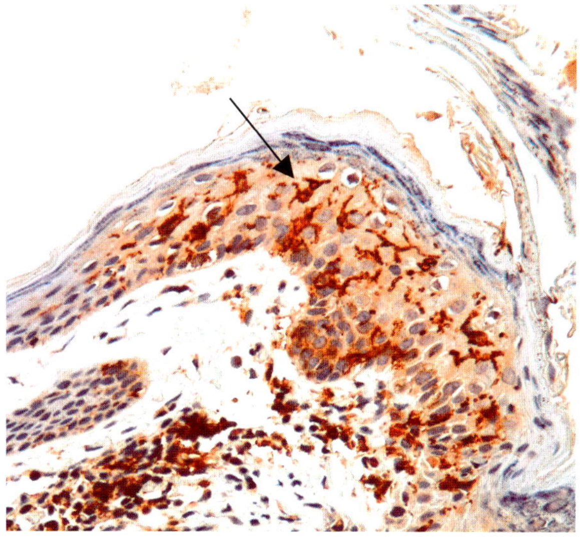

▲ **Figures 2.19, 2.20** This en-face RCM image (0.5 mm × 0.5 mm) taken at the level of the stratum spinosum is from an area of chronically sun-damaged skin. The honeycomb pattern is preserved, but numerous delicate refractile dendritic cells (white arrows) are seen in addition to small bright cells and particles (rectangle). Corresponding CD1a immunohistochemically stained histology (20×) reveals numerous activated dendritic Langerhans cells (arrow) and patchy chronic inflammation. Melan-A immunohistochemical stain (not shown) confirmed the absence of dendritic or pagetoid melanocytes, which can be difficult to distinguish from activated Langerhans cells with RCM.

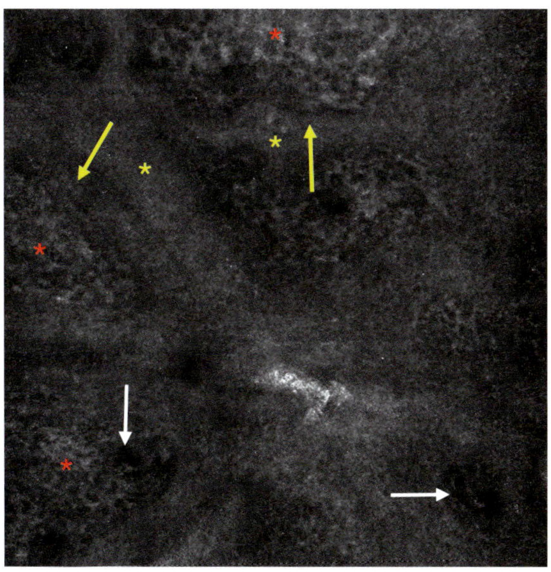

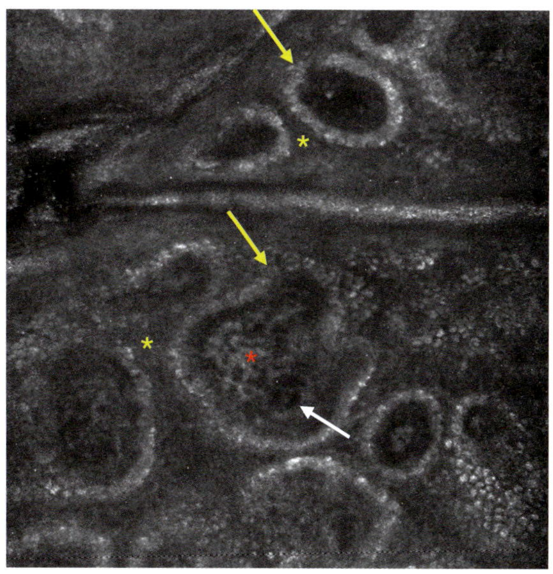

▲ **Figures 2.21, 2.22** En-face RCM images (0.5 mm × 0.5 mm) at the level of the dermal–epidermal junction/papillary dermis. Left panel: in this skin phototype I individual, the dermal papillary rings (yellow arrows) are difficult to distinguish from the rete meshwork (yellow asterisks) and appear dark relative to the dermal papillary fibrillar collagen, which is arranged in a reticulated pattern (red asterisks). Right panel: in this skin phototype III individual, dermal papillary rings (yellow arrows) are easily seen and generally appear brighter than the reticulated collagen (red asterisks) and the rete meshwork (yellow asterisks). Curved dark canalicular structures, corresponding to capillary loops, are seen in the papillary dermis of each image (white arrows).

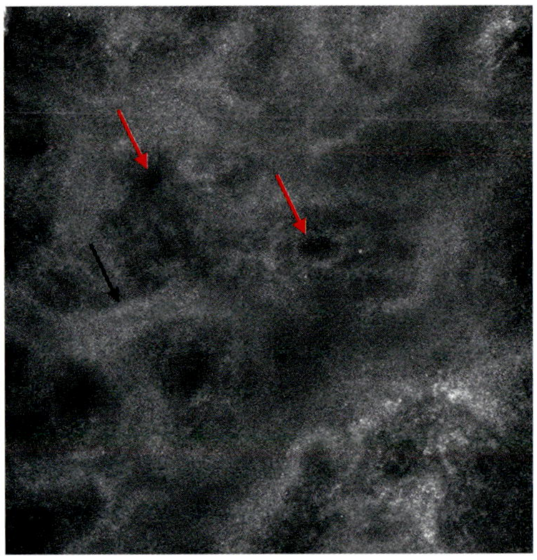

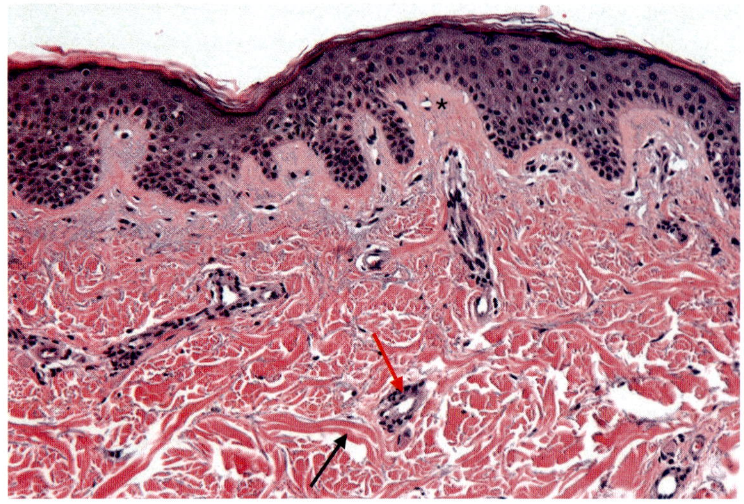

▲ **Figures 2.23, 2.24** En-face RCM image (0.5 mm × 0.5 mm) at the level of the superficial reticular dermis demonstrates moderately refractile bundles of collagen (black arrow) arranged in interwoven fascicles between which dark lumina (red arrows), corresponding to blood vessels, are seen. On vertical formalin-fixed histology (10×), the thick interwoven bundles of collagen (black arrow) form a similar pattern around small blood vessels (red arrow). The collagen in the dermal papillae (asterisks) is much thinner and more delicate than that in the reticular dermis (black arrow).

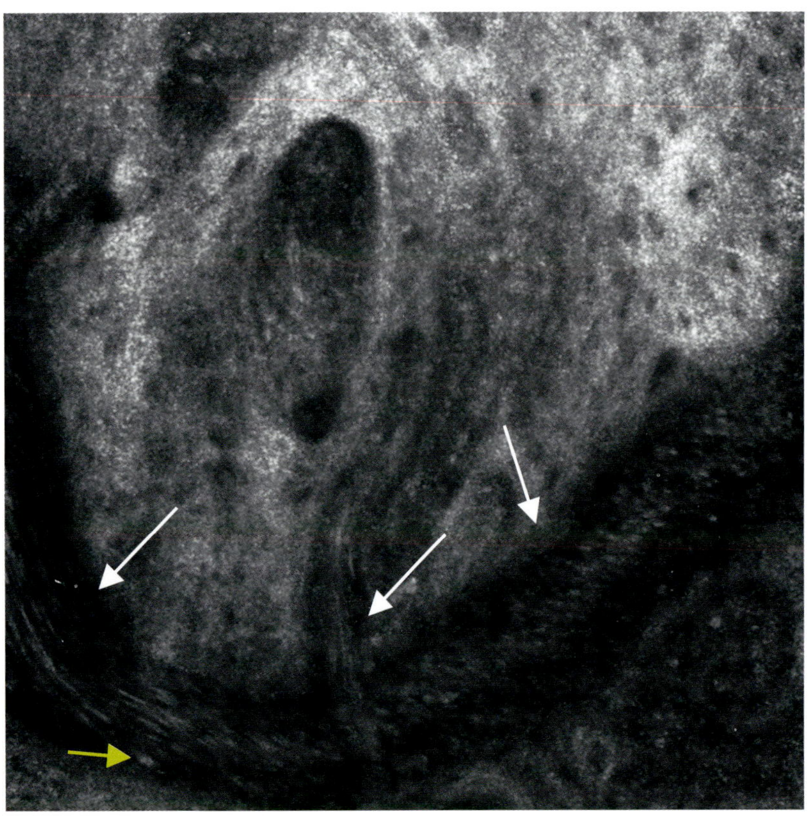

◀ **Figure 2.25**

This en-face RCM image (0.5 mm × 0.5 mm) demonstrates two anastomosing blood vessels (white arrows). In real time or video capture, numerous weakly refractile and brightly refractile small, round cells, corresponding to red and white blood cells, can be seen moving through these dark canalicular structures. A leukocyte rolling along the endothelial wall is captured in this image (yellow arrow).

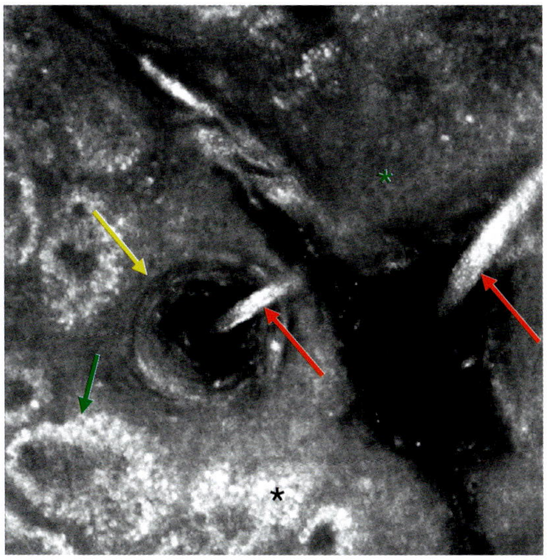

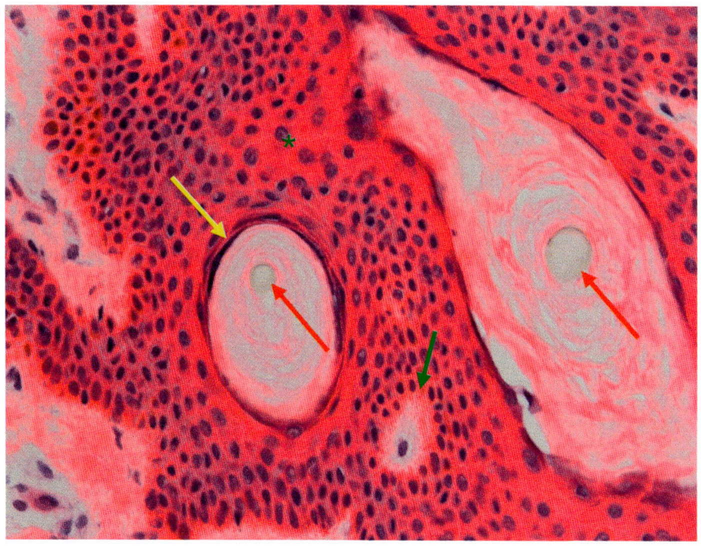

▲ **Figures 2.26, 2.27** This en-face RCM image (0.5 mm × 0.5 mm) at the level of the basal layer/ superficial DEJ demonstrates two hair shafts (red arrows): one emerging from a recognizable follicular orifice (yellow arrow); the other from the intersection of skin folds, for which the follicular orifice is not visible at this imaging depth. The confocal appearance of the epithelial wall of the follicle (yellow arrow) and the emerging hair shaft (orange arrow) can be appreciated. The small diameter of the hair shafts is consistent with vellous, rather than terminal hairs. In this RCM image, the honeycomb pattern of stratum spinosum (green asterisk), the cobblestone pattern of the superficial stratum basalis (black asterisk), and a few dermal papillary rings (green arrow) of the DEJ can be seen. Horizontal frozen section histology (40×) from a less-pigmented individual shows almost identical findings, but the hair shafts (red arrows) have been cut by the microtome and are seen in cross section rather than bent to the side.

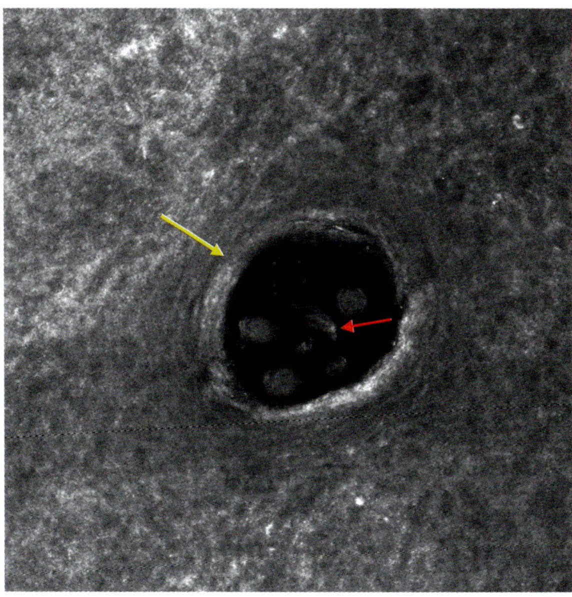

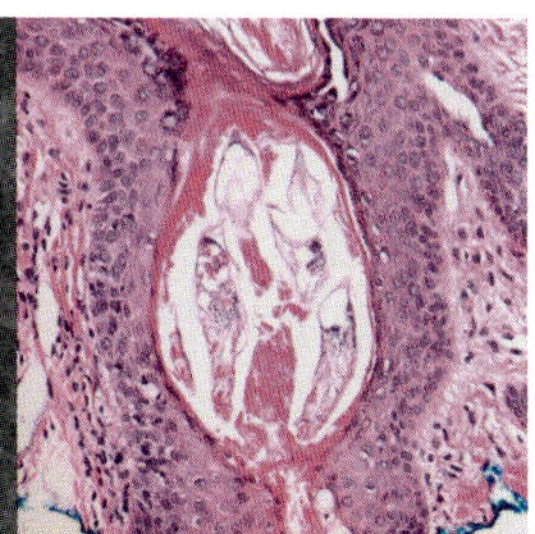

▲ **Figures 2.28, 2.29** This en-face RCM image (0.475 mm × 0.500 mm) shows sun-damaged skin at the level of the stratum spinosum with a central follicle. The epithelial layers of this follicle can be seen (yellow arrow) in addition to numerous moderately refractile structures within the follicular lumen. The tapered end of one such structure (red arrow), suggests these probably represent *Demodex* mites. Vertical formalin-fixed histology (40×) shows *Demodex* mites within a follicle for comparison.

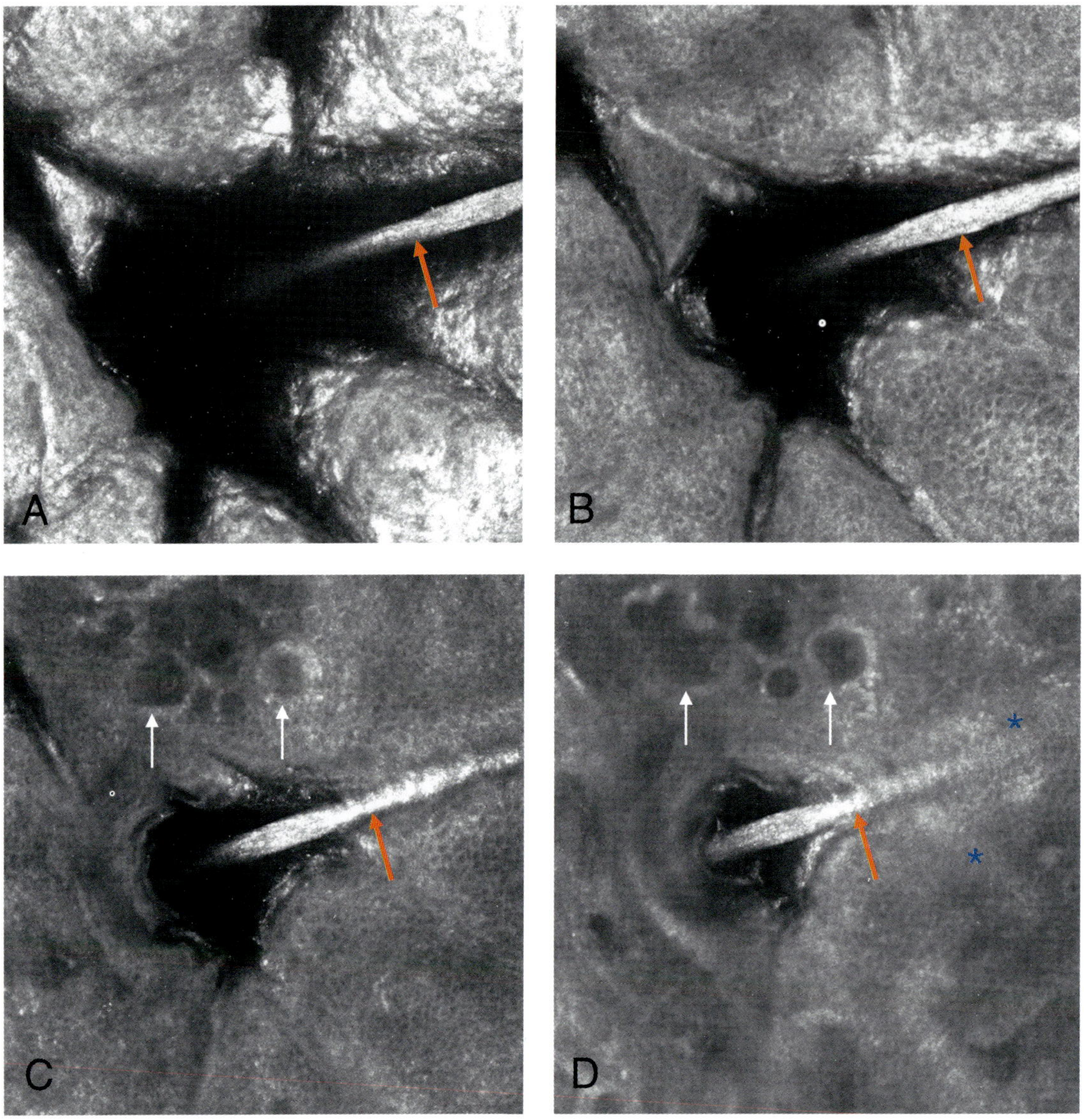

▲ **Figure 2.30A–D** These en-face RCM images (0.5 mm × 0.5 mm) of the same hair shaft (orange arrows) and follicle demonstrate their appearance at progressively deeper depths: corneal layer (A); granular/upper spinous layer (B); spinous layer with focal superficial DEJ (white arrows) (C); and DEJ/papillary dermis (white arrows) with focal deep spinous layer (blue asterisks) (D). The dark crevice-like skin folds, prominent in the superficial epidermis, disappear gradually with each level.

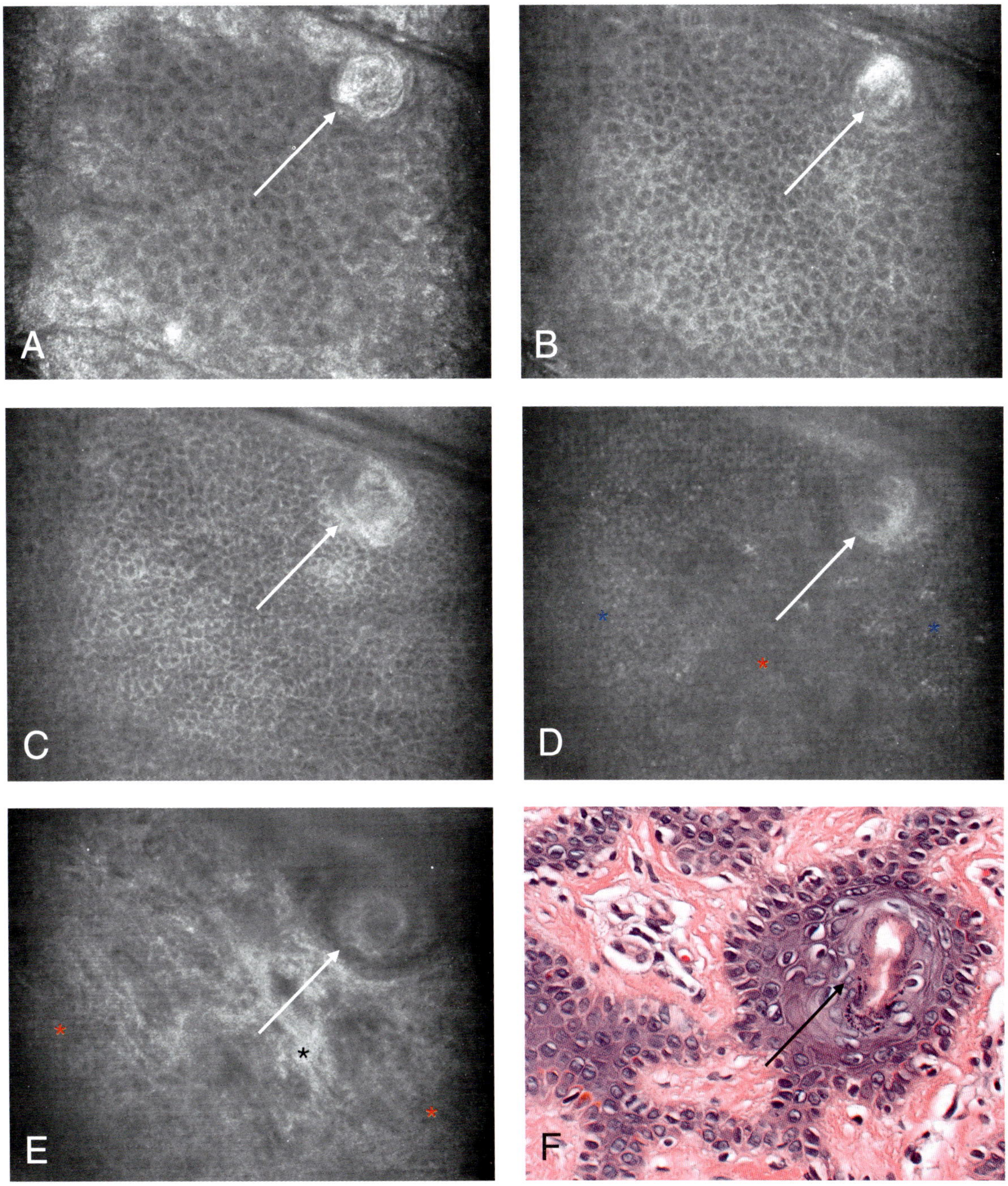

▲ **Figure 2.31A–F** These en-face RCM images (0.45 mm × 0.34 mm) of the eccrine duct (arrows) demonstrate its appearance at progressively deeper depths: stratum corneum/stratum granulosum (A), stratum granulosum (B), stratum spinosum (C), basal layer (blue asterisks)/DEJ/papillary dermis (red asterisks)(D), and deep papillary (red asterisks)/upper reticular dermis (black asterisk)(E). The acrosyngium, or intraepidermal duct, appears as a spiraling brightly refractile structure, whereas the intradermal duct is somewhat less refractile and develops a 'donut' shape. Horizontal formalin-fixed histology (40×) shows an eccrine duct at the level of the DEJ. Note the abrupt transition from stratum spinosum to papillary dermis in the RCM images (C to D), a phenomenon seen in skin with flattened rete ridges. By contrast, 'dermal papillary rings' are visible in the histologic section which comes from an area with preserved rete.

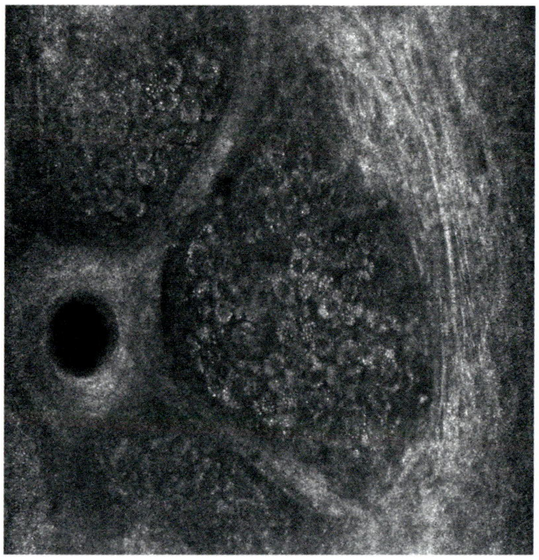

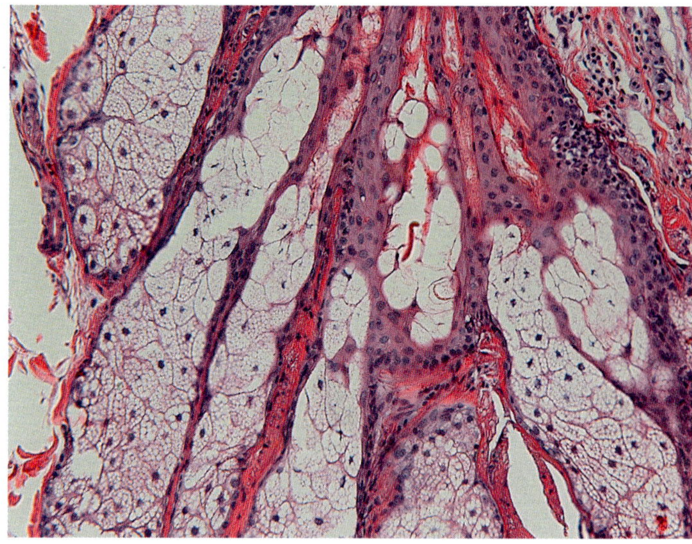

▲ **Figure 2.32, 2.33** This en-face RCM image (0.5 mm × 0.5 mm) demonstrates the morular appearance of sebaceous glands in the context of sebaceous hyperplasia. Vertical formalin-fixed histology (20×) demonstrates an example of prominent sebaceous glands.

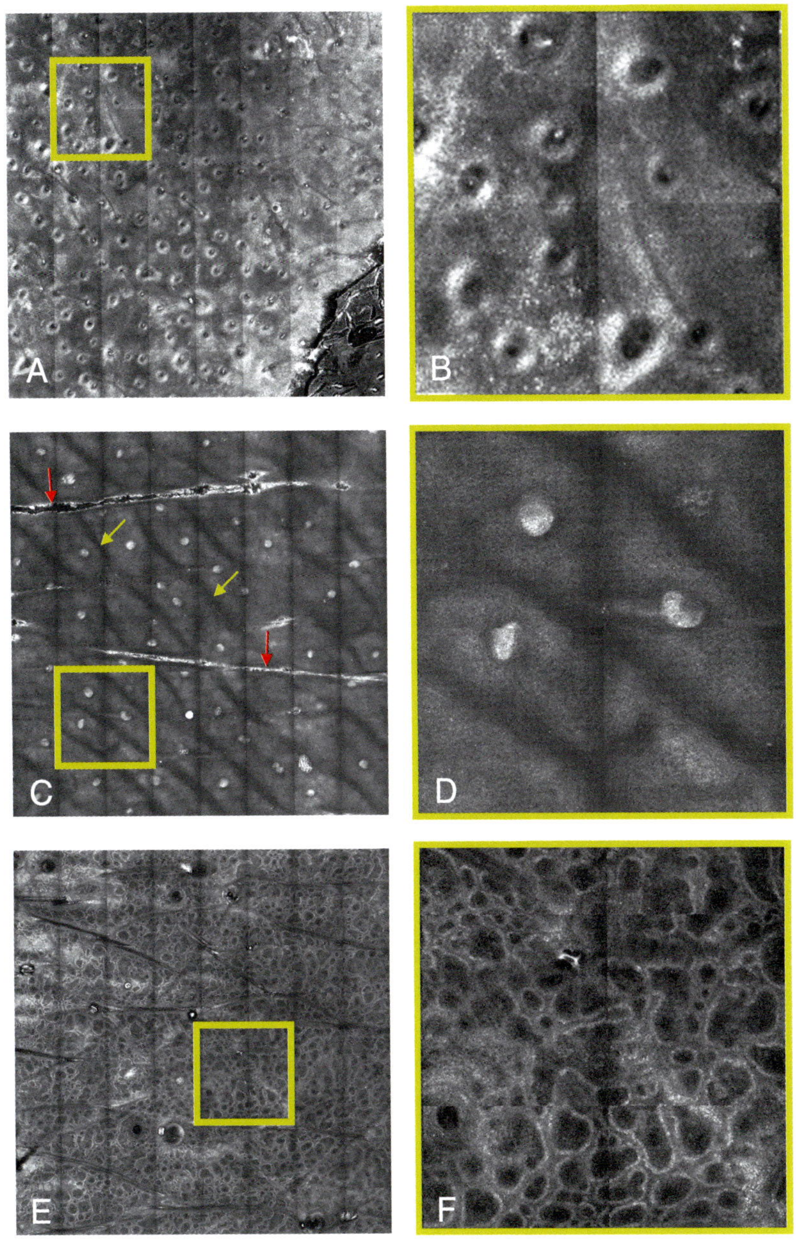

▲ **Figure 2.34A–F** Unique characteristics of various topographic sites are shown using RCM mosaics (4 mm × 4 mm) and submosaics (1 mm × 1 mm). The face (A and B) shows an increased density of pilosebaceous units containing small vellous hairs. The skin folds are barely visible in these images taken from the deep stratum spinosum. The palm, like the sole, (C and D) is characterized by the absence of pilosebaceous units, an increased concentration of eccrine ducts, a thickened epidermis, and the presence of dermatoglyphs (yellow arrows), which create a striped pattern on RCM rather than the diamond shapes created by skin folds on non-glabrous skin. A few palmar creases (red arrows) containing refractile keratin can also be seen. The back (E and F) has notable decreased density of pilosebaceous units and eccrine ducts as compared to the face and palm, respectively. Also note the diamond-shaped pattern of the skin folds, which are still visible at the DEJ.

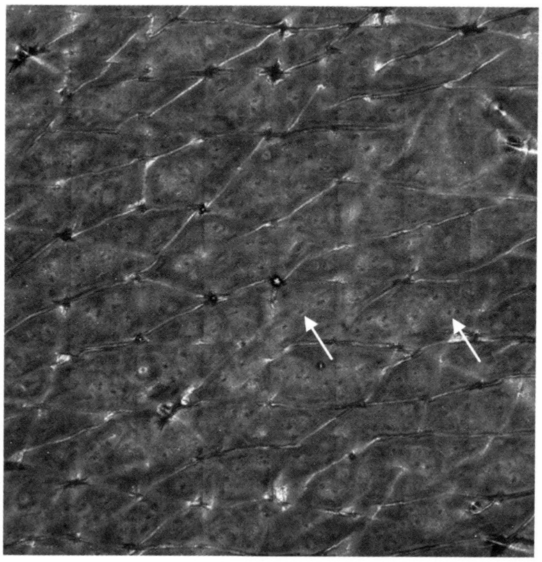

◀ **Figure 2.35** En-face RCM mosaic (4 mm × 4 mm) at the level of the DEJ of normal skin on the inner forearm of an individual with skin phototype I. Note the overall lack of contrast; dermal papillary rings are barely perceptible (arrows).

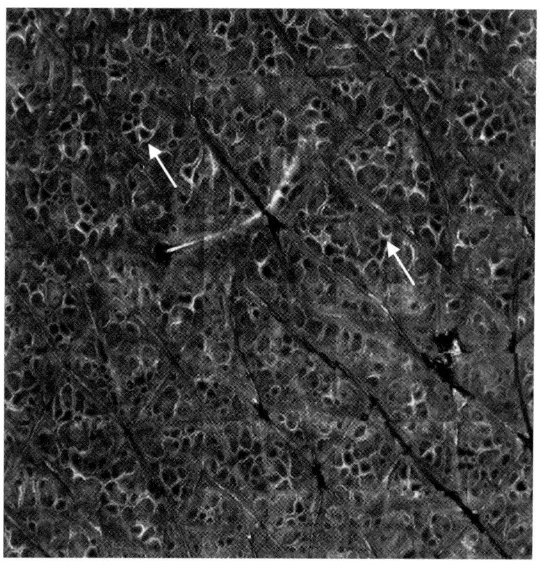

◀ **Figure 2.36** En-face RCM mosaic (4 mm × 4 mm) at the level of the DEJ of normal skin on the inner forearm of an individual with skin phototype III. Melanin pigment in the basal layer provides adequate contrast to allow for easy detection of the dermal papillary rings (white arrows).

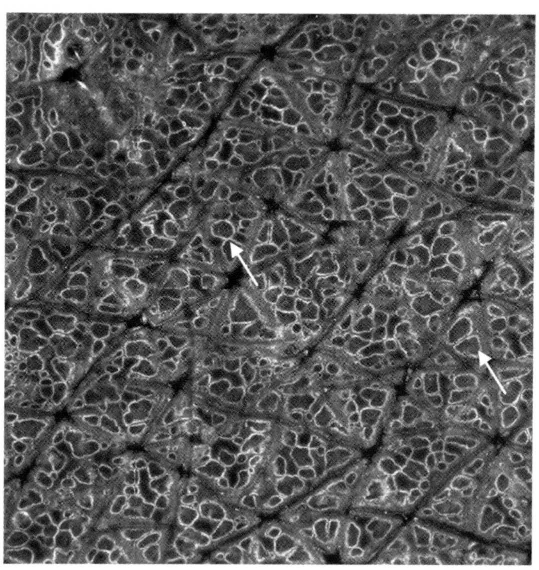

◀ **Figure 2.37** En-face RCM mosaic (4 mm × 4 mm) at the level of the DEJ of normal skin on the inner forearm of an individual with skin phototype V. More abundant melanin pigment in the basal layer causes the dermal papillary rings to be brightly refractile (white arrows).

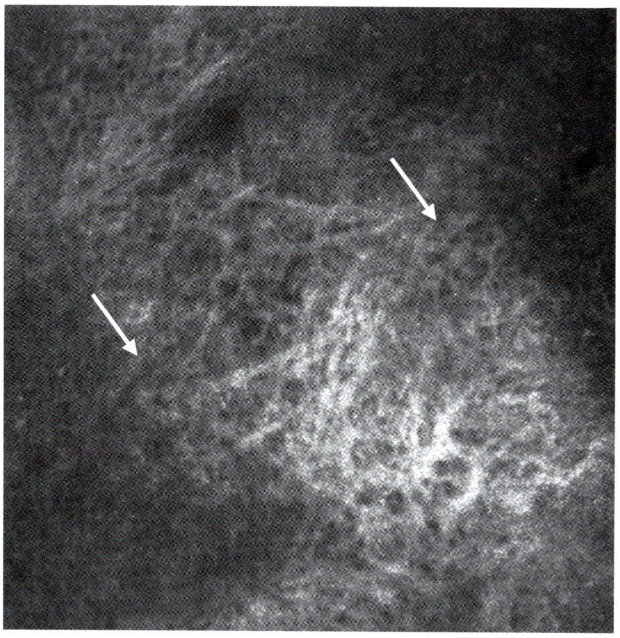

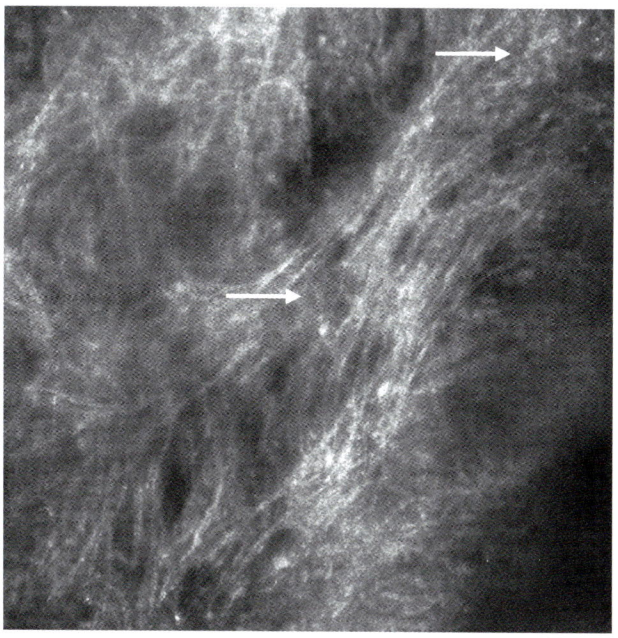

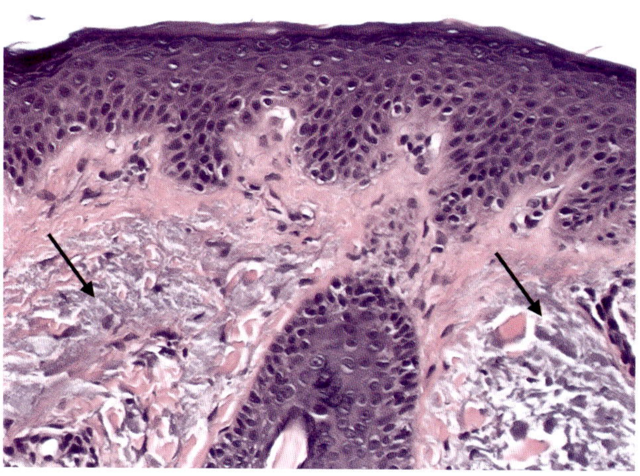

◀ **Figures 2.38–2.40**

Upper RCM image (0.5 mm × 0.5 mm) through intact overlying epidermis at the level of the upper reticular dermis shows ragged, moderately refractile lacy structures (arrows), compatible with solar elastosis, admixed with some straight, brightly refractile collagen bundles. Confocal imaging (lower RCM image, 0.5 mm × 0.5 mm) of these ragged, moderately refractile, lacy dermal structures (arrows), which both cluster and interdigitate with straight refractile collagen bundles, is facilitated by shaving off the epidermis prior to imaging. Vertical formalin-fixed histology (20×) shows extensive blue amorphous solar elastotic material (arrows) between collagen bundles in the dermis.

CHAPTER 3a

Seborrheic keratosis

Marco Ardigo, Alon Scope, Ruby Delgado, Salvador González, and Melissa Gill

Seborrheic keratosis (SK) is a benign epithelial lesion commonly found in adults over the age of 30 years. SK most frequently occurs on the trunk, but can appear anywhere on the cutis. Clinically, early lesions are light to dark brown, oval or round macules with well-demarcated borders.[1] More well-developed seborrheic keratoses range from small papules to plaques with a characteristic 'stuck on' appearance and a waxy, warty, keratotic surface often containing follicular plugs[1] (Figures 3.1, 3.9). Dermoscopic examination of SK usually reveals a sharply demarcated border, variably cerebriform surface with ridges and fissures, comedo-like openings, milia-like cysts, and hairpin vessels, typical of keratinizing lesions[2,3] (Figures 3.2, 3.10). The diagnosis is usually straightforward, but flat seborrheic keratosis may harbor clinical and dermoscopic features of solar lentigo, and pigmented SK can clinically simulate malignant melanoma.[4,5]

Reflectance confocal microscopic (RCM) examination of seborrheic keratosis shows several features which correlate closely with findings on dermoscopy and histology. RCM mosaic of the epidermis reveals a well-demarcated lesion with striking cerebriform architecture (Figure 3.4). Dark areas, resembling the sulci of the brain, contain variable amounts of refractile material and correspond to fissures on dermoscopy and keratin-filled surface invaginations on histology (Figures 3.3, 3.4). Gray anastomosing ribbons, resembling the gyri of the brain, correspond to ridges on dermoscopy and interwoven, acanthotic cords and tongues of basaloid cells on histology (Figures 3.3, 3.4, 3.7, 3.8). Comedo-like openings and milia-like cysts on dermoscopy, corresponding to horn cysts on histology, appear on RCM as well-defined, round, whorled collections of brightly refractile material surrounded by cords of keratinocytes[6,7] (Figures 3.5, 3.6); these have been recently termed cystic inclusions.[8] RCM of the stratum spinosum shows crowded, basaloid cells (Figures 3.6, 3.8).

In general, the basaloid keratinocytes forming a seborrheic keratosis contain a greater amount of refractile melanin pigment as compared to normal skin.[8] In pigmented SK, the stratum spinosum has a cobblestone pattern composed of monomorphic, polygonal bright cells with distinct cellular borders, corresponding to pigmented keratinocytes on histology (Figures 3.11–3.14). Confocal examination of the dermal–epidermal junction finds enlarged and distorted dermal papillary rings often lined by brightly refractile cells, corresponding to pigmented basal keratinocytes on histology (Figures 3.7, 3.8, 3.11, 3.12). Within dermal papillae, RCM reveals occasional large, single or clustered, plump, brightly refractile round or polygonal cells, representing melanophages, on histology[6] (Figures 3.15, 3.16).

Key RCM features of seborrheic keratosis

- Cerebriform architecture of the epidermis
- Keratin-filled cystic inclusions
- Plump, bright round or polygonal cells in the upper dermis (melanophages)
- Bright cobblestone pattern of stratum spinosum (pigmented SK)

REFERENCES

1. Ho V, McLean D. Benign epithelial tumors. In: Freeberg IM, Wolff K, Austen KF et al. eds. Fitzpatrick's Dermatology in General Medicine. New York: McGraw-Hill, 1999: 873–76.

2. Elgart GW. Seborrheic keratoses, solar lentigines, and lichenoid keratoses. Dermatoscopic features and correlation to histology and clinical signs. Dermatol Clin 2001; 19(2):347–57.

3. Wang S, Rabinovitz H, Oliviero M. Dermoscopic pattern of solar lentigines and seborrheic keratoses. In: Marghoob AA, Braun RP, Kopf AW, eds. Atlas of Dermoscopy. Abingdon, UK: Taylor & Francis; 2005: 60.

4. Braun RP, Rabinovitz HS, Krischer J et al. Dermoscopy of pigmented seborrheic keratosis: a morphological study. Arch Dermatol 2002; 138(12):1556–60.

5. Sahin MT, Ozturkcan S, Ermertcan AT, Gunes AT. A comparison of dermoscopic features among lentigo senilis/initial seborrheic keratosis, seborrheic keratosis, lentigo maligna and lentigo maligna melanoma on the face. J Dermatol 2004; 31(11):884–9.

6. Busam KJ, Charles C, Lee G, Halpern AC. Morphologic features of melanocytes, pigmented keratinocytes, and melanophages by in vivo confocal scanning laser microscopy. Mod Pathol 2001; 14(9):862–8.

7. Kirkham N. Tumors and cysts of the epidermis. In: Elder DE, Elenitzas R, Johnson BL Jr, Murphy GF, eds. Lever's Histopathology of the Skin. Philadelphia: Lippincott, Williams & Wilkins; 2005: 809.

8. Gerger A, Koller S, Weger W et al. Sensitivity and specificity of confocal laser-scanning microscopy for in vivo diagnosis of malignant skin tumors. Cancer 2006; 107(1):193–200.

SEBORRHEIC KERATOSIS

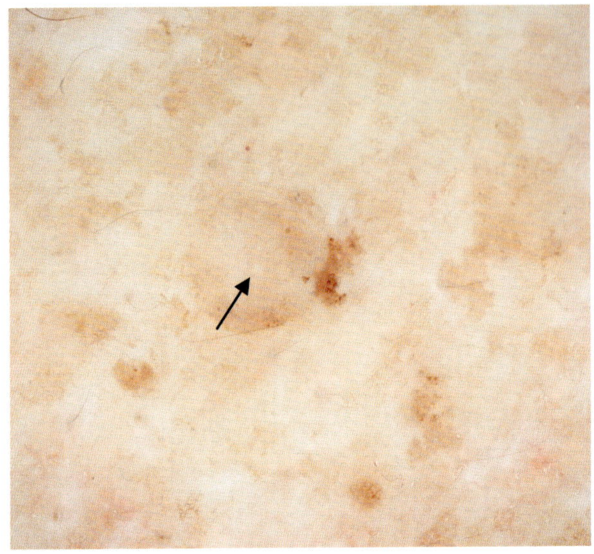

▲ **Figures 3.1, 3.2** Clinical photograph of a 5 mm, flesh-colored, round, papule with well-demarcated borders and a slightly verrucous surface on the left shoulder. Dermoscopically, this is a sharply circumscribed lesion with central milia-like cysts (arrow) and peripheral globule-like structures on a pigmented background.

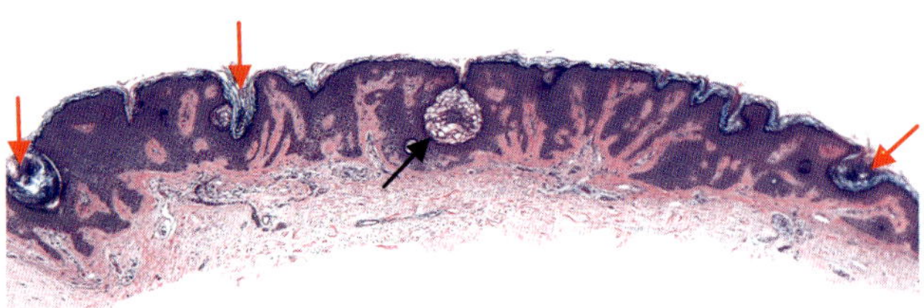

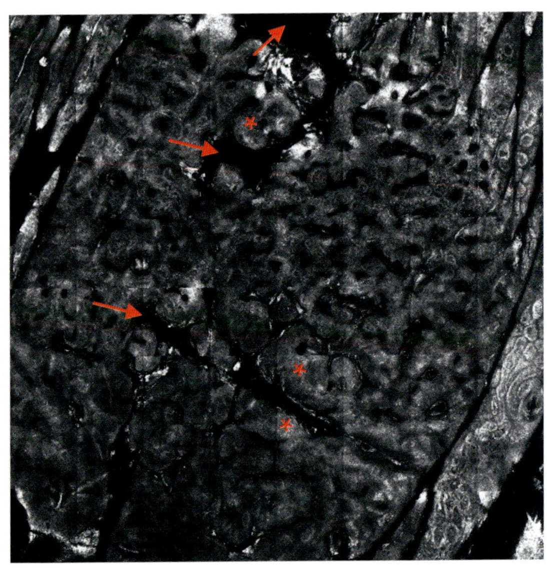

▲ **Figures 3.3, 3.4** Histology (4×) shows hyperkeratosis, papillated and reticulated epidermal hyperplasia, keratin-filled surface invaginations (red arrows) and horn cysts (black arrow), corresponding to the milia-like cysts seen on dermoscopy. RCM mosaic (4 mm × 4 mm) at the level of the mid stratum spinosum discloses a well-demarcated lesion with striking cerebriform architecture. Black 'sulcus-like' (arrows) and gray 'gyrus-like' (asterisks) areas correspond to keratin-filled surface invaginations and anastomosing tongues of epidermis, respectively.

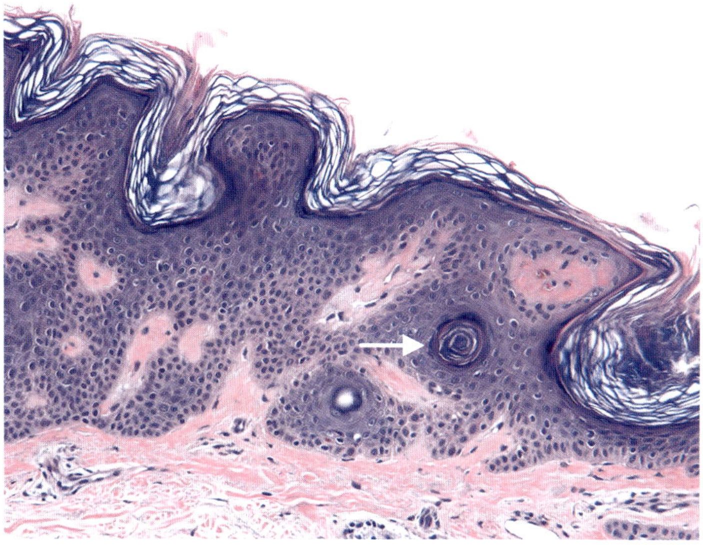
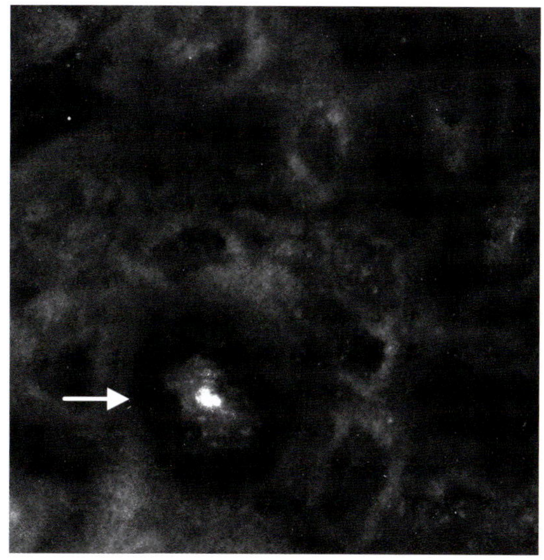

▲ **Figures 3.5, 3.6** Keratinocytes of the stratum spinosum are small, organized, and basaloid in appearance on histology (20×) and confocal. Horn cysts seen on histology (arrow) are easily identified using RCM (0.5 mm × 0.5 mm) as well-defined, round, black areas filled with whorled, brightly refractile material (keratin) and edged by cords of keratinocytes (arrow).

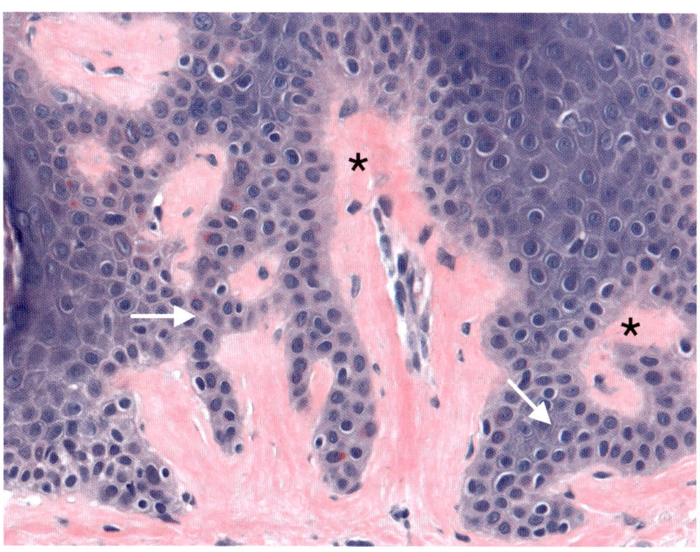
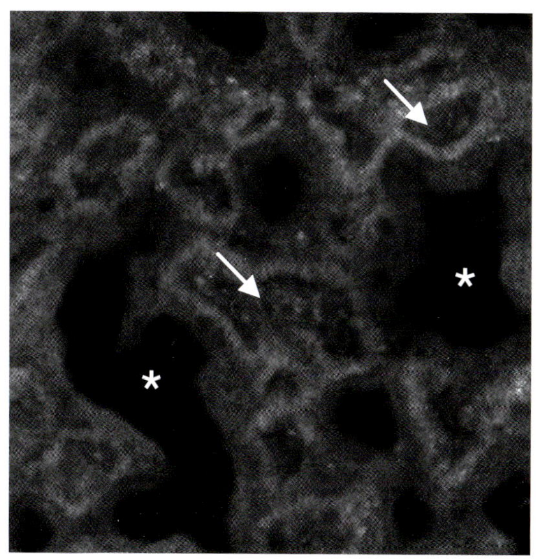

▲ **Figures 3.7, 3.8** Histology (40×) shows cords and tongues of basaloid cells (arrows), corresponding to the gray anastomosing ribbons (arrows), resembling brain gyri, that can be seen on RCM (0.5 mm × 0.5 mm). Dermal papillae, distorted by the tumor, are irregular in size and shape with curvilinear, invaginated borders (asterisks).

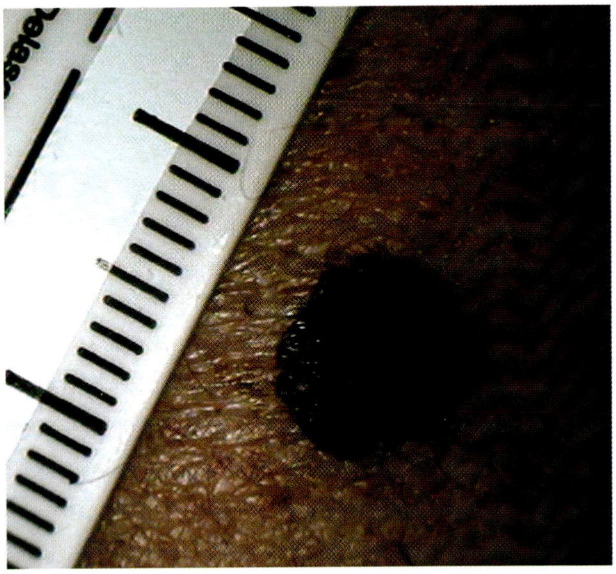

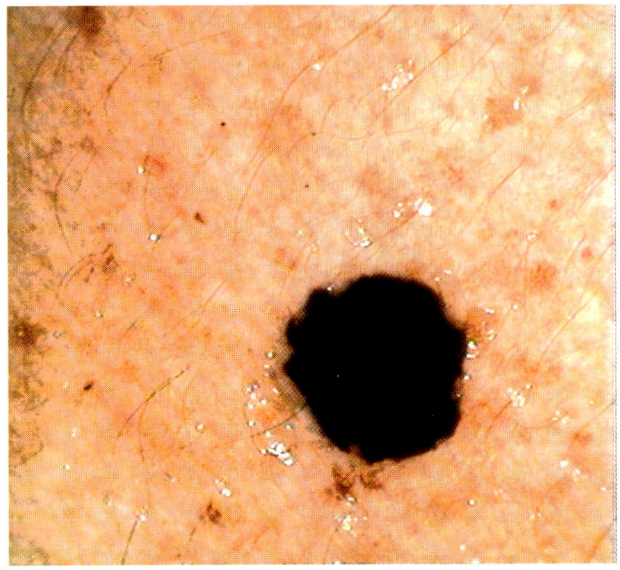

▲ **Figures 3.9, 3.10** Clinical photograph of a 6 mm, dark brown, dome-shaped papule with a 'stuck on' appearance. Corresponding dermoscopy shows a uniformly dark, well-circumscribed lesion with comedo-like openings on its surface.

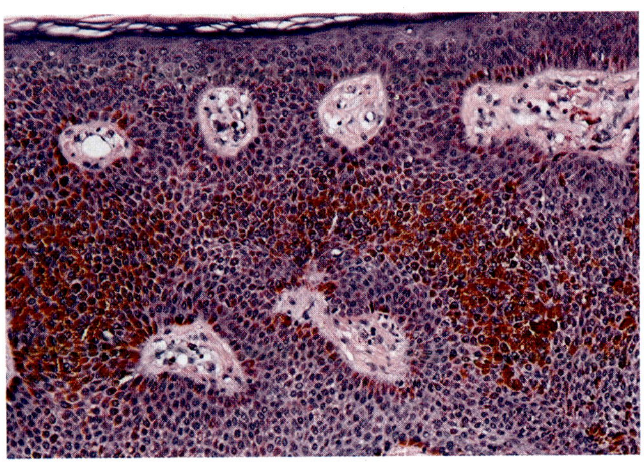

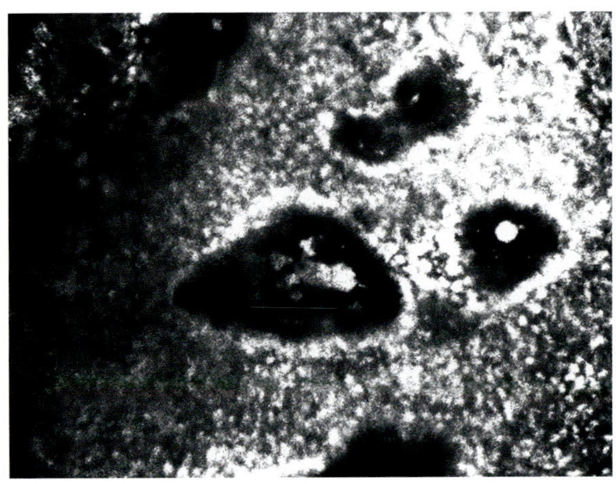

▲ **Figures 3.11, 3.12** Histology (20×) shows numerous pigmented basaloid keratinocytes throughout the strata spinosum and basalis, corresponding to a 'cobblestone' pattern composed of brightly refractile cells with distinct cellular borders on RCM (0.45 mm × 0.34 mm).

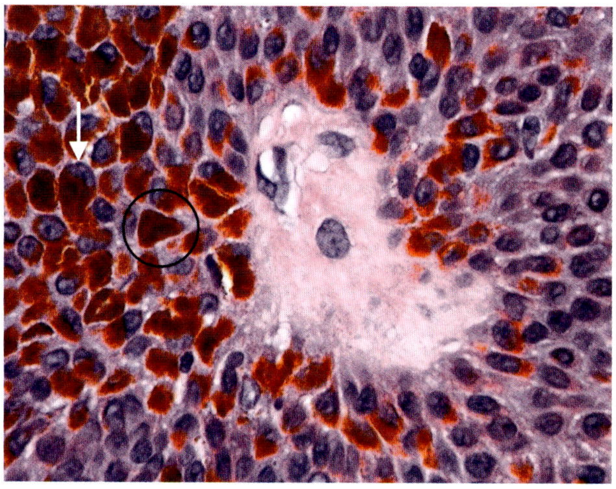

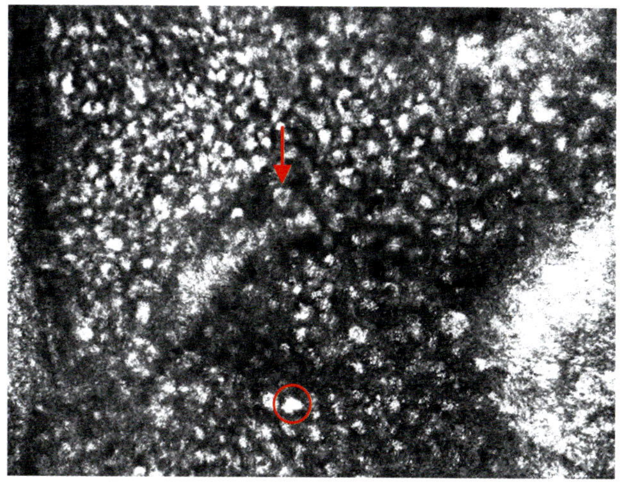

▲ **Figures 3.13, 3.14** On higher-power histology (40×), melanin is seen filling the cytoplasms of the tumor cells, causing some cells to achieve larger polygonal shapes. The cytoplasmic melanin is so abundant that some sections transect only cytoplasm, missing the nucleus altogether (circle). In other cells (arrow), both cytoplasm and nucleus are seen. Corresponding RCM (0.45 mm × 0.34 mm) optical section reveals a similar phenomenon: occasionally, dark regular nuclei can be seen within the bright cobblestone-like cells (arrow), but sometimes only the bright melanin-filled cytoplasm is seen (circle).

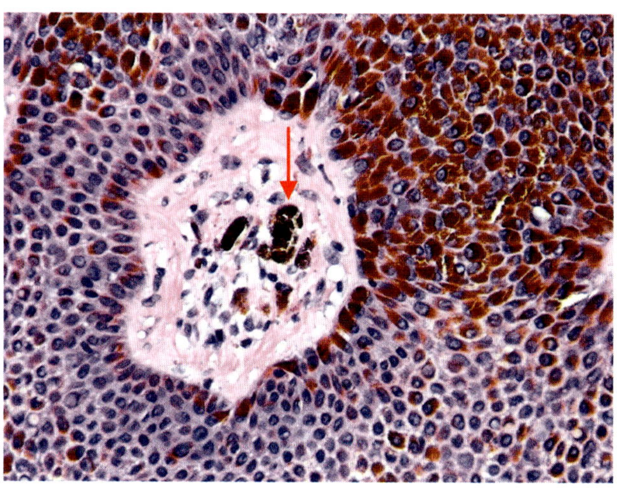

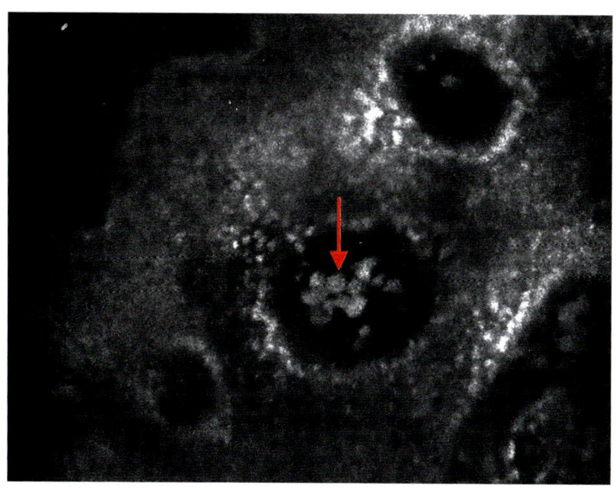

▲ **Figures 3.15, 3.16** On histology (40×), dermal papillae contain clusters of melanophages (arrow), which appear as plump, bright cells (arrow) on RCM (0.45 mm × 0.34 mm).

CHAPTER 3b

Clear cell acanthoma

Alon Scope, Marco Ardigo, Ashfaq A Marghoob, and Melissa Gill

Clear cell acanthoma (CCA), also known as Degos' acanthoma or pale cell acanthoma, is an uncommon benign epidermal tumor occurring in adults with no gender predisposition.[1] The etiology is still unknown; however, the expression of markers, such as involucrin and epithelial membrane antigens, suggests that CCA derives from suprabasal keratinocytes.[2,3] The typical lesion is a slowly growing, sharply marginated, pink to brown, blanchable, dome-shaped nodule or plaque ranging from 1 to 2 cm in diameter, but reaching up to 5 cm or more (Figures 3.17, 3.21).[4,5] A wafer-like scale forming a peripheral collarette may be present (Figure 3.17). CCA usually occurs as a solitary lesion on the leg or less commonly on the trunk. Interestingly, an eruptive variant with up to 50 lesions has also been reported.[6] CCA shows pinpoint or globular vessels[7] distributed in a serpiginous pattern on dermoscopy (Figures 3.18, 3.22).[8]

Reflectance confocal microscopic (RCM) examination of clear cell acanthoma finds many features that have been described using histology and dermoscopy. Confocal mosaic images show a sharply demarcated lesion often surrounded by a collarette of refractile scale with prominent glomeruloid vessels following serpiginous lines (Figures 3.19, 3.20, 3.23, 3.24). Examination of the stratum corneum shows refractile areas with flattened, elongated nuclei corresponding to parakeratosis on histopathology (Figures 3.25, 3.26). The stratum spinosum shows disarray and loss of the normal honeycomb pattern in areas where, on histology, the characteristic pale keratinocytes filled with glycogen are identified (Figures 3.27, 3.28). Broadened areas between dermal papillae and increased epidermal thickness correspond to psoriasiform acanthosis on histology. The dermal papillae are enlarged and contain dilated glomeruloid capillaries (Figures 3.29, 3.30).[9]

Key RCM features of clear cell acanthoma

- Sharp lateral circumscription
- Often surrounded by collarette of refractile scale
- Glomeruloid vessels expanding the dermal papillae

REFERENCES

1. Degos R, Delort J, Civatte J, Poiares Baptista A. Epidermal tumor with an unusual appearance: clear cell acanthoma. Ann Dermatol Syphiligr (Paris) 1962; 89:361–71.
2. Hashimoto T, Inamoto N, Nakamura K. Two cases of clear cell acanthoma: an immunohistochemical study. J Cutan Pathol 1988; 15(1):27–30.
3. Ohnishi T, Watanabe S. Immunohistochemical characterization of keratin expression in clear cell acanthoma. Br J Dermatol 1995; 133(2):186–93.
4. Fine RM, Chernosky ME. Clinical recognition of clear-cell acanthoma (Degos'). Arch Dermatol 1969; 100(5):559–63.
5. Murphy R, Kesseler ME, Slater DN. Giant clear cell acanthoma. Br J Dermatol 2000; 143(5):1114–15.
6. Innocenzi D, Barduagni F, Cerio R, Wolter M. Disseminated eruptive clear cell acanthoma – a

case report with review of the literature. Clin Exp Dermatol 1994; 19(3):249–53.

7. Blum A, Metzler G, Bauer J, Rassner G, Garbe C. The dermatoscopic pattern of clear-cell acanthoma resembles psoriasis vulgaris. Dermatology 2001; 203(1):50–2.

8. Malvehy J, Puig S, Braun R, Marghoob A, Kopf A. Handbook of Dermoscopy. London: Taylor & Francis; 2006.

9. Kirkham N. Tumors and cysts of the epidermis. In: Elder DE, Elenitzas R, Johnson BL, Murphy GF, eds. Lever's Histopathology of the Skin, 9th edn. Philadelphia: Lippincott Williams & Wilkins; 2005: 813–14.

CLEAR CELL ACANTHOMA

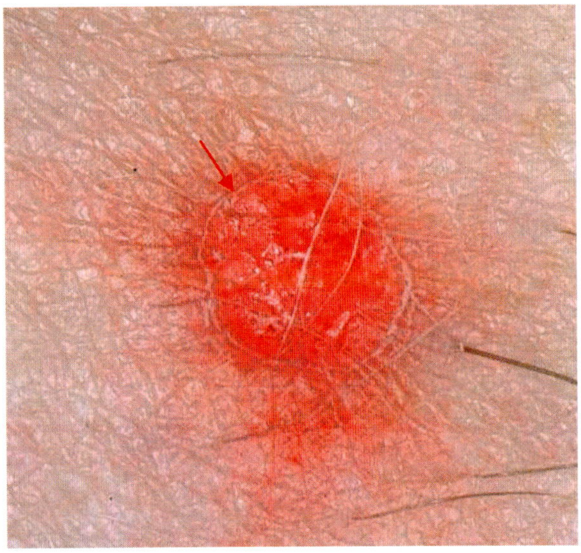
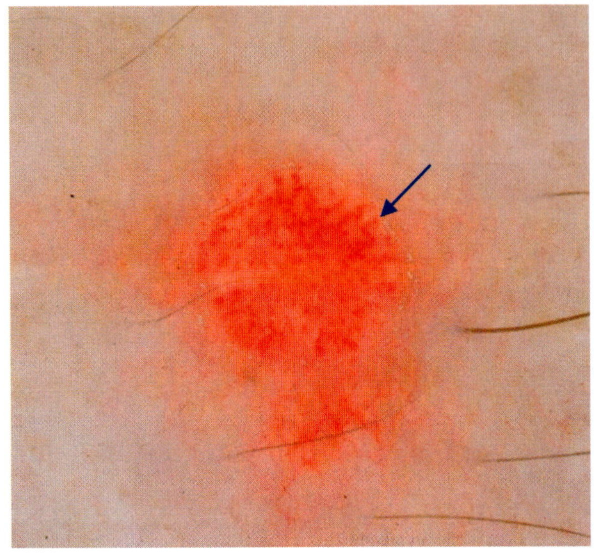

▲ **Figures 3.17, 3.18** Case 1: clinical photograph of a 4 mm, scaly, pink, blanchable, dome-shaped nodule with wafer-like peripheral collarette of scale (red arrow) on the thigh. Dermoscopic photograph reveals pinpoint or globular vessels distributed in a serpiginous pattern (blue arrow).

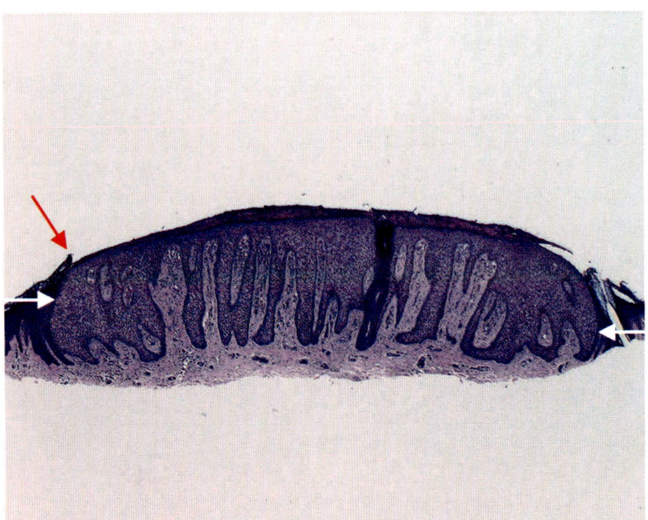
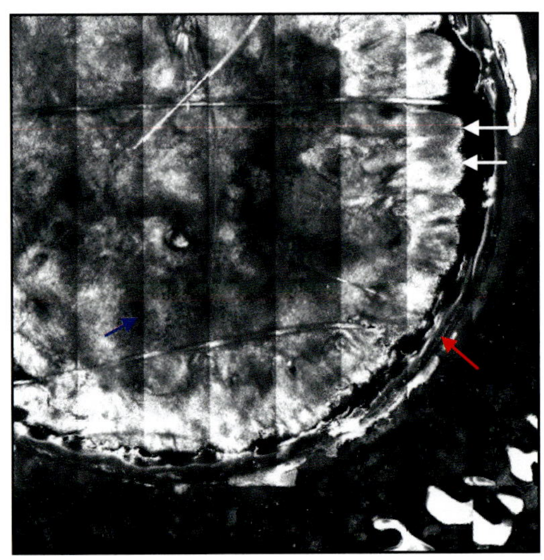

▲ **Figures 3.19, 3.20** Case 1: histology (2×) shows characteristic sharp lateral demarcation with abrupt transition from lesional clear cells to normal epidermis (white arrows) and a collarette of scale (red arrow). Acanthosis of the epidermis and an increased number of enlarged dermal papillae are evident at low power. RCM mosaic (4 mm × 4 mm) at the level of the superficial epidermis reveals the same sharp lateral demarcation (white arrows) with a refractile peripheral collarette (red arrow) as seen on histology. The tips of a few dermal papillae are just emerging and contain glomeruloid vessels (blue arrow).

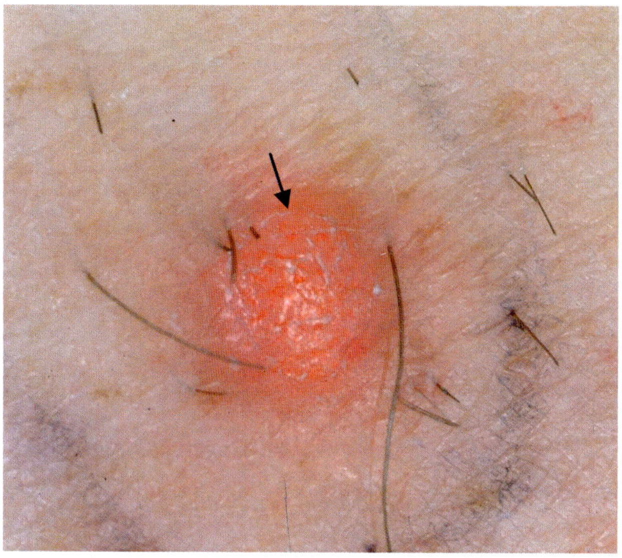

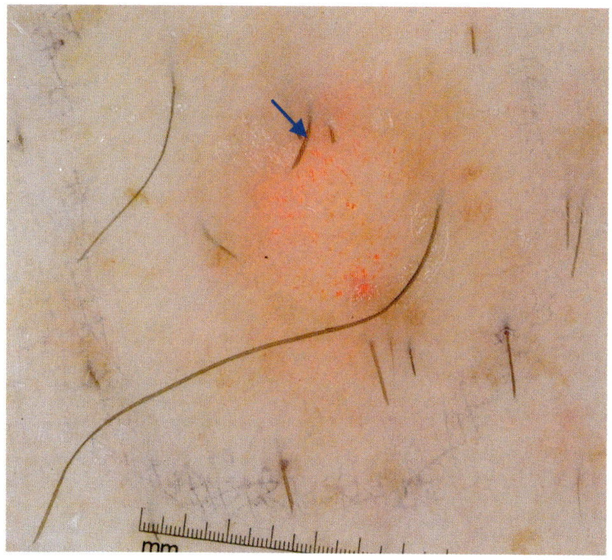

▲ **Figures 3.21, 3.22** Case 2: clinical and confocal photographs of this 4 mm clear cell acanthoma on the thigh are similar to Case 1, but the peripheral collarette of scale is incomplete (arrow) and the characteristic vascular pattern seen on dermoscopy is much more subtle (blue arrow).

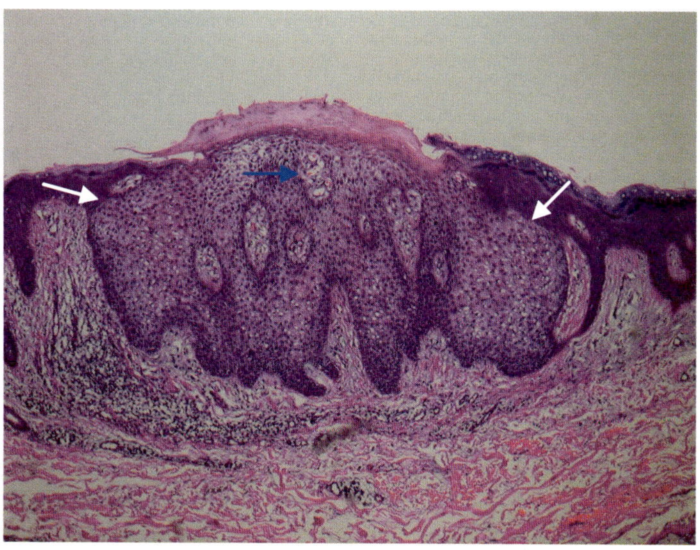

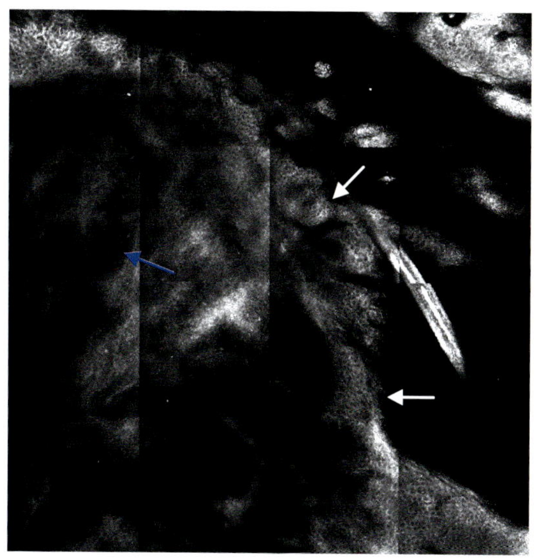

▲ **Figures 3.23, 3.24** Case 2: histology (4×) and RCM mosaic (2 mm × 2 mm) at the level of the dermal–epidermal junction, however, clearly capture both the sharp lateral demarcation (white arrows) and the dermal papillae, expanded by glomeruloid vessels (blue arrows). This case nicely illustrates how RCM may aid in diagnosis when dermoscopic findings are subtle.

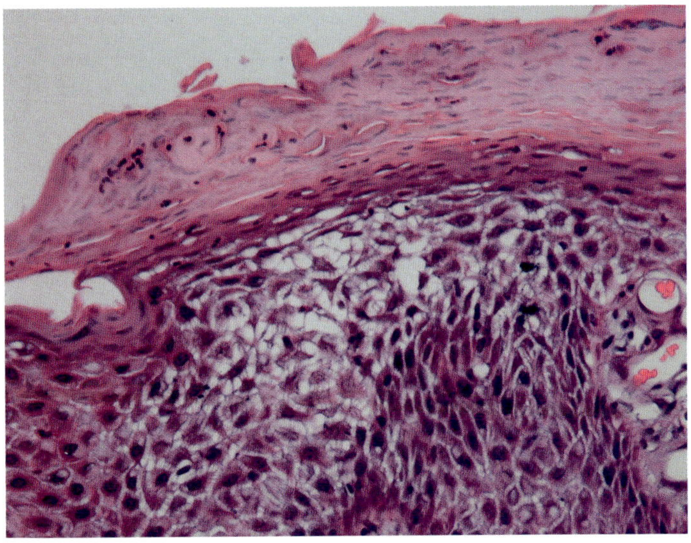

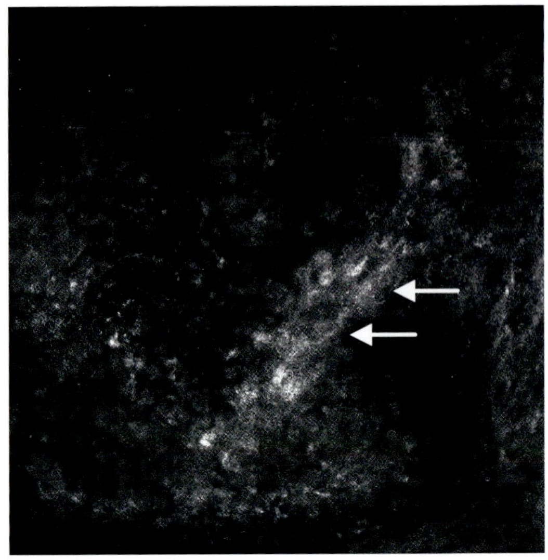

▲ **Figures 3.25, 3.26** Case 2: histology (40×) of the stratum corneum shows parakeratosis with scattered neutrophils. RCM (0.5 mm × 0.5 mm) of the stratum corneum shows refractile areas containing elongated dark spaces (white arrows), consistent with parakeratosis.

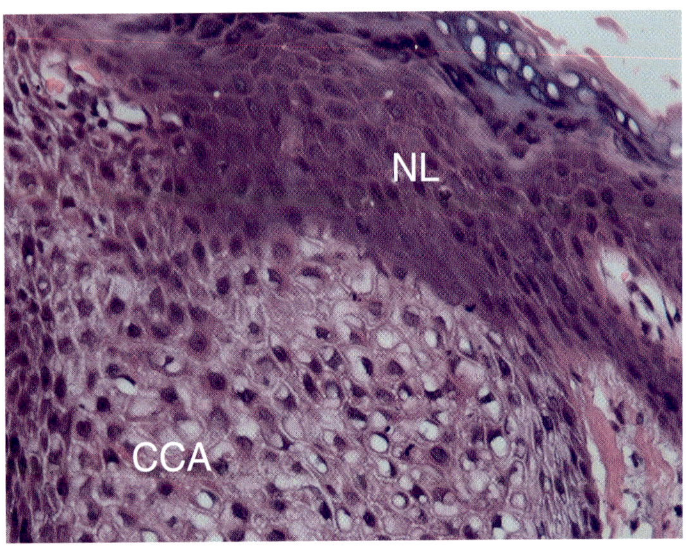

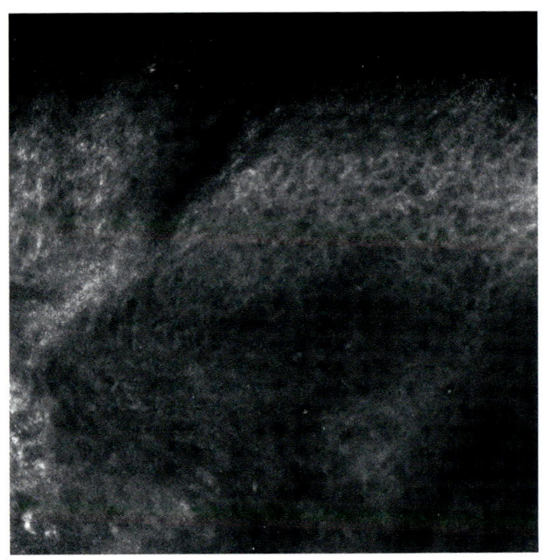

▲ **Figures 3.27, 3.28** Case 2: histology (40×) of the stratum spinosum shows keratinocytes with abundant pale pink to clear cytoplasm (CCA), which contrast with adjacent normal keratinocytes (NL). Corresponding RCM (0.5 mm × 0.5 mm) from the center of the lesion is remarkable for disarray with loss of the normal honeycomb pattern.

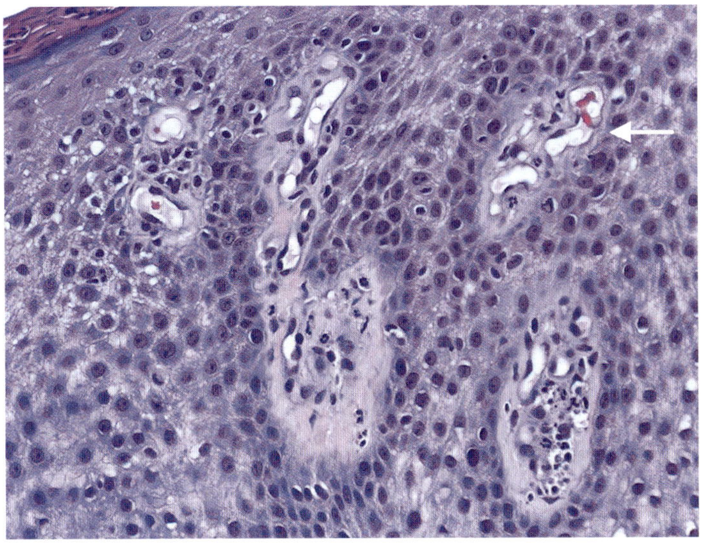

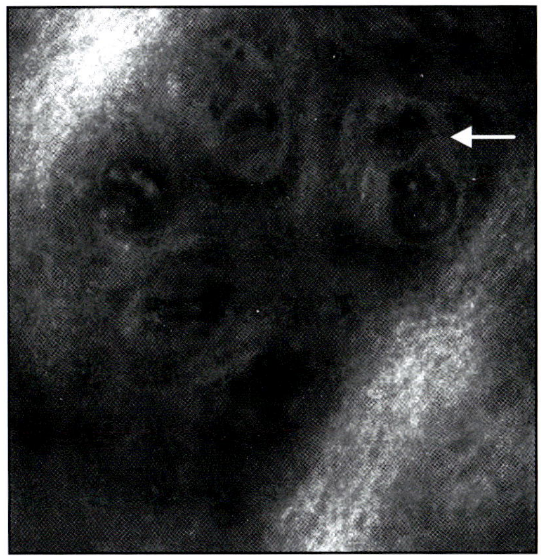

▲ **Figures 3.29, 3.30** Case 1: dermal papillae expanded by glomeruloid vessels (arrows) are evident on histology (20×) and RCM (0.5 mm × 0.5 mm) at the level of the dermal–epidermal junction.

CHAPTER 3c

Porokeratosis

Susanne Astner, Martina Ulrich, Jesus Cuevas, and Salvador González

Porokeratosis is a histopathologic entity referring to a group of five phenotypically distinct disorders of keratinization:

- the classical variant, porokeratosis of Mibelli
- linear porokeratosis
- porokeratosis punctata palmaris et plantaris
- porokeratosis palmaris, plantaris et disseminata
- disseminated superficial (actinic) porokeratosis (Figure 3.31).[1–4]

Porokeratosis may occur anywhere on the body, but commonly presents on acral areas and distal aspects of extremities; disseminated superficial actinic porokeratosis (DSAP) predominates on sun-exposed body areas. A genetic predisposition has been described,[5] and there is a male preponderance. Skin lesions generally start as small, brownish keratotic papules or plaques with a well-demarcated, raised, hyperkeratotic, ridge-like border (Figure 3.32). Depending on the subtype, size may vary from a few millimeters to several centimeters in diameter. An association of porokeratosis with skin tumors is rare, yet the development of in-situ and invasive squamous cell carcinoma and basal cell carcinoma has been reported.[6,7] Dermoscopically, these lesions show a circumferential, yellowish-brown to skin-colored hyperkeratosis at their periphery, also referred to as 'white track pattern'. In thin lesions, increased vascularity may be noted dermoscopically as pinpoint vessels, red dots, globules, or lines. Furthermore, features of dyspigmentation with no pigment network and various degrees of erythema can be observed.[8,9] The histologic hallmark of all subtypes of porokeratosis is the presence of a cornoid lamella, or tower of parakeratosis, at the periphery of the lesion (Figures 3.33, 3.35, 3.37). Beneath the cornoid lamella, attenuation of the granular layer, dyskeratotic spinous keratinocytes, and vacuolated basal keratinocytes are commonly seen (Figures 3.35, 3.37, 3.39). The subjacent papillary dermis often shows a lymphocytic infiltrate around dilated capillaries[10] (Figure 3.41). The center of the lesion may be unremarkable, atrophic, show changes of lichen planus-like keratosis, or rarely show variable degrees of keratinocytic atypia, resembling an actinic keratosis.[10,11]

Owing to the clinical resemblance of DSAP and actinic keratosis (AK), differential diagnosis is often difficult based on clinical findings alone. Reflectance confocal microscopy (RCM) has been used for the non-invasive evaluation and differentiation of porokeratosis from AK in a pilot study.[12] Confocal examination of DSAP shows distinct features that correlate well with those observed on histology. A highly refractile structure sharply demarcated from the surrounding normal skin, resembling a cornoid lamella (Figures 3.34, 3.36), is characteristically found at the periphery of the lesion. Within this refractile structure, superficial disruptive changes in the stratum corneum (Figure 3.36) and retention of nuclei in the stratum corneum, or parakeratosis, are commonly found. The subjacent epidermis shows severe architectural disarray associated with a loss of the granular layer (Figure 3.38), while the remainder of the lesion may show only mild epidermal disarray. The presence of bright, round cells within the epidermis may correspond to exocytosis (Figure 3.40). Furthermore, a superficial dermal inflammatory infiltrate and blood vessel dilatation with increased capillary tortuosity may be detected using RCM (Figure 3.42).

Key RCM features of disseminated superficial actinic porokeratosis

- Cornoid lamella at the periphery
- Sharp demarcation from surrounding skin
- Mild superficial disruption of the stratum corneum with focal parakeratosis
- Pleomorphism of the granular/spinous layer
- Architectural disarray of the epidermis

REFERENCES

1. Ayres S Jr. Porokeratosis of Mibelli. Arch Dermatol Syphilology 1949; 60(6):1218.
2. Dover JS, Miller JA, Levene GM. Linear porokeratosis of Mibelli and DSAP. Clin Exp Dermatol 1986; 11(1):79–83.
3. Rahbari H, Cordero AA, Mehregan AH. Linear porokeratosis. A distinctive clinical variant of porokeratosis of Mibelli. Arch Dermatol 1974; 109(4):526–8.
4. Reed RJ, Leone P. Porokeratosis – a mutant clonal keratosis of the epidermis. I. Histogenesis. Arch Dermatol 1970; 101(3):340–7.
5. Anderson DE, Chernosky ME. Disseminated superficial actinic porokeratosis. Genetic aspects. Arch Dermatol 1969; 99(4):408–12.
6. Goerttler EA, Jung EG. Porokeratosis [correction of Parakeratosis] Mibelli and skin carcinoma: a critical review. Humangenetik 1975; 26(4):291–6.
7. Maubec E, Duvillard P, Margulis A et al. Common skin cancers in porokeratosis. Br J Dermatol 2005; 152(6):1389–91.
8. Delfino M, Argenziano G, Nino M. Dermoscopy for the diagnosis of porokeratosis. J Eur Acad Dermatol Venereol 2004; 18(2):194–5.
9. Zaballos P, Puig S, Malvehy J. Dermoscopy of disseminated superficial actinic porokeratosis. Arch Dermatol 2004; 140(11):1410.
10. Weedon D. Disorders of epidermal maturation and keratinisation. In: Weedon D, ed. Skin Pathology. New York: Churchill Livingstone, Elsevier Science, Limited; 2002: 292–4.
11. McKee PH, Calonje E, Granter SR. Disorders of keratinization. In: McKee PH, Calonje E, Granter SR, eds. Pathology of the Skin with Clinical Correlations. Vol. 1, 3rd edn. Philadelphia: Elsevier Mosby; 2005: 76–7.
12. Ulrich M, Forschner T, Rowert-Huber J et al. Differentiation between actinic keratoses and disseminated superficial actinic porokeratosis with reflectance confocal microscopy. Br J Dermatol 2007; 156(Suppl 3):47–52.

POROKERATOSIS

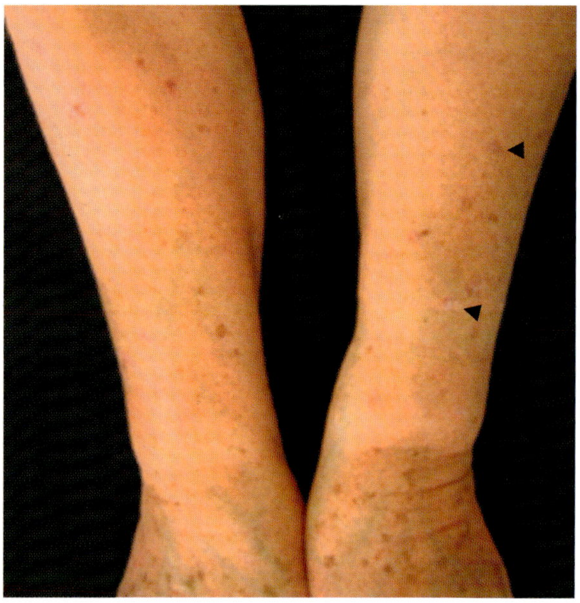

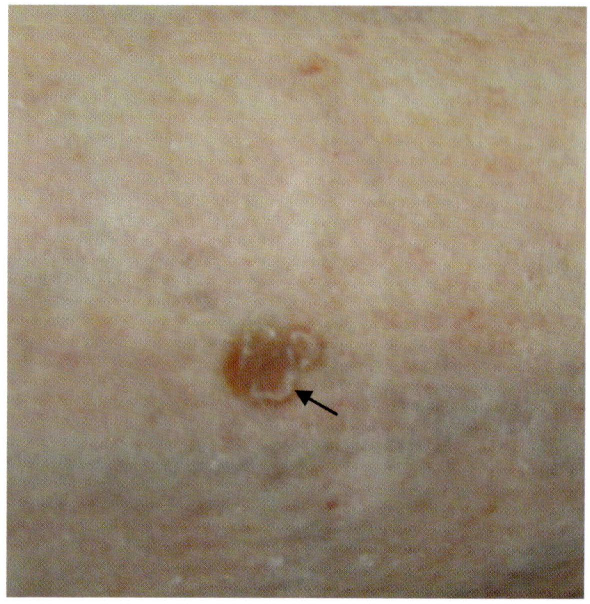

▲ **Figures 3.31, 3.32** Case 1: the clinical photograph shows multiple, 0.5–1.0 cm in diameter, sharply demarcated, hyperkeratotic, centrally atrophic plaques (arrowheads) of disseminated superficial actinic porokeratosis (DSAP) on the forearms of a 62-year-old female. The hyperkeratotic ridge-like border (arrow) on this well-demarcated plaque is evident in the close-up photograph of a representative lesion. Reproduced with permission of The British Journal of Dermatelogy from Ulrich M, Forschner T, Röwert-Huber S, Gonzalez S, et al. Differentiation between actinic keratoses and disseminated actinic porokeratoses with reluctance confocal microscopy. 2007 May 156.3.47–52. Reproduced with permission of Blackwall from referance 12.

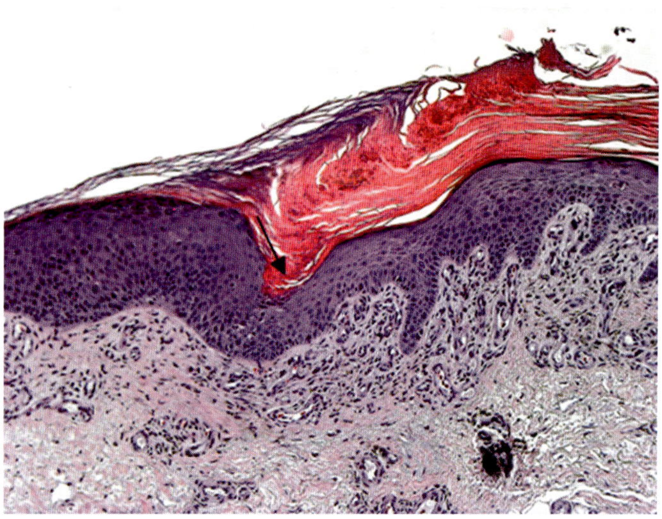

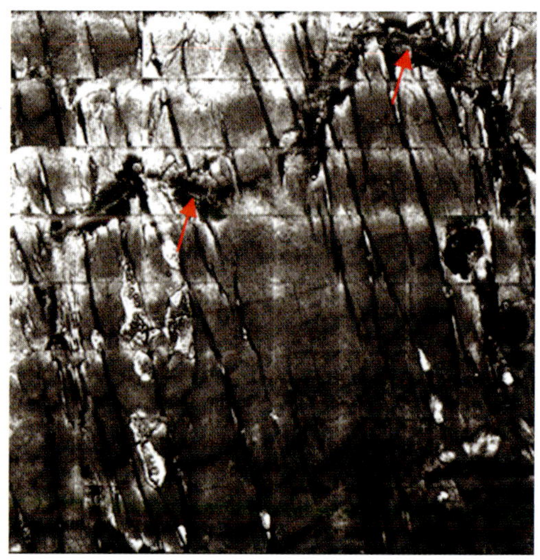

▲ **Figures 3.33, 3.34** Case 1: histology (10×) shows the characteristic leaning tower of parakeratosis, or cornoid lamella, with subjacent depression of the epidermal surface and loss of the granular layer (arrow). On the RCM mosaic (4 mm × 4 mm) at the level of the granular layer, a hyporefractile granular ridge corresponding to the cornoid lamella is easily seen (red arrows).

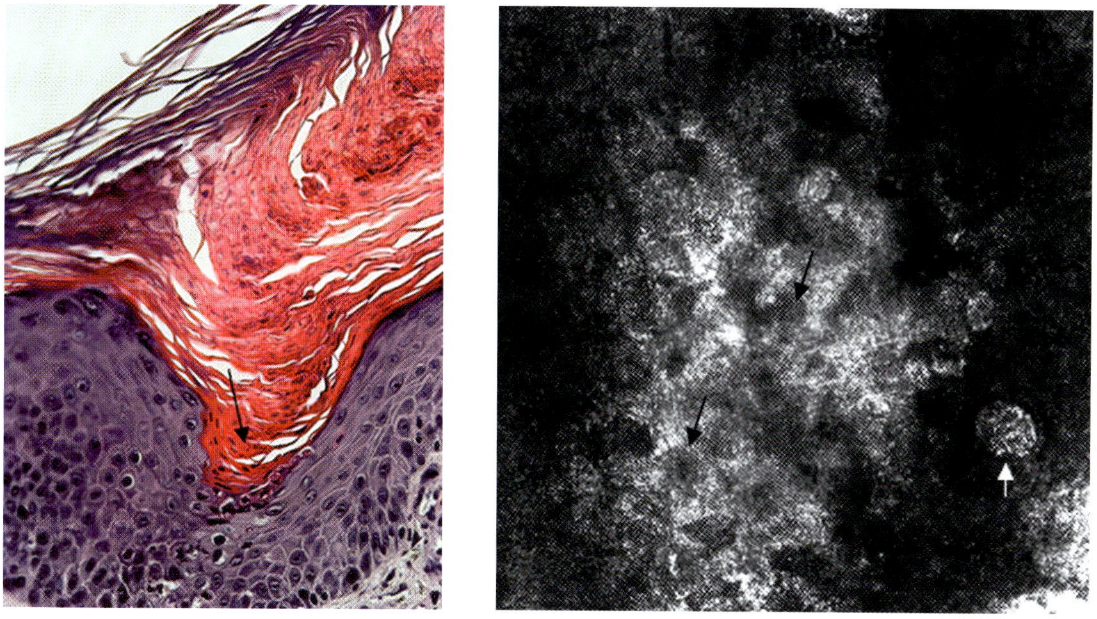

▲ **Figures 3.35, 3.36** Case 1: high-power histology (40×) again showing the well-demarcated vertical stack of parakeratosis forming the cornoid lamella (black arrow). Corresponding RCM (0.5 mm × 0.5 mm) at the level of the skin surface reveals a disruption of the normal stratum corneum by a focal zone of bright, granular refractility with regularly sized and spaced dark nuclei (black arrows) and individual detached keratinocytes (white arrow). Reproduced with permission of The British Journal of Dermatelogy from Ulrich M, Forschner T, Röwert-Huber S, Gonzalez S, et al. Differentiation between actinic keratoses and disseminated actinic porokeratoses with reluctance confocal microscopy. 2007 May 156.3.47–52. Reproduced with permission of Blackwall from referance 12.

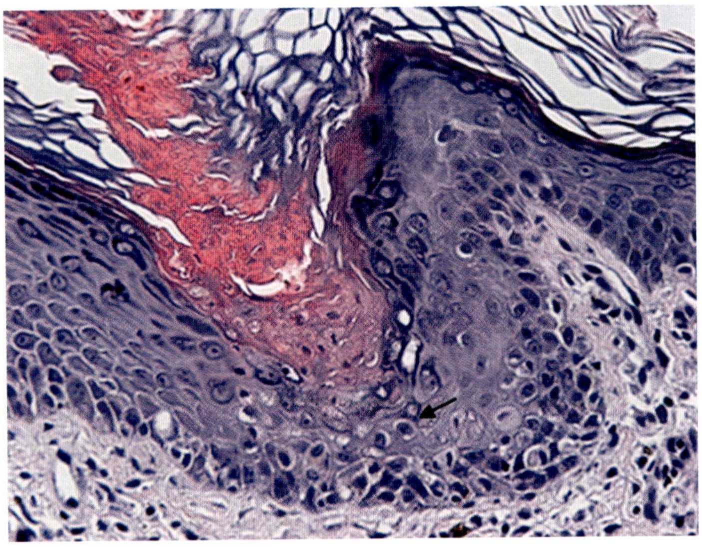

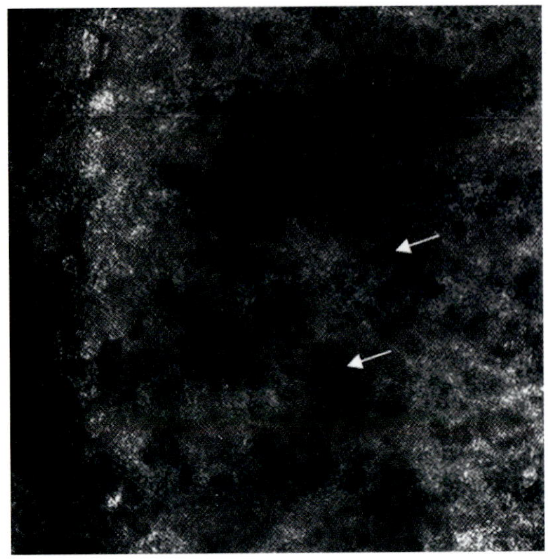

▲ **Figures 3.37, 3.38** Case 2: histology (40×) showing another example of a cornoid lamella. In this cut, the dell or depression of the surface of the epidermis below the cornoid lamella is prominent (black arrow). A few subjacent dyskeratotic keratinocytes and a few mildly atypical basal and suprabasal keratinocytes are seen, but the granular layer is preserved. Corresponding RCM (0.5 mm × 0.5 mm) at the level of the stratum granulosum reveals architectural disarray, with a darker zone showing loss of the normal honeycomb pattern and mild variation in keratinocytic nuclear size (white arrows). Dark zones may be due to their location under areas with hyperkeratosis, allowing less light penetration. Reproduced with permission of The British Journal of Dermatelogy from Ulrich M, Forschner T, Röwert-Huber S, Gonzalez S, et al. Differentiation between actinic keratoses and disseminated actinic porokeratoses with reluctance confocal microscopy. 2007 May 156.3.47–52. Reproduced with permission of Blackwall from referance 12.

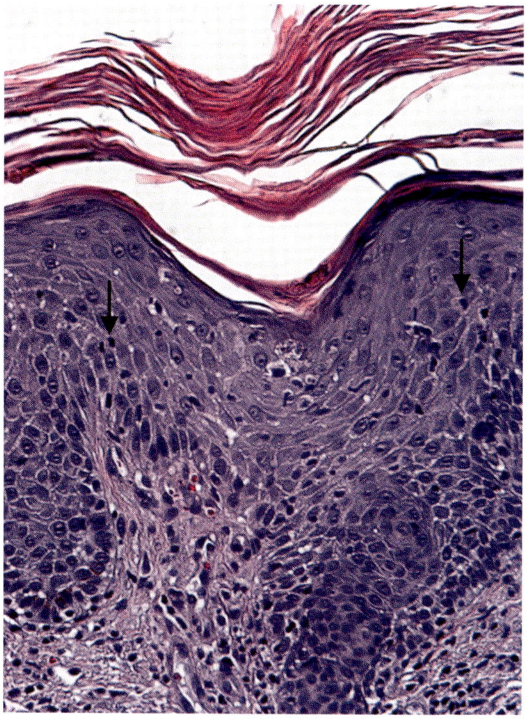

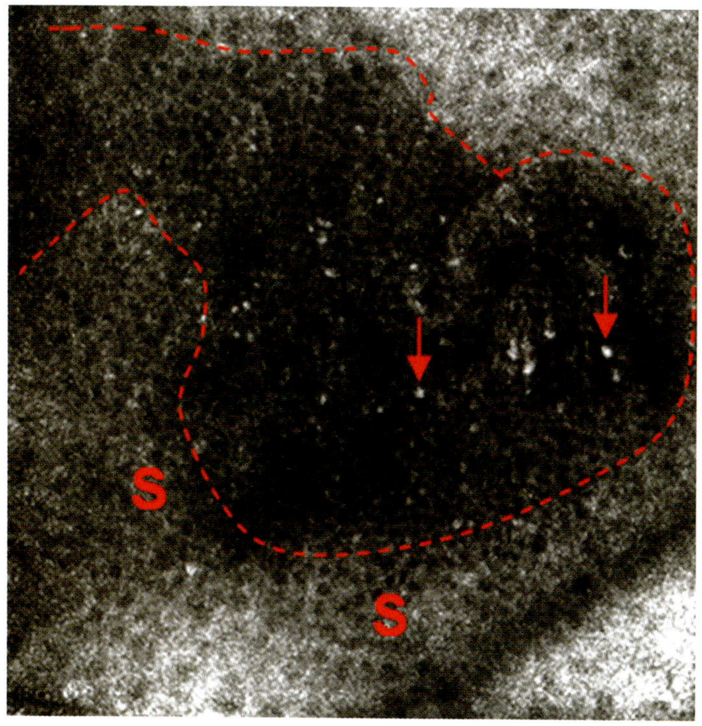

▲ **Figures 3.39, 3.40** Case 2: histology (40×) shows epidermis beneath the cornoid lamella in an area with more subtle changes. A small dell in the surface contour of the epidermis with a thin stratum granulosum and a few dyskeratotic cells are present. In addition, slight spongiosis and mild exocytosis of lymphocytes (arrows) are noticeable. On RCM (0.5 mm × 0.5 mm) at the level of the stratum spinosum, the honeycomb architecture is preserved, but somewhat distorted by partially thickened and blurred intercellular demarcations, indicative of spongiosis (S), and scattered small, round bright cells (red arrows), representing inflammation. The epidermis directly beneath the cornoid lamella corresponds to the well-demarcated dark zone (dashed red line) in the center of the optical image.

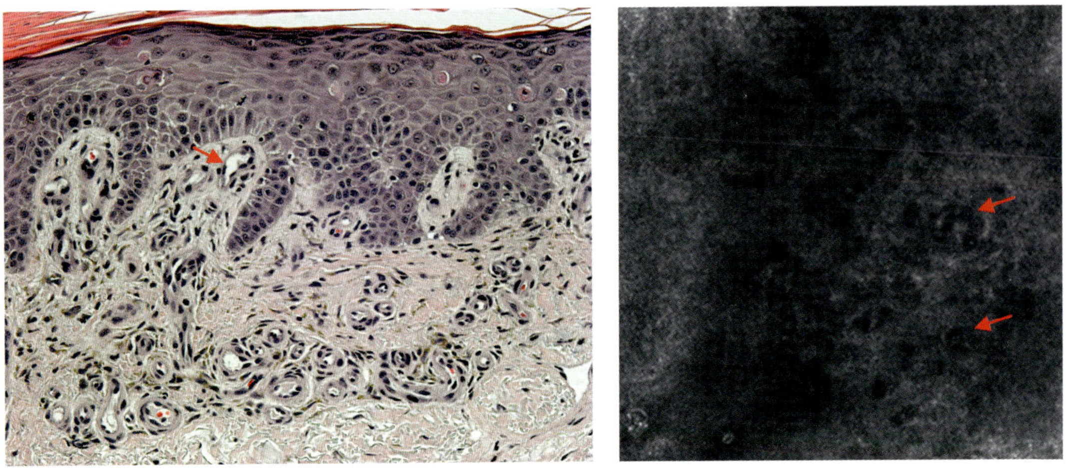

▲ **Figures 3.41, 3.42** Case 2: on histology (20×), this lesion shows an increased number of lobulated, tortuous, small blood vessels in the papillary dermis, which are seen on corresponding RCM (0.5 mm × 0.5 mm) at the level of the superficial dermis as coiling black canalicular structures containing variably refractile cells (red arrows). Reproduced with permission of The British Journal of Dermatelogy from Ulrich M, Forschner T, Rowert-Huber S, Gonzalez S, et al. Differentiation between actinic keratoses and disseminated actinic porokeratoses with reluctance confocal microscopy. 2007 May 156.3.47–52. Reproduced with permission of Blackwall from referance 12.

CHAPTER 3d

Squamous neoplasia

Susanne Astner, Martina Ulrich, Jesus Cuevas, and Salvador González

Actinic keratosis (AK) and squamous cell carcinoma (SCC) are among the most common cutaneous malignancies.[1,2] Predisposing risk factors include skin phototypes (SPT) I–III, a history of blistering sunburns and long-standing sun exposure, and a positive family history. Clinically, they present as erythematous, hyperkeratotic macules, papules, and plaques occurring on sun-exposed areas of the face, scalp, forearms, upper back, hands, and lower legs, and lesions are often better felt than seen (Figure 3.43). Although they generally occur as single lesions (Figure 3.45), the concept of field cancerization suggests that large areas with actinic damage will show similar histologic changes in areas surrounding the clinically visible lesion such that entire anatomic areas may be affected (Figures 3.47, 3.63). Generally, clinical diagnosis does not pose a significant problem; however, the gold standard for diagnosis remains histologic evaluation.

ACTINIC KERATOSIS

Histopathologically, AKs are usually characterized by parakeratosis and hypogranulosis overlying keratinocytic dysmaturation and atypia, including nuclear enlargement, pleomorphism, and hyperchromasia, with sparing of the acrosyringia and acrotrichia and subjacent solar elastosis (Figures 3.44, 3.46, 3.48).[3] The architecture, extent of squamous atypia, and presence of associated inflammation vary among the many described histopathologic subtypes. Dermoscopic findings are non-specific and include focal hyperkeratosis, hemorrhagic or serous crusting, and increased vasculature, or fine telangiectases that may appear as pinpoint or hairpin-like vessels.[4]

Characteristic features of AK are readily detected by reflectance confocal microscopy (RCM) and correlate well with routine histology.[5] In the stratum corneum, superficial disruption and detached individual corneocytes are seen as bright, highly refractile cells of polygonal morphology (Figures 3.49, 3.50). The presence of parakeratosis, seen as dark, round, well-demarcated, centrally placed structures (retention of nuclei) within corneocytes of 15–20 μm in diameter, is also frequently observed (Figures 3.51, 3.52). Various degrees of architectural disarray and cellular pleomorphism at the level of the spinous and granular layers correspond to different levels of dysplasia in routine histology (Figures 3.55–3.58). Inflammation in the epidermal and upper dermal compartment may be present and may also correlate with superficial impetiginization (Figures 3.53, 3.54, 3.57, 3.58). Solar elastosis is easily visualized, owing to its moderate refractility and particular amorphous lace-like morphology (Figures 3.59–3.62). The detection of dilated blood vessels as elongated or tortuous superficial dermal vascular structures with marked blood flow corresponds to the increased vascularity associated with neoplastic growth (Figures 3.59–3.62). The detection of dermal RCM features of AK, however, may be limited by the presence of significant hyperkeratosis which does not permit their optical resolution with increased depths of penetration. A recent study aimed at evaluating the RCM criteria of AK for clinical and histomorphologic correlation suggests that RCM is a valuable tool for AK detection.[6] Future studies are needed to test the clinical applicability.

Key RCM features of actinic keratosis

- Superficial disruption of the stratum corneum with detached corneocytes and parakeratosis
- Pleomorphism of the epidermis
- Architectural disarray of the epidermis

SQUAMOUS CELL CARCINOMA

Squamous cell carcinoma is the second most common subtype of non-melanoma skin cancer (NMSC).[7] Besides chronic ultraviolet (UV) exposure, a history of long-standing immunosuppression, radiation therapy, arsenic exposure, chronic wounds, and genetic aberrations have been discussed as etiologic factors.[8,9] Several distinct subtypes have been described, and the majority of SCCs develop from precursor lesions such as AK.[10] Clinically, SCC presents as irritated, hyperkeratotic, superficially erosive or ulcerated papules or plaques with recurrent episodes of bleeding. The increased vulnerability and friability of the tissue may indicate the progression from AK to SCC. Examination of surrounding skin reveals actinic field damage in the majority of patients (Figure 3.63). Histopathologically, SCC is defined by proliferation of atypical squamous cells, containing abundant eosinophilic cytoplasm and a large nucleus, which extends from the epidermis into the dermis (Figure 3.64). Overlying hyperkeratosis and parakeratosis and associated inflammation are often seen.[3,11] SCC may arise in association with full-thickness keratinocytic atypia or may be connected to a near-normal overlying epidermis. Dermoscopic findings are non-specific and may reveal patterns of increased keratinization around hairpin vessels and hemorrhagic or serous crusting. Atypical reticular and globular pigment patterns may not permit the differentiation from melanocytic skin lesions.[12,13]

Using RCM, characteristic features of SCC may only be detected if hyperkeratosis is limited and does not interfere with the evaluation. Mild curettage or the use of keratolytic agents may facilitate the imaging process. When imaging the superficial layers, changes are comparable to those observed with AK but are generally more severe. The presence of superficial disruption, detached individual corneocytes, and parakeratosis are characteristically found (Figures 3.65, 3.66). Architectural disarray and cellular pleomorphism at the level of the basal, spinous, and granular layers reflect the severe cellular atypia and dysplasia described by routine histopathology (Figures 3.65, 3.67, 3.68). Inflammation in the epidermal and upper dermal compartments may be identified (Figures 3.67–3.70). With the increased hyperkeratosis and acanthosis of progressing SCC, it may be difficult to determine the morphology of the dermal component, including islands of invasive tumor, increased vasculature, and solar elastosis (Figures 3.69–3.72). Due to limited light penetration, the absence of these features may indicate to the operator that the dermis is not being reached by RCM. In that regard, the *horizontal* sections obtained by RCM may not permit the detection of dermal invasion in individual lesions. Moreover, RCM in its current configuration is not ideal for determining the *vertical* extent of SCC invasion.

Key RCM features of squamous cell carcinoma

- Superficial disruption of the stratum corneum
- Pleomorphic parakeratosis
- Severe atypical pleomorphism of the epidermis
- Severe architectural disaray of the epidermis
- Atypical aggregates of keratinocytes in the dermis (if light penetration possible)

REFERENCES

1. Cockerell CJ. Histopathology of incipient intraepidermal squamous cell carcinoma ("actinic keratosis"). J Am Acad Dermatol 2000; 42:11–17.
2. Montgomery H, Dorffler J. Verruca seniles and keratoma senile. Arch Dermatol Syph (Berlin) 1932; 166:635.
3. James C, Crawford RI, Martinka M et al. Actinic keratosis. In: LeBoit PE, Burg G, Weedon D, Sarasin A, eds. World Health Organization Classification of Tumors. Pathology and Genetics of the Skin Tumors. Lyon: IARC Press; 2006: 30–2.
4. Zalaudek I, Giacomel J, Argenziano G et al. Dermoscopy of facial nonpigmented actinic keratosis. Br J Dermatol 2006; 155:951–6.

5. Aghassi D, Anderson RR, Gonzalez S. Confocal laser microscopic imaging of actinic keratoses in vivo: a preliminary report. J Am Acad Dermatol 2000; 43:42–8.

6. Ulrich M, Maltusch A, Rowert-Huber J et al. Actinic keratoses: non-invasive diagnosis for field cancerisation. Br J Dermatol 2007; 156(Suppl 3):13–7.

7. Skidmore RA Jr, Flowers FP. Nonmelanoma skin cancer. Med Clin North Am 1998; 82:1309–23,vi.

8. Dodson JM, DeSpain J, Hewett JE et al. Malignant potential of actinic keratoses and the controversy over treatment. A patient-oriented perspective. Arch Dermatol 1991; 127:1029–31.

9. Johnson TM, Rowe DE, Nelson BR et al. Squamous cell carcinoma of the skin (excluding lip and oral mucosa). J Am Acad Dermatol 1992; 26:467–84.

10. Marks R, Rennie G, Selwood TS. Malignant transformation of solar keratoses to squamous cell carcinoma. Lancet 1988; 1:795–7.

11. Rinker MH, Fenske NA, Scalf LA et al. Histologic variants of squamous cell carcinoma of the skin. Cancer Control 2001; 8:354–63.

12. Stante M, de Giorgi V, Massi D et al. Pigmented Bowen's disease mimicking cutaneous melanoma: clinical and dermoscopic aspects. Dermatol Surg 2004; 30:541–4.

13. Zalaudek I, Citarella L, Soyer HP et al. Dermoscopy features of pigmented squamous cell carcinoma: a case report. Dermatol Surg 2004; 30:539–40.

ACTINIC KERATOSIS

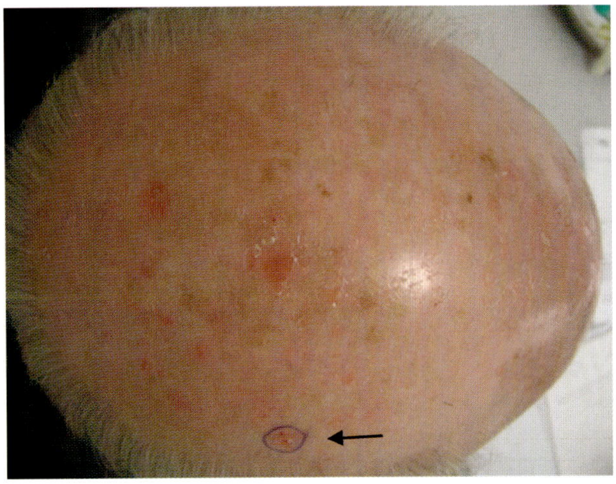

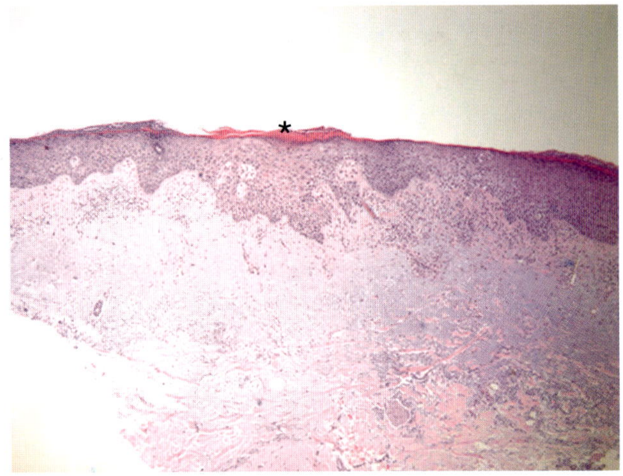

▲ **Figures 3.43, 3.44** Case 1: the clinical photograph shows the scalp of a 65-year-old male (SPT II), which harbors numerous erythematous macules with fine hyperkeratotic scale, marked dyspigmentation, and skin atrophy, consistent with multiple actinic keratoses (AKs). The AK selected for RCM imaging (black arrow) measured 10 mm × 12 mm. Corresponding histopathology (4×) reveals hyperkeratosis (asterisk), parakeratosis, partial-thickness keratinocytic atypia, and marked solar elastosis.

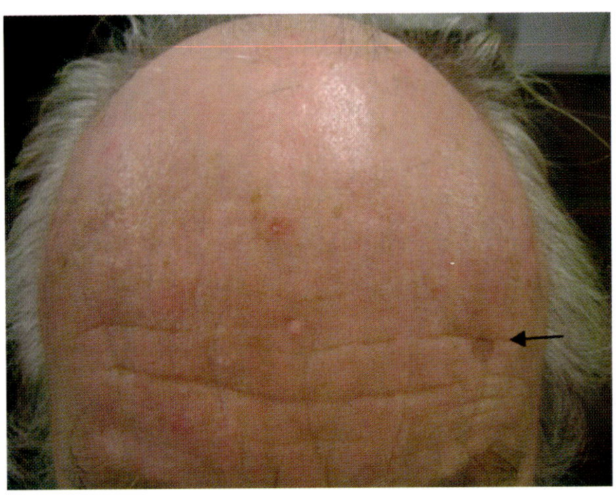

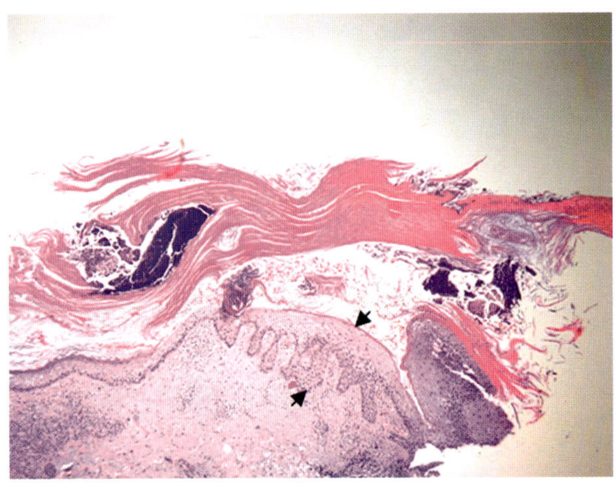

▲ **Figures 3.45, 3.46** Case 2: the clinical photograph shows the forehead of a 69-year-old male (SPT II), which harbors multiple erythematous macules with hyperkeratotic scale and irregular surface structure. An 8 mm × 9 mm flat erythematous papule with fine hyperkeratotic scale and an irregular surface located on the left temple (black arrow) was selected for RCM imaging. Corresponding histopathology (4×) reveals marked hyperkeratosis, parakeratosis, acanthosis (arrows), partial-thickness keratinocytic atypia, and extensive solar elastosis.

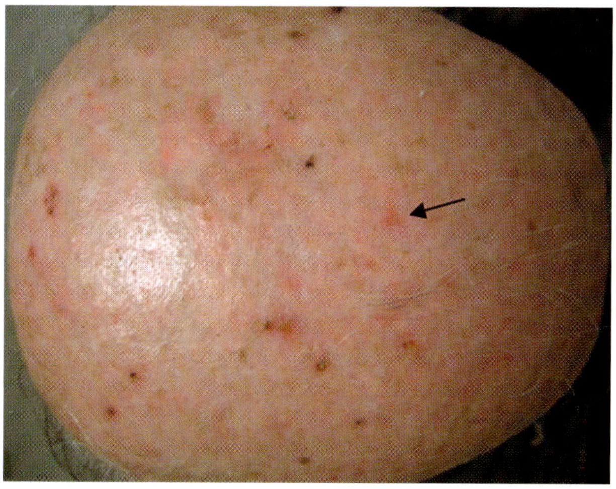

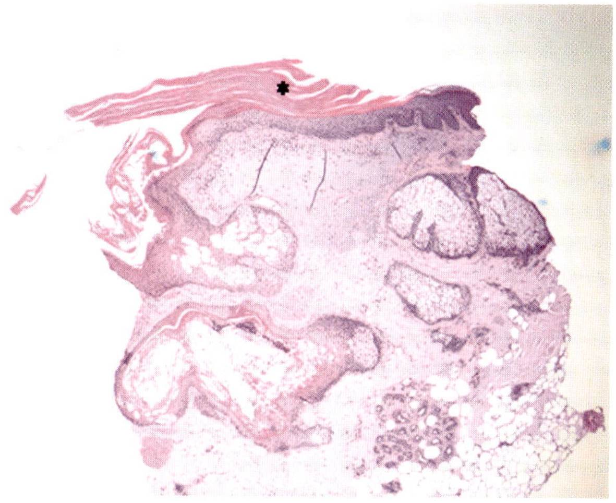

▲ **Figures 3.47, 3.48** Case 3: the clinical photograph of the scalp of a 72-year-old male (SPT II) with actinic field cancerization shows multiple erythematous, partially erosive macules, papules, and plaques with hyperkeratotic scale or serosanguinous crusting. A 7 mm erythematous papule with hyperkeratotic scale (arrow) was selected for imaging and biopsy. Corresponding low-power histology (4×) reveals an actinic keratosis with marked RCM hyperkeratosis (asterisk), parakeratosis, and partial-thickness keratinocytic atypia.

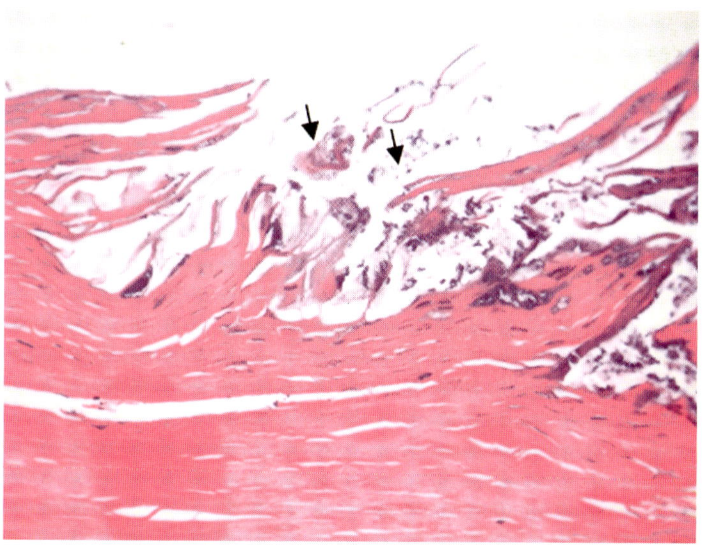

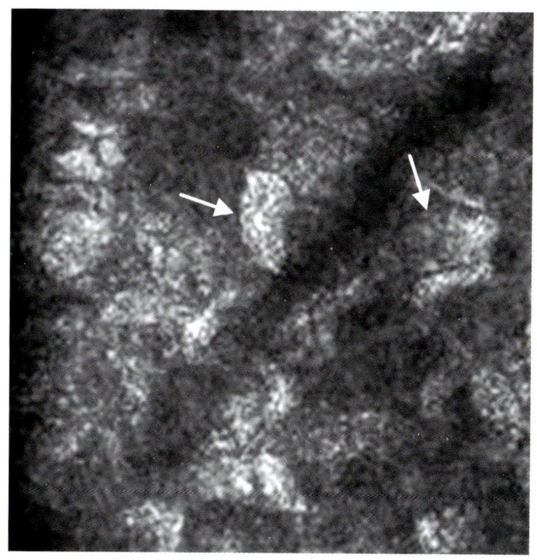

▲ **Figures 3.49, 3.50** Case 1: histology (40×) of the stratum corneum with extensive parakeratosis and foci of orthokeratosis. Disruption of the stratum corneum is seen (arrows). Corresponding RCM (0.5 mm × 0.5 mm) shows detached individual corneocytes (white arrows) that are indicative of disruption of this layer. Reproduced with permission of Blackwell publishing from Ulrich M, Maltasch A, Rius-Diaz et al. Clinical applicability of in vivo reflectance confocal microscopy for the diagnosis of actinic keratoses. Dermatol Surg. in press.

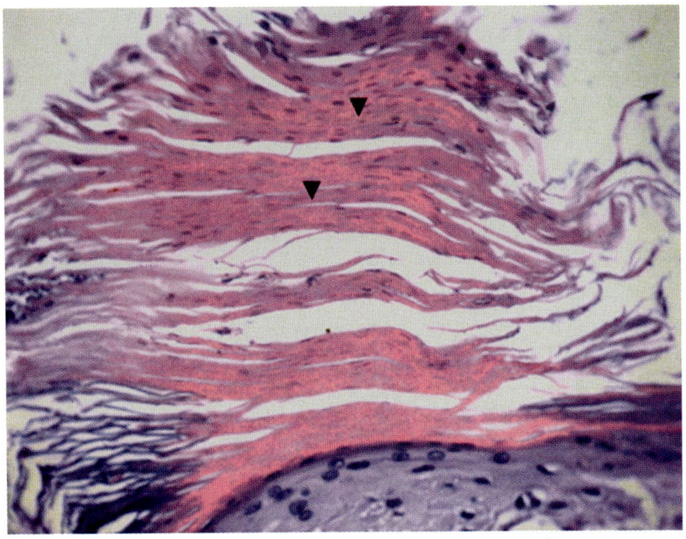

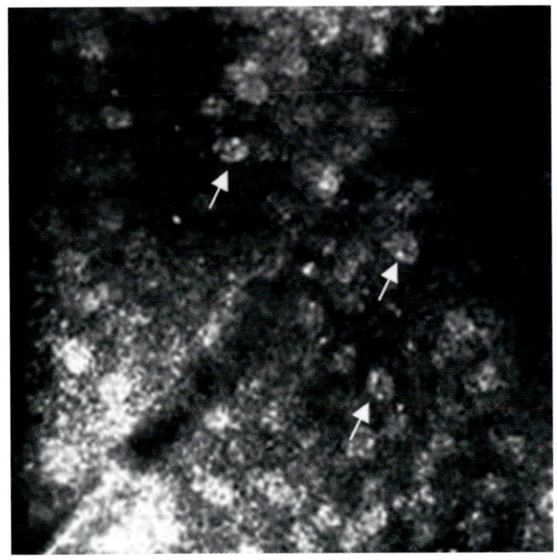

▲ **Figures 3.51, 3.52** Case 3: histology (40×) shows alternating orthokeratosis (lower left) and parakeratosis (arrowheads) of the stratum corneum, characteristic of AK. Corresponding RCM (0.5 mm × 0.5 mm) shows numerous brightly refractile corneocytes with central dark areas (white arrows) compatible with parakeratosis. Reproduced with permission of Blackwell publishing from Ulrich M, Maltasch A, Rius-Diaz et al. Clinical applicability of in vivo reflectance confocal microscopy for the diagnosis of actinic keratoses. Dermatol Surg. in press.

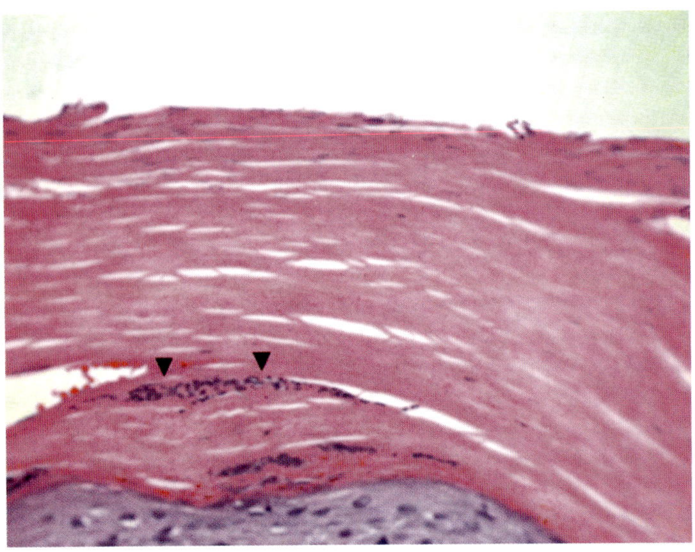

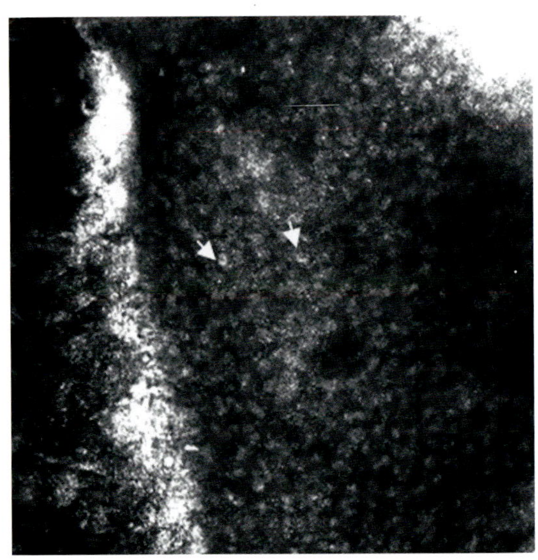

▲ **Figures 3.53, 3.54** Case 3: on histology (40×), clusters of neutrophils (arrowheads) are seen within the stratum corneum, consistent with focal impetiginization. Corresponding RCM (0.5 mm × 0.5 mm) reveals numerous, bright, round-to-oval structures resembling inflammatory cells (white arrows) within the stratum corneum. Reproduced with permission of Blackwell publishing from Ulrich M, Maltasch A, Rius-Diaz et al. Clinical applicability of in vivo reflectance confocal microscopy for the diagnosis of actinic keratoses. Dermatol Surg. in press.

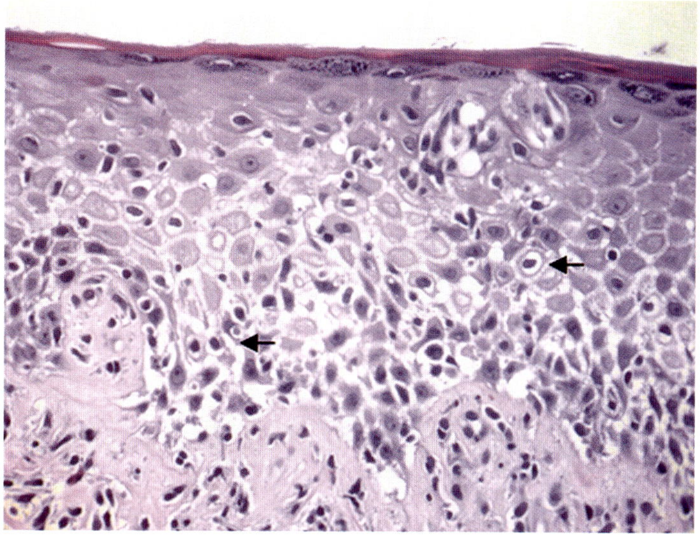

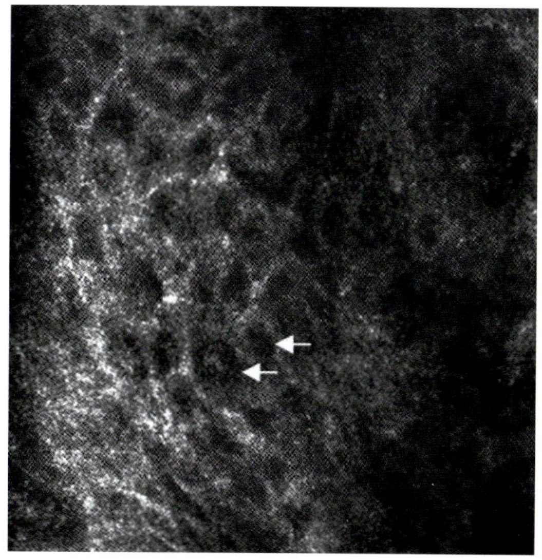

▲ **Figures 3.55, 3.56** Case 3: histology (40×) shows keratinocytic atypia, including increased nuclear-to-cytoplasmic ratio and nuclear pleomorphism, mainly limited to lower half of the epidermis (black arrows). The granular layer is notably intact. Also present is mild exocytosis of lymphocytes with mild-to-moderate associated spongiosis. Corresponding RCM (0.5 mm × 0.5 mm) at the level of the stratum granulosum reveals a distorted architecture, with an altered honeycombed pattern demonstrating increased thickness and brightness of intercellular demarcations, consistent with spongiosis. Focal variation in nuclear size (pleomorphism) indicates focal keratinocytic atypia (white arrows). Reproduced with permission of Blackwell publishing from Ulrich M, Maltasch A, Rius-Diaz et al. Clinical applicability of in vivo reflectance confocal microscopy for the diagnosis of actinic keratoses. Dermatol Surg. in press.

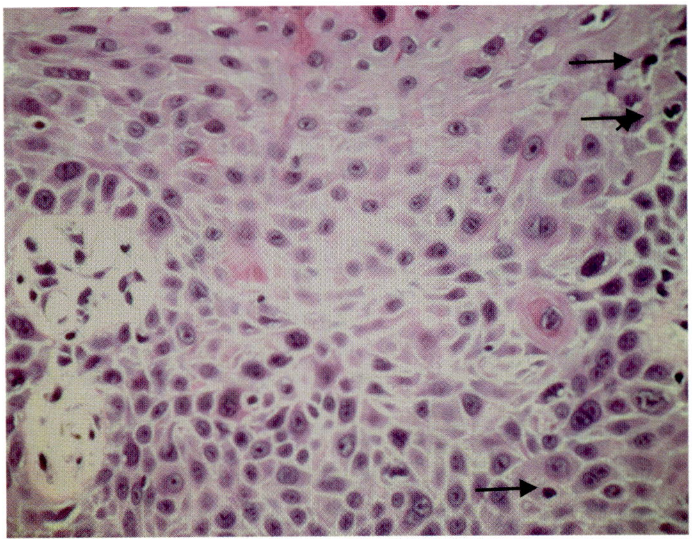

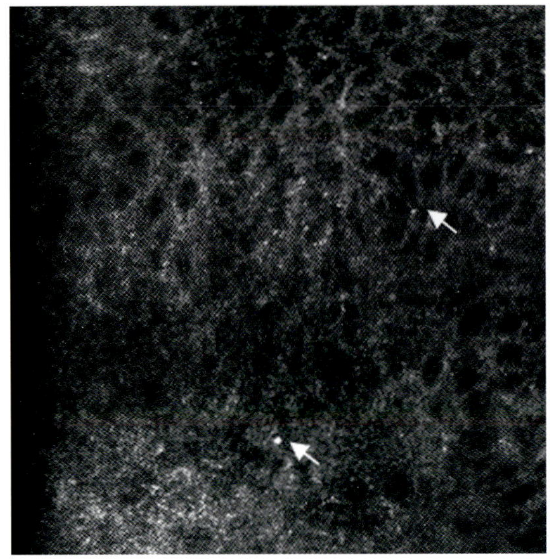

▲ **Figures 3.57, 3.58** Case 3: on histology (40×), moderate keratinocytic atypia, mild-to-moderate spongiosis and scattered lymphocytes (black arrows) are seen in the stratum spinosum. Keratinocytic nuclear pleomorphism is easy to identify. Corresponding RCM (0.5 mm × 0.5 mm) at the level of the stratum spinosum reveals variation in size and shape of keratinocytic nuclei and severe disruption of the epidermal architecture, including complete loss of the honeycomb pattern in the lower half of the optical section and brightened and thickened intercellular demarcations, indicating spongiosis, in the upper half of the optical section. Scattered small, round bright cells (white arrows), compatible with inflammatory cells, are seen. Reproduced with permission of Blackwell publishing from Ulrich M, Maltasch A, Rius-Diaz et al. Clinical applicability of in vivo reflectance confocal microscopy for the diagnosis of actinic keratoses. Dermatol Surg. in press.

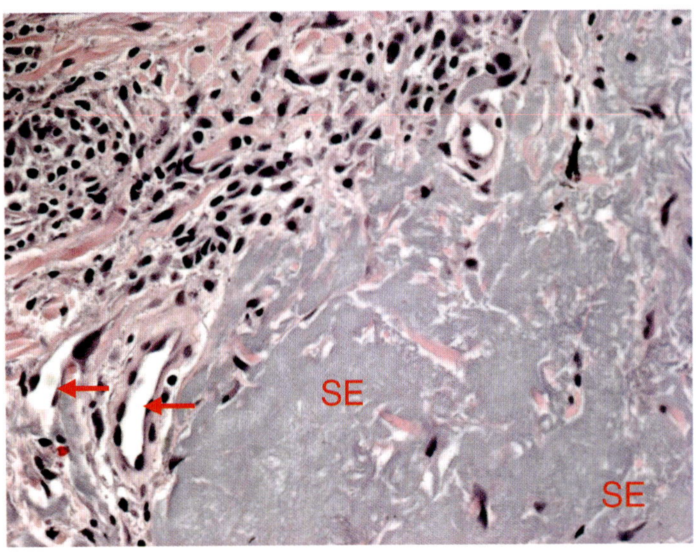

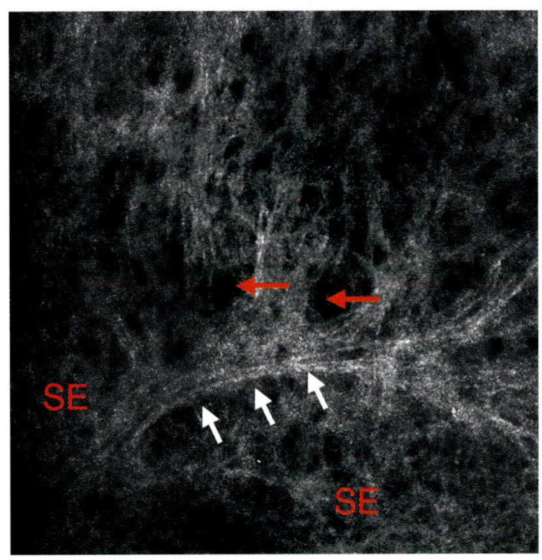

▲ **Figures 3.59, 3.60** Case 2: histology (40×) shows dilated small blood vessels (red arrows), chronic inflammation, and extensive solar elastosis (SE) in the upper dermis. Corresponding RCM (0.5 mm × 0.5 mm) at the level of the superficial dermis shows prominent, refractile bundled collagen (white arrows), prominent blood vessels (red arrows), and lace-like amorphous moderately refractile material (SE). Reproduced with permission of Blackwell publishing from Ulrich M, Maltasch A, Rius-Diaz et al. Clinical applicability of in vivo reflectance confocal microscopy for the diagnosis of actinic keratoses. Dermatol Surg. in press.

SQUAMOUS CELL CARCINOMA

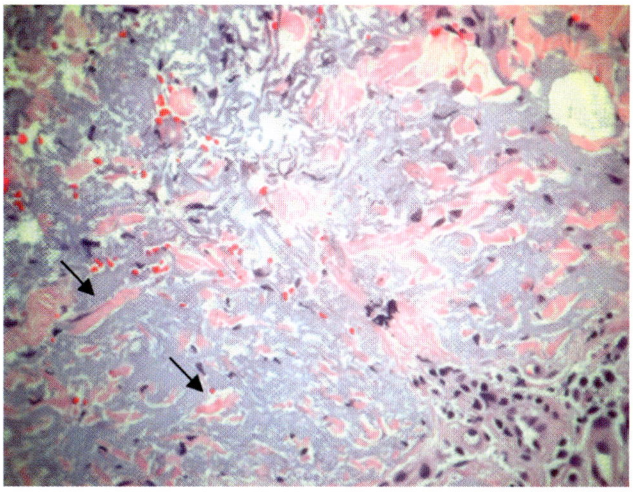

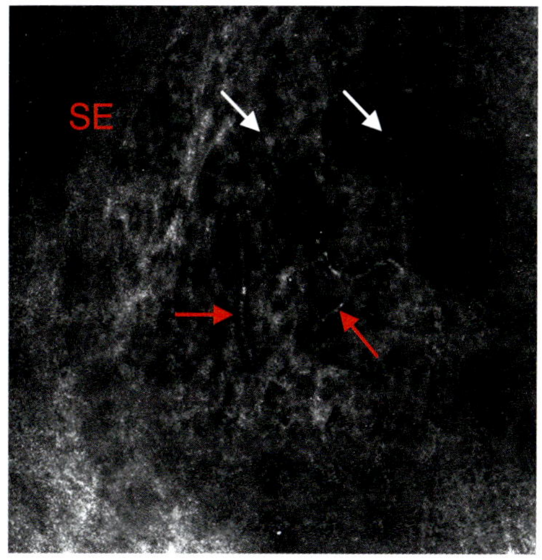

▲ **Figures 3.61, 3.62** Case 1: on histology (40×), solar elastosis appears as homogenized, thick wavy blue fibers interspersed among pink collagen fibers (arrows). A few prominent vessels and sparse associated inflammation are seen in the lower right corner. RCM (0.5 mm × 0.5 mm) at the level of the superficial dermis reveals prominent and tortuous small canalicular structures containing refractile cells (red arrows), corresponding to blood vessels; scattered round-to-oval refractile cells (white arrows), suggestive of inflammatory cells; and a thickened, moderately refractile lacy background stroma, compatible with solar elastosis (SE). Reproduced with permission of Blackwell publishing from Ulrich M, Maltasch A, Rius-Diaz et al. Clinical applicability of in vivo reflectance confocal microscopy for the diagnosis of actinic keratoses. Dermatol Surg. in press.

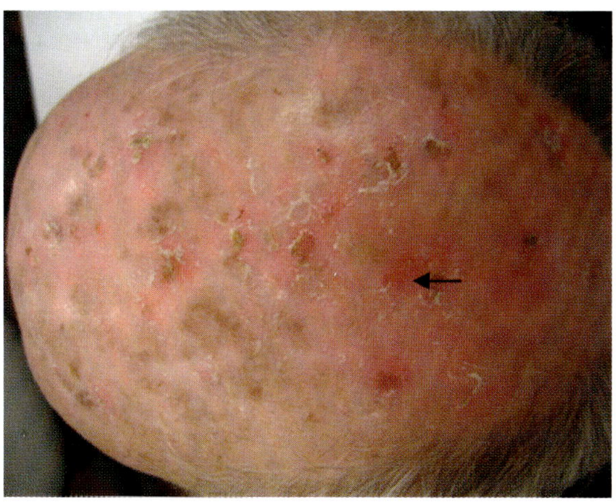

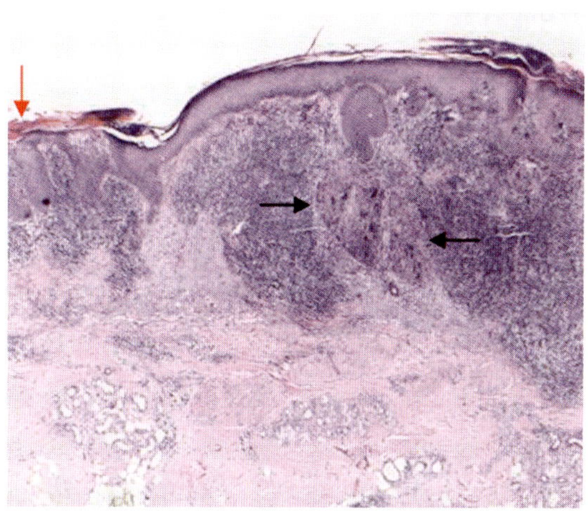

▲ **Figures 3.63, 3.64** Case 1: the clinical photograph shows the scalp of a 71-year-old male (SPT II) with numerous erythematous macules, papules, and plaques with thick attached scale, marked dyspigmentation, and skin atrophy consistent with multiple actinic keratoses and diffuse actinic field damage. A superficially erosive, erythematous plaque with increased tissue vulnerability is clinically suspicious for squamous cell carcinoma (SCC; black arrow). Low-power histology (4×) shows invasive SCC. Notably, the intraepidermal component ranges from atypia only within the lower portion over the frankly invasive tumor (black arrows) to near carcinoma in situ (red arrow) lateral to the invasive component. Marked hyperkeratosis and parakeratosis are also seen.

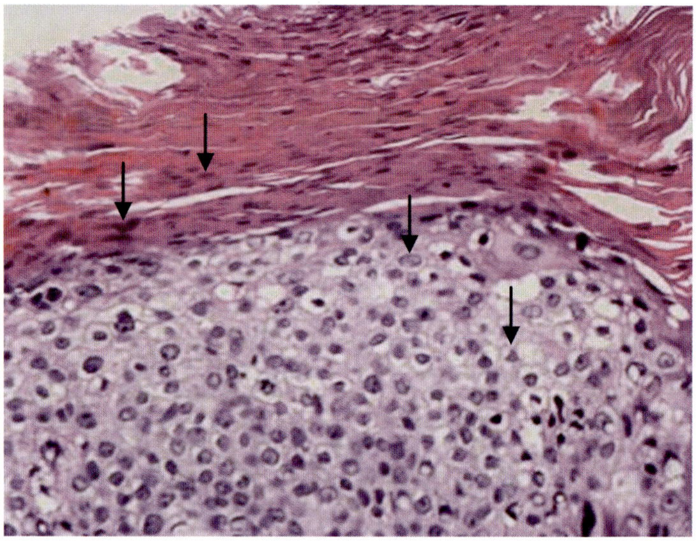

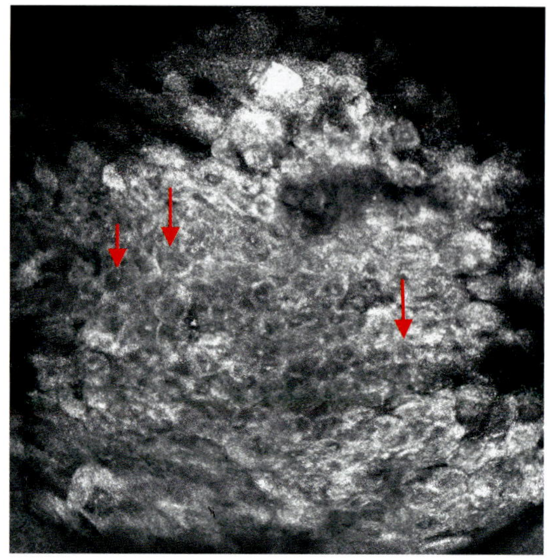

▲ **Figures 3.65, 3.66** Case 1: high-power histology (40×) shows near to focal full-thickness keratinocytic atypia with overlying parakeratosis. The increased nuclear-to-cytoplasmic ratio and nuclear pleomorphism is easily appreciated both in the stratum spinosum and within the parakeratosis (black arrows). Stratum granulosum is absent. Corresponding RCM (0.5 mm × 0.5 mm) at the level of the stratum corneum shows rounded granular highly refractile cells. The central darker areas within the cells, corresponding to the parakeratotic pyknotic nuclei, vary in size (red arrows).

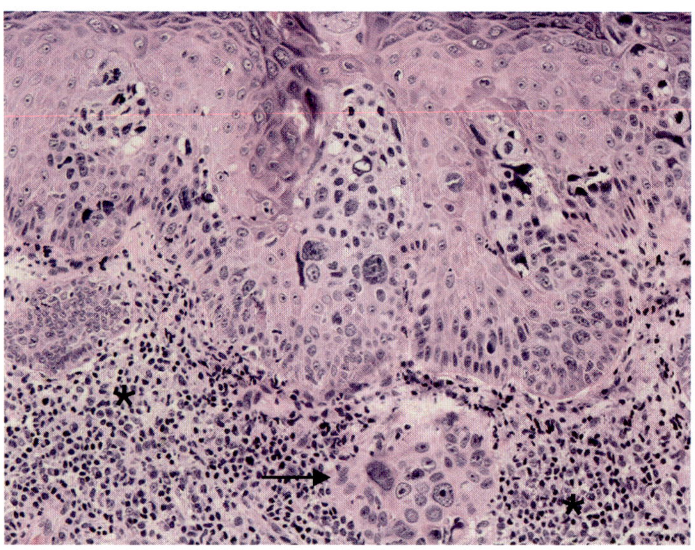

▲ **Figures 3.67, 3.68** Case 1: histology (40×) shows aggregates of enlarged atypical keratinocytes with marked nuclear pleomorphism and quite abundant pink cytoplasm in the epidermis and the superficial dermis (black arrow) with associated chronic inflammation (asterisks). Corresponding RCM (0.5 mm × 0.5 mm) of the upper epidermis reveals severe disruption of the epidermal architecture, with haphazard distribution of keratinocytes, nuclear pleomorphism and atypia, spongiosis, and bright round cells (white arrowheads), corresponding to exocytosis.

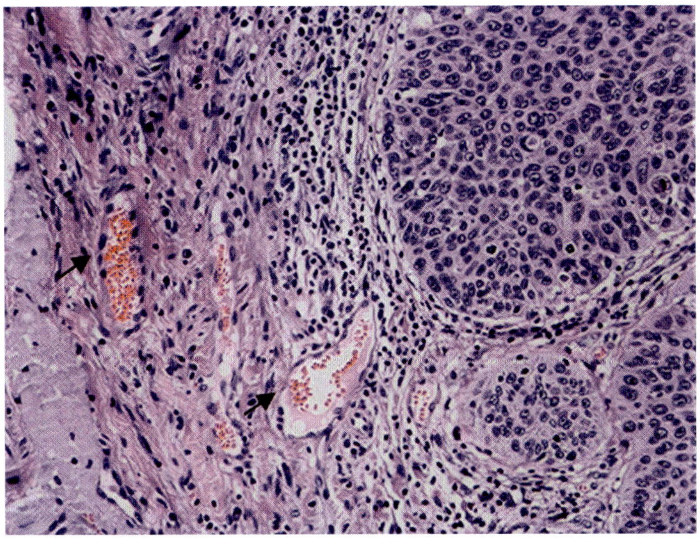

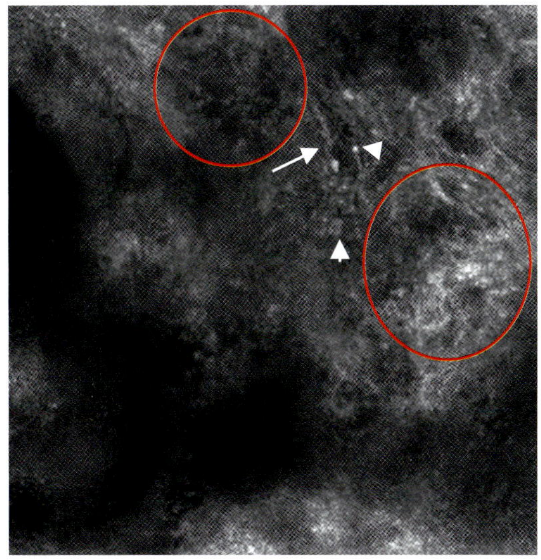

▲ **Figures 3.69, 3.70** Case 1: histology (40×) shows islands of invasive SCC with peritumoral inflammation and increased vascularity (black arrows). RCM (0.5 mm × 0.5 mm) of the upper dermis reveals brighter zones within which subtle outlines of atypical keratinocytes (red circles) can be seen, corresponding to invasive tumor. Subtle vascular dilatation and elongation (white arrow) and scattered refractile round inflammatory cells (white arrowheads) can be seen.

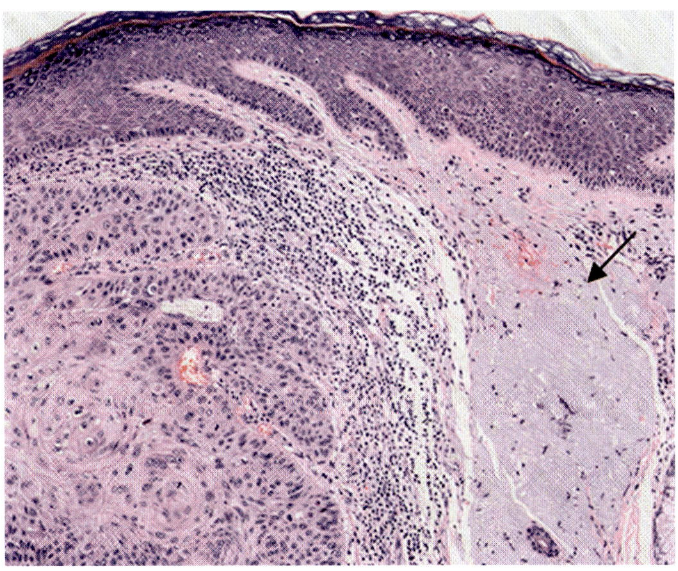

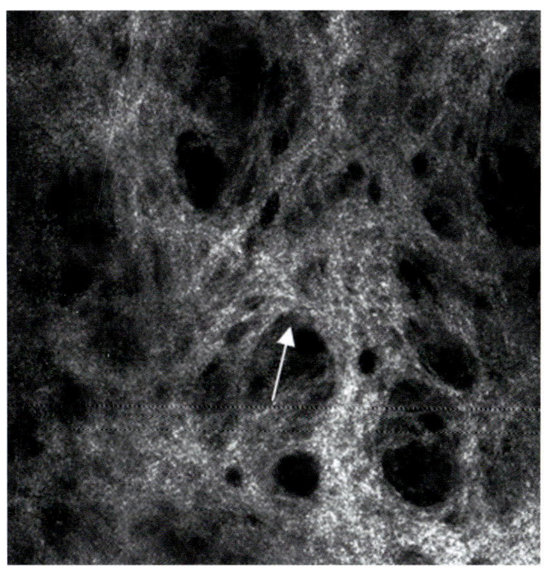

▲ **Figures 3.71, 3.72** Case 1: histology (20×) illustrates severe solar elastosis (black arrow) adjacent to the SCC. Corresponding RCM image (0.5 mm × 0.5 mm) of the upper dermis adjacent to the tumor reveals extensive amorphous moderately refractile lacy material obscuring aberrant fibrotic bundles (white arrow).

CHAPTER 3e

Basal cell carcinoma

Anna Liza C Agero, Jesus Cuevas, Pedro Jaen, Ashfaq A Marghoob, Melissa Gill, and Salvador González

Basal cell carcinoma (BCC) is the most common malignant skin tumor, constituting approximately 80% of the non-melanoma skin cancers.[1] BCCs are derived from non-keratinizing cells which originate from the epidermal basal cell layer; its pathogenesis involves factors such as exposure to ultraviolet light and ionizing radiation, regulatory gene mutations, and altered immunosurveillance.[2] BCCs typically arise on the sun-exposed areas of light-skinned individuals, most frequently on the head and neck. Lesions commonly occur in older adults (4th decade and older), with a slight male predominance. However, BCCs may also occur in younger patients, particularly in the setting of genodermatoses and immune compromise.[3] BCCs are known to be slow-growing tumors that exhibit local invasion, although cases of metastasis have been reported.[4]

Clinical characteristics of BCCs may vary according to the histopathologic subtypes. Classic nodular BCC is the most common subtype and appears as a well-circumscribed pearly pink or translucent papule or nodule with a rolled border and telangiectasias, often accompanied by bleeding, crusting, and ulceration (Figure 3.73). Nodular BCC can clinically simulate dermal nevi and amelanotic melanoma. Superficial BCC, the second most common subtype, presents as an erythematous scaly patch or plaque usually located on the trunk, and may be clinically confused with an eczematous dermatitis (Figure 3.83). Morpheaform/sclerosing/infiltrative BCCs are aggressive variants of BCC that may appear as erythematous or whitish, depressed scar-like plaques (Figure 3.91).[1–3] Pigmentation may also occur in BCCs, most commonly in the nodular, micronodular, and superficial subtypes (Figures 3.99, 3.105, 3.109).[5] Heavily pigmented BCCs occasionally may cause clinical difficulty in differentiation from other pigmented lesions. In pigmented BCC, dermoscopic examination reveals key features, such as absence of a pigment network and presence of one or more of the following: blue-gray ovoid nests and globules, leaf-like or spoke-wheel areas, ulceration, and arborizing telangiectasia (tree-like branching of blood vessels) (Figures 3.100, 3.106, 3.110). Dermoscopy is most useful when distinguishing pigmented BCC from other pigmented lesions, but non-pigmented BCC lesions likewise show the characteristic arborizing vascular pattern.[6]

BCCs are characterized histopathologically by aggregates of atypical basaloid cells organized into nodules/lobules, islands, cords, or elongated strands; the architectural pattern determines the histologic subtype of BCC (Figures 3.74, 3.84, 3.92, 3.101, 3.107, 3.111). Tumor cells have large oval or elongated nuclei with relatively scant cytoplasm (Figures 3.75, 3.79, 3.85, 3.87, 3.95, 3.103, 3.107, 3.111, 3.115). Commonly, tumor aggregates show peripheral palisading of nuclei (Figures 3.79, 3.84, 3.85, 3.103, 3.111). The epidermis surrounding intraepidermal BCC or overlying superficial dermal BCC often shows mild spongiosis, mild keratinocytic atypia, and/or overlying parakeratosis (Figures 3.77, 3.84, 3.87, 3.93). Peritumoral clefting (retraction artifact) and peritumoral mucin deposition are usually seen at least focally (Figures 3.79, 3.101,

3.103, 3.107). Surrounding aggregates of tumor is a specialized stroma, which ranges from well-vascularized, mucin-rich, loose, and cellular, containing numerous fibroblasts and inflammatory cells, to more densely fibrotic, as in the case of morpheaform BCC (Figures 3.79, 3.81, 3.89, 3.92, 3.97, 3.101, 3.103).[2,7]

Reflectance confocal microscopy (RCM) of BCCs, regardless of the subtype, has demonstrated the following common confocal features:

- The presence of elongated monomorphic nuclei (Figures 3.76, 3.86, 3.88, 3.96).
- Polarization of these elongated nuclei along the same axis of orientation, often manifested as (1) streaming, when an entire aggregate of tumor shows nuclei oriented along the same axis, or as (2) peripheral palisading, when a single outer layer of tumor cells are oriented parallel to each other and perpendicular to the border of the tumor aggregate (Figures 3.80, 3.104, 3.108, 3.112).
- Prominent associated inflammatory cell infiltrate (Figures 3.82, 3.90, 3.98).
- Increased vascularity with vascular dilatation and tortuosity and active leukocyte trafficking (visualized best in real time or on video capture) (Figures 3.82, 3.90).
- Pleomorphism of the overlying epidermis compatible with actinic damage, including features such as retention of nuclei in the stratum corneum (parakeratosis) and mild variation in keratinocyte nuclear size (Figures 3.78, 3.88, 3.94).[8–10]

A recent large retrospective, multicenter study involving 152 lesions, 83 of which were BCC, suggested that these five specific confocal features are both sensitive and specific in diagnosing BCC in vivo; the presence of two or more confocal criteria had 100% sensitivity, and the presence of four or more criteria had a specificity of 95.7% and a sensitivity of 82.9%. The presence of monomorphic elongated nuclei was the most sensitive (100%) of the five criteria, while the presence of polarized nuclei was both sensitive (91.6%) and specific (97.1%). Interestingly, the presence of the two aforementioned criteria simultaneously produced almost identical sensitivity (91.6%) and specificity (97%) to the presence of polarized nuclei alone. Notably, this study revealed little variability in RCM findings across BCC subtypes (superficial, nodular, and infiltrative) that were included in the evaluation.[9]

Key RCM features of BCC

- Elongated monomorphic nuclei
- Polarization of elongated nuclei along the same axis of orientation:
  - Streaming: polarization of nuclei in an entire aggregate of tumor cells
  - Peripheral palisading of nuclei: peripheral monolayer of tumor cells oriented parallel to each other and perpendicular to the stroma
- Prominent inflammatory cell infiltrate
- Increased vascularity
- Variable epidermal disarray (nucleated corneocytes, loss of the honeycomb pattern, and keratinocytic nuclear pleomorphism)

NODULAR BASAL CELL CARCINOMA

Nodular basal cell carcinoma, which accounts for half of all BCC subtypes, is characterized histopathologically by variably sized nodules of tumor cells in the dermis and may show involvement of the overlying epidermis (Figure 3.74).[2] On RCM, this subtype exhibits the key confocal features of BCCs in general, as described above. In addition, the architecture of the tumor cell aggregates in the epidermis and upper dermis, in particular, can be visualized.[8,11,12] The tumor appears as distinct aggregates of tightly packed refractile cells often with elongated, monomorphic nuclei forming lobulated nodules, islands, or trabeculae (Figures 3.76, 3.80, 3.102, 3.104, 3.108, 3.112, 3.116). Peripheral palisading of nuclei, or the polarization of a single layer of elongated nuclei along the same axis in a parallel arrangement around the periphery of tumor cell aggregates, can also be detected (Figures 3.80, 3.104). Peritumoral cleft-like dark spaces, corresponding to peritumoral mucin or peritumoral clefting on histology, are usually seen at least focally (Figures 3.80, 3.102, 3.104).[13] Surrounding the tumor is variably refractile stroma, which often contains refractile round cells, corresponding to inflammatory cells, and an increased number of prominent vessels.

Key RCM features of nodular basal cell carcinoma

- Lobulated nodules, islands, or trabeculae of tightly packed refractile cells
- Peripheral palisading of elongated monomorphic nuclei
- Peritumoral cleft-like dark spaces
- Variably refractile stroma

SUPERFICIAL BASAL CELL CARCINOMA

Superficial basal cell carcinomas are characterized microscopically by atypical basaloid cells forming intraepidermal aggregates and/or forming aggregates which emanate from the lower portion of the epidermis and bulge into the dermis (Figure 3.84).[2] RCM of superficial BCC reveals intraepidermal or immediately subepidermal aggregates of tumor cells with elongated monomorphic nuclei. These aggregates often show streaming, or polarization of the aggregate's cells along the same en-face axis (Figures 3.86, 3.88). The surrounding epidermis often shows some degree of architectural disarray by features such as retention of corneocyte nuclei (parakeratosis) and focal loss of the normal honeycomb or cobblestone pattern due to factors such as bright and thickened or lost intercellular demarcations (spongiosis) (Figure 3.88), permeation by small refractile round cells (inflammation), and pleomorphism of keratinocytes (mild atypia). Juxtaposed to the tumor is variably refractile stroma containing numerous weakly refractile round cells, corresponding to inflammatory infiltrates, together with an increased number of dilated blood vessels showing active leukocyte trafficking (Figures 3.90).[8]

Key RCM features of superficial basal cell carcinoma

- Intraepidermal or immediately subepidermal aggregates of cells with elongated monomorphic nuclei
- Streaming, or polarization of aggregated tumor cells along the same axis
- Peritumoral weakly refractile round cells
- Abundant, dilated peritumoral blood vessels with active leukocyte trafficking

INFILTRATIVE BASAL CELL CARCINOMA

Infiltrative basal cell carcinomas are characterized histopathologically by islands and cords of tumor cells showing jagged pointed contours embedded in a cellular, often mucin-rich, fibrous stroma (Figures 3.92, 3.95, 3.97). Peripheral palisading of nuclei is uncommon.[2,7] On RCM, this subtype often exhibits some degree of epidermal architectural disarray by features such as retention of corneocyte nuclei (parakeratosis) and focal loss of the normal honeycomb or cobblestone pattern due to factors such as bright and thickened or lost intercellular demarcations (spongiosis), permeation by small refractile round cells (inflammation), and pleomorphism of keratinocytes (mild atypia) (Figure 3.94).[9] Dermal tumor aggregates are composed of refractile cells with elongated monomorphic nuclei, which often show streaming (Figure 3.96). The borders of the tumor aggregates are jagged or may be poorly defined, merging with the stroma (Figure 3.96), which is characteristically cellular, containing numerous refractile round cells and prominent blood vessels (Figure 3.98).[9,13]

Key RCM features of infiltrative basal cell carcinoma

- Dermal aggregates of cells with elongated monomorphic nuclei
- Streaming, or polarization of aggregated tumor cells along the same axis
- Jagged or poorly defined tumor aggregate borders
- Abundant, dilated peritumoral blood vessels with active leukocyte trafficking
- Peritumoral weakly refractile round cells
- Architectural disarray of the epidermis

PIGMENTED BASAL CELL CARCINOMA

Pigmented basal cell carcinomas are characterized by colonization of tumor cells by benign, heavily pigmented, dendritic melanocytes, which may transfer melanin to tumor cells. Around 75% of BCCs contain melanocytes, but melanin is seen in only approximately 25% and abundant melanin is rare.[14] As previously mentioned, any subtype of BCC may be pigmented, but it is most commonly present in nodular, micronodular, and superficial types. One therefore finds the previously described RCM characteristics corresponding to the histologic architectural subtype in addition to features related to pigmentation in areas corresponding to blue-gray ovoid areas on dermoscopy and pigmented tumor cell aggregates on histopathology. On RCM, highly refractile nucleated dendritic cells (oval, plump cell bodies with slender peripheral branching processes) can be seen within BCC tumor nests (Figures 3.108, 3.114), corresponding to melanized, dendritic melanocytes (Figures 3.107, 3.113). Bright dot and granular structures are also found scattered among the tumor cells, which may represent transferred melanin-filled melanosomes within tumor cells or melanocyte dendrites seen in cross section (Figures 3.104, 3.108, 3.113).[15,16] Numerous bright plump or oval- to stellate-shaped structures with indistinct borders, corresponding to melanophages, are present in the tumoral stroma (Figures 3.104, 3.108, 3.116).[11,17]

Key RCM features of pigmented BCC

- Brightly refractile nucleated dendritic cells within tumor aggregates
- Brightly refractile dots and granular structures scattered among tumor cells
- Brightly refractile plump oval- to stellate-shaped cells in the tumoral stroma
- RCM features characteristic of the histologic architectural subtype of BCC

REFERENCES

1. Rubin AI, Chen EH, Ratner D. Basal-cell carcinoma. N Engl J Med 2005; 353:2262–9.
2. Carucci J, Leffell DJ. Basal cell carcinoma. In: Freedberg IM, Eisen AZ, Wolff K et al, eds. Fitzpatrick's Dermatology in General Medicine. New York: McGraw-Hill; 2003: 747–54.
3. Crowson AN. Basal cell carcinoma: biology, morphology and clinical implications. Mod Pathol 2006; 19 (Suppl 2):S127–47.
4. Ting PT, Kasper R, Arlette JP. Metastatic basal cell carcinoma: report of two cases and literature review. J Cutan Med Surg 2005; 9:10–5.
5. Maloney ME, Jones DB, Sexton FM. Pigmented basal cell carcinoma: investigation of 70 cases. J Am Acad Dermatol 1992; 27:74–8.
6. Polsky D. Pigmented basal cell carcinoma. In: Marghoob AA, Braun RP, Kopf AW, eds. Atlas of Dermoscopy. London: Taylor & Francis; 2005: 55–9.
7. Brenn T, McKee P. Tumors of the surface epithelium. Basal cell carcinoma. In: McKee PH, Calonje E, Granter SR, eds. Pathology of the Skin with Clinical Correlations, 3rd edn, Vol. 2. Philadelphia: Elsevier Mosby; 2005: 1167–84.
8. Gonzalez S, Tannous Z. Real-time, in vivo confocal reflectance microscopy of basal cell carcinoma. J Am Acad Dermatol 2002; 47:869–74.
9. Nori S, Rius-Diaz F, Cuevas J et al. Sensitivity and specificity of reflectance-mode confocal microscopy for in vivo diagnosis of basal cell carcinoma: a multicenter study. J Am Acad Dermatol 2004; 51:923–30.
10. Sauermann K, Gambichler T, Wilmert M et al. Investigation of basal cell carcinoma by confocal laser scanning microscopy in vivo. Skin Res Technol 2002; 8:141–7.
11. Charles CA, Marghoob AA, Busam KJ et al. Melanoma or pigmented basal cell carcinoma: a clinical-pathologic correlation with dermoscopy, in vivo confocal scanning laser microscopy, and routine histology. Skin Res Technol 2002; 8:282–7.
12. Agero AL, Dusza SW, Benvenuto-Andrade C et al. Dermatologic side effects associated with the epidermal growth factor receptor inhibitors. J Am Acad Dermatol 2006; 55:657–70.
13. Chung VQ, Dwyer PJ, Nehal KS et al. Use of ex vivo confocal scanning laser microscopy during Mohs surgery for nonmelanoma skin cancers. Dermatol Surg 2004; 30:1470–8.
14. Kirkham N. Tumors and cysts of the epidermis. Basal cell carcinoma. In: Elder DE, Elenitsas R, Johnson BJ, Murphy GF, eds. Lever's Histopathology of the Skin. Philadelphia: Lippincott Williams & Wilkins; 2005: 837–49.
15. Langley RG, Rajadhyaksha M, Dwyer PJ et al. Confocal scanning laser microscopy of benign and malignant melanocytic skin lesions in vivo. J Am Acad Dermatol 2001; 45:365–76.
16. Middelkamp-Hup MA, Park HY, Lee J et al. Detection of UV-induced pigmentary and epidermal changes over time using in vivo reflectance confocal microscopy. J Invest Dermatol 2006; 126:402–7.
17. Agero AL, Busam KJ, Benvenuto-Andrade C et al. Reflectance confocal microscopy of pigmented basal cell carcinoma. J Am Acad Dermatol 2006; 54:638–43.

NODULAR BASAL CELL CARCINOMA

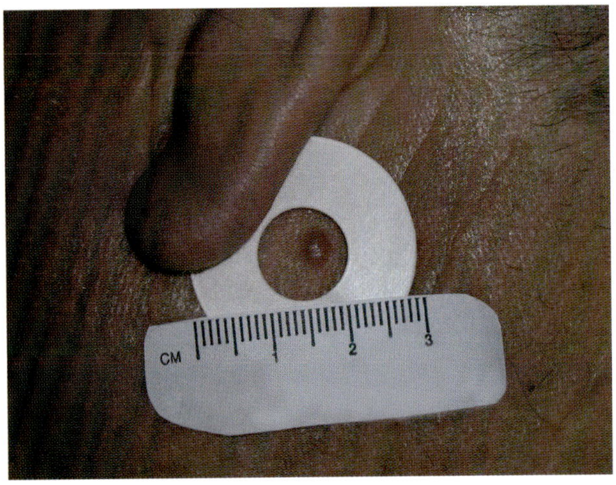

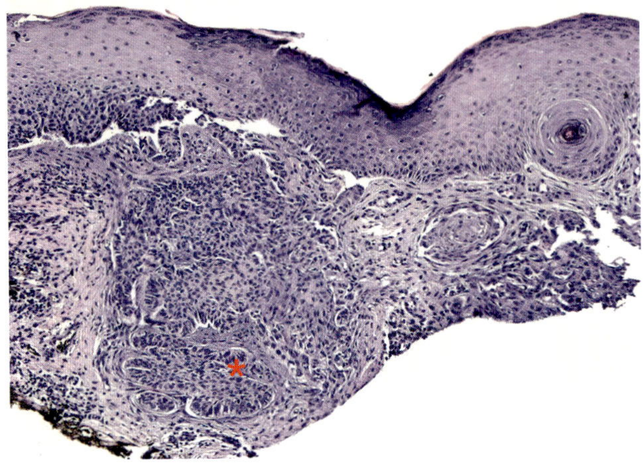

▲ **Figures 3.73, 3.74** Case 1: clinical photograph of a 5 mm pink pearly papule located in the retroauricular area of a 71-year-old male. Histology (10×) shows a proliferation of basaloid cells (asterisk) expanding the lower epidermis and forming nodular aggregates in the dermis.

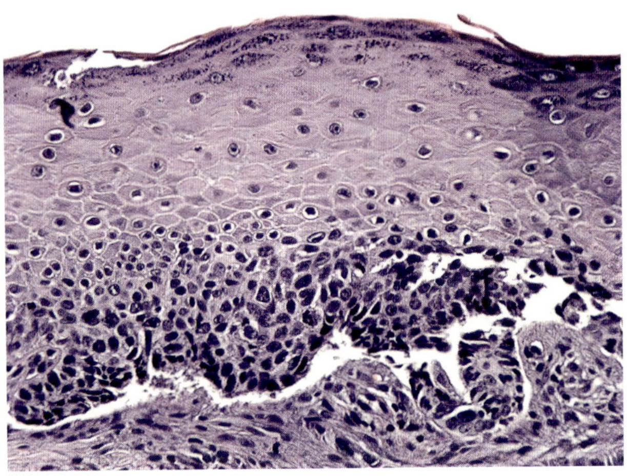

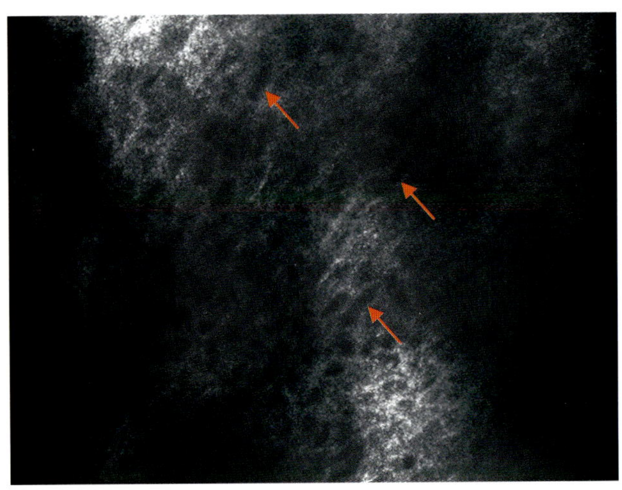

▲ **Figures 3.75, 3.76** Case 1: histology (40×) shows a proliferation of atypical basaloid cells in the lower epidermis. RCM (0.45 mm × 0.34 mm) at the level of the lower stratum spinosum discloses packed cells with discrete large, elongated nuclei (red arrows), many of which are oriented along the same axis.

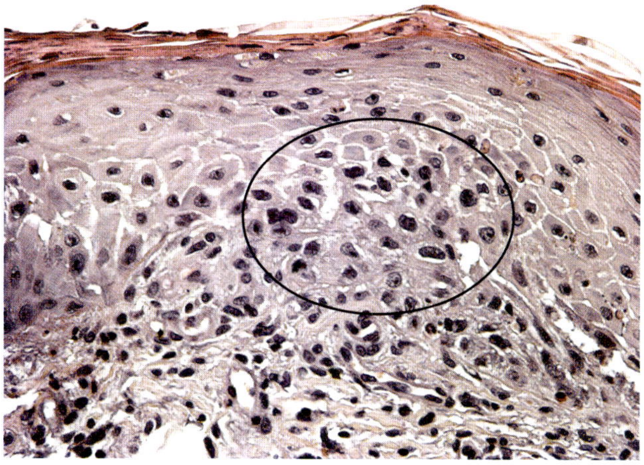

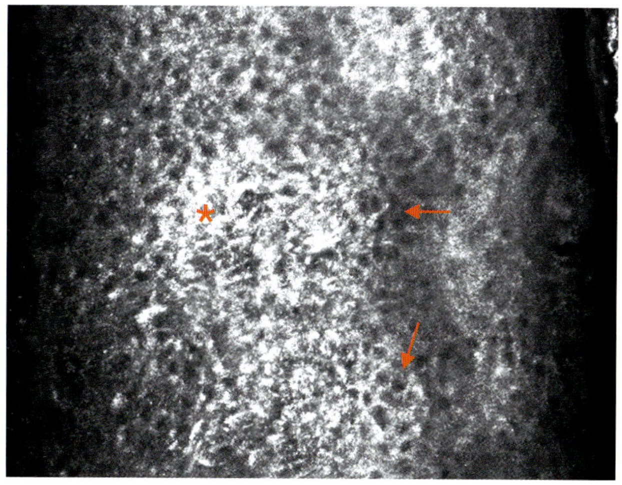

▲ **Figures 3.77, 3.78** Case 1: histology (40×) of an area of the epidermis overlying the BCC shows parakeratosis, mild spongiosis, and minimal focal keratinocytic atypia (circle). RCM (0.45 mm × 0.34 mm) at the level of stratum granulosum/upper stratum spinosum reveals focal loss of the normal honeycomb pattern by bright thickened or effaced intercellular demarcations (asterisks) and focal pleomorphism and disorganization of keratinocytes (red arrows).

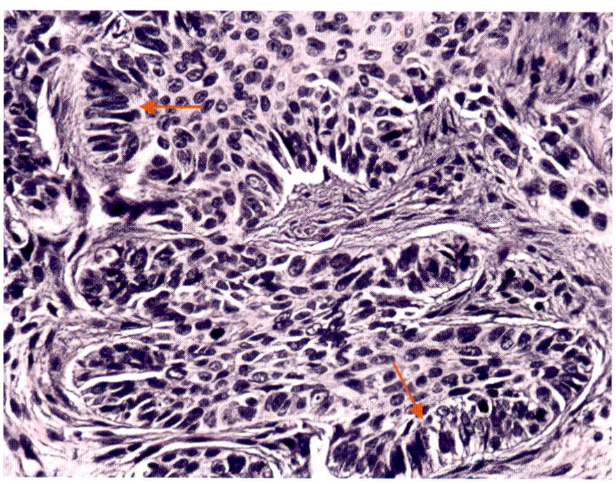

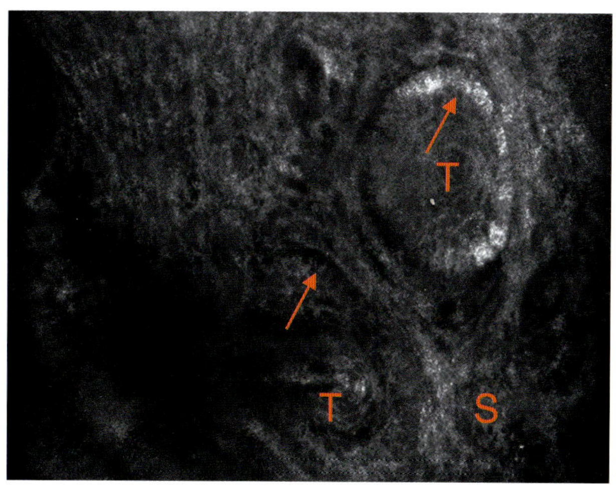

▲ **Figures 3.79, 3.80** Case 1: histology (40×) shows dermal islands of atypical basaloid cells with focal peripheral palisading of nuclei (red arrows) surrounded by cellular fibrous stroma. Subtle peritumoral clefting is also seen. RCM (0.45 mm × 0.34 mm) at level of the dermis reveals tumor islands (T) composed of tightly packed, weakly to moderately refractile cells with peripheral palisading of nuclei (red arrows) surrounded by moderately refractile stroma (S). Peritumoral cleft-like dark spaces are also seen.

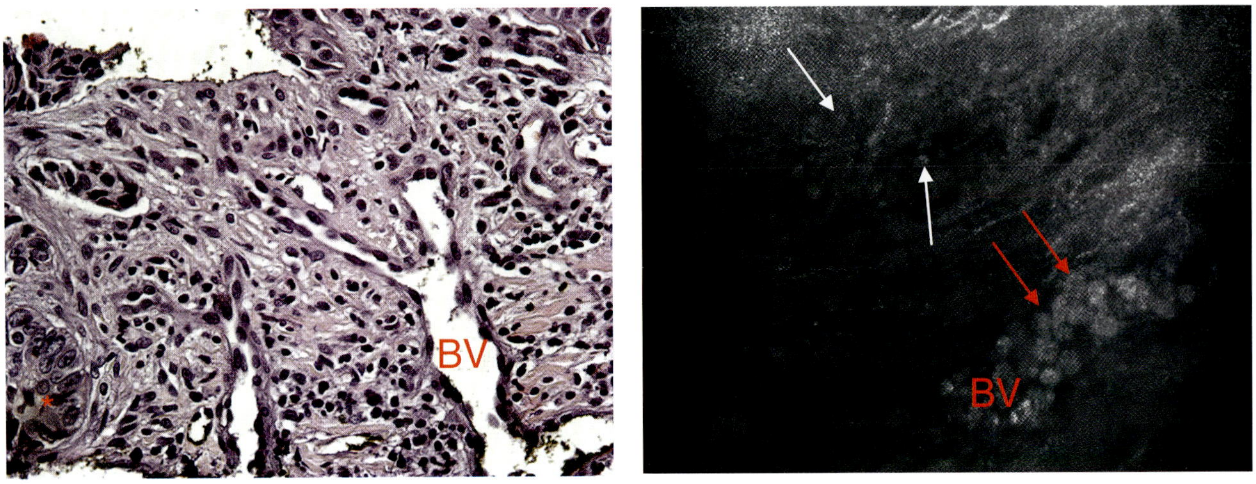

▲ **Figures 3.81, 3.82** Case 1: histology (40×) shows increased number of dilated blood vessels (BV) and an inflammatory cell infiltrate adjacent to tumor islands (asterisk) within the dermis. RCM (0.45 mm × 0.34 mm) at the level of the dermis demonstrates the presence of stromal inflammatory cells (white arrows) and a dilated blood vessel (BV) containing leukocytes (red arrows).

SUPERFICIAL BASAL CELL CARCINOMA

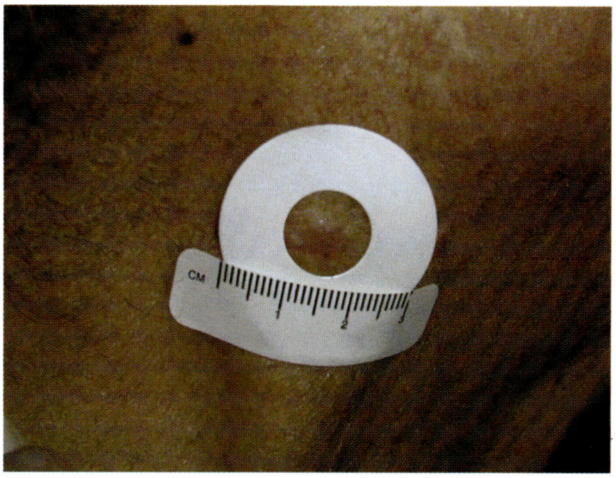

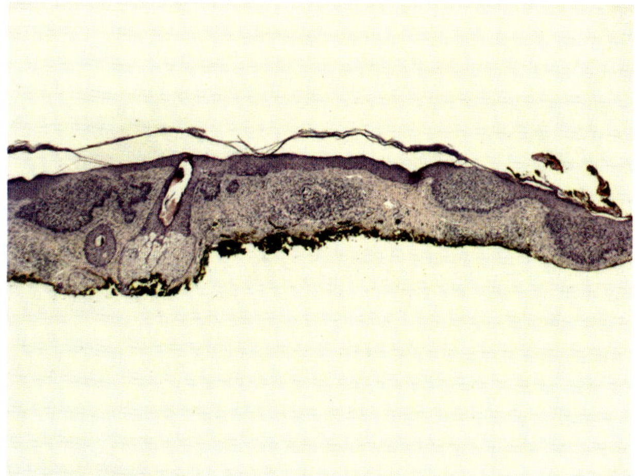

▲ **Figures 3.83, 3.84** Case 2: clinical photograph of a 7 mm scaly erythematous lesion located on the lateral side of the neck of a 59-year-old male. Histology (4×) shows hyperkeratosis, parakeratosis, and aggregates of atypical basaloid cells emanating from the lower portion of the epidermis and bulging into the dermis. Peripheral palisading of nuclei can be appreciated even at this low magnification.

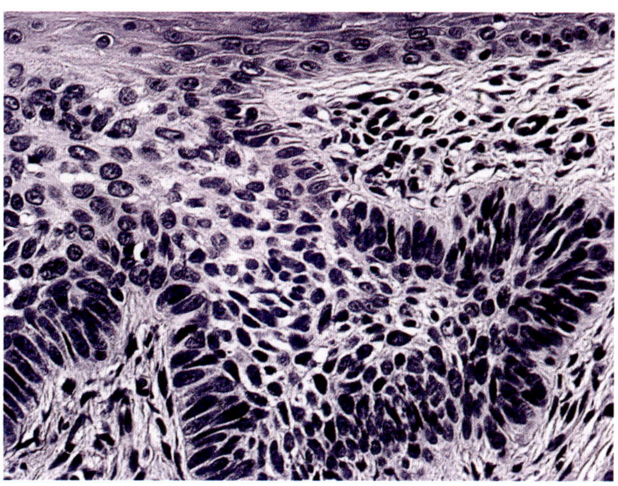

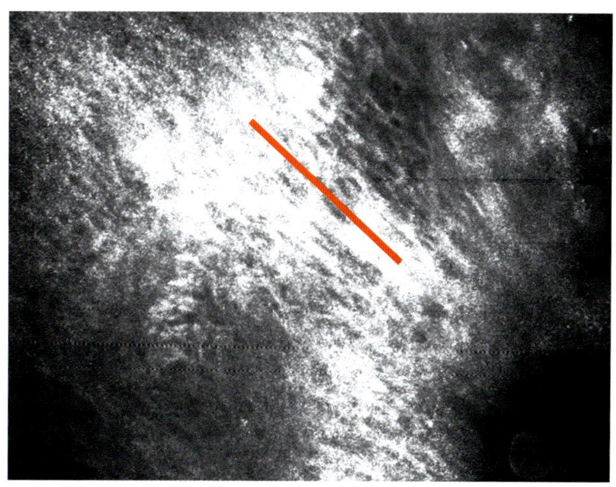

▲ **Figures 3.85, 3.86** Case 2: histology (40×) shows an aggregate of uniformly atypical cells with increased nuclear-to-cytoplasmic ratio and elongated basophilic nuclei, which are often arranged parallel to one another in a polarized fashion. Peripheral nuclei show palisading. RCM (0.45 mm × 0.34 mm) at the level of the epidermis shows a population of large cells with elongated monomorphic nuclei polarized along the same axis (red line), or streaming.

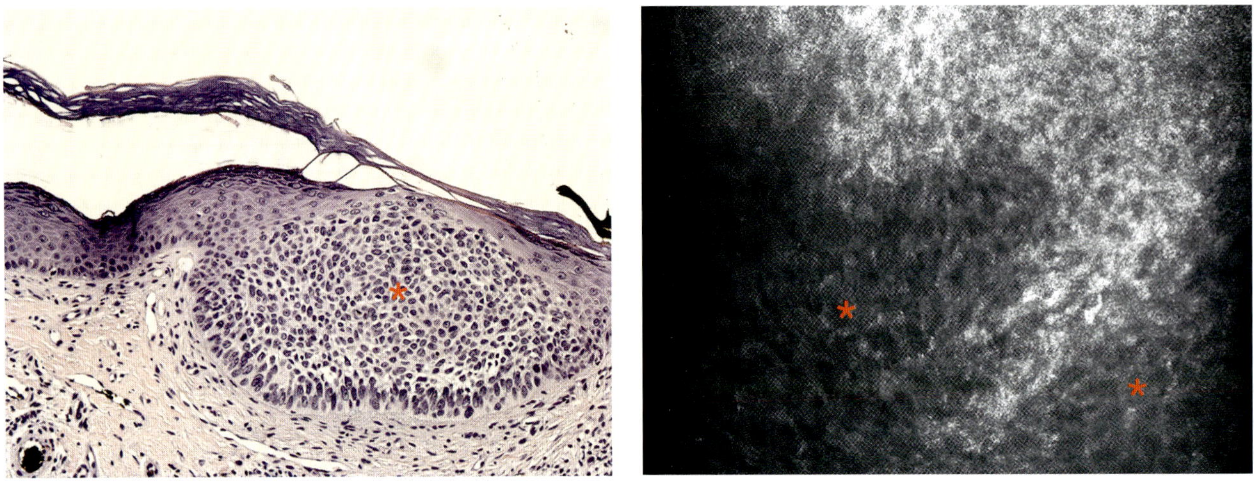

▲ **Figures 3.87, 3.88** Case 2: histology (20×) shows an intraepidermal aggregate of basal cell carcinoma (asterisk), which occupies almost the entire thickness of the epidermis and bulges into the papillary dermis. The hyperkeratotic scale is replaced by a focus of parakeratosis immediately above the tumor. Immediately adjacent to the tumor, slight reactive keratinocytic changes are seen. RCM (0.45 mm × 0.34 mm) at the level of the stratum spinosum reveals zones containing darker, weakly refractile cells with nuclear streaming, corresponding to BCC (asterisks), and zones of brighter cells with slight breakdown of the normal honeycomb pattern.

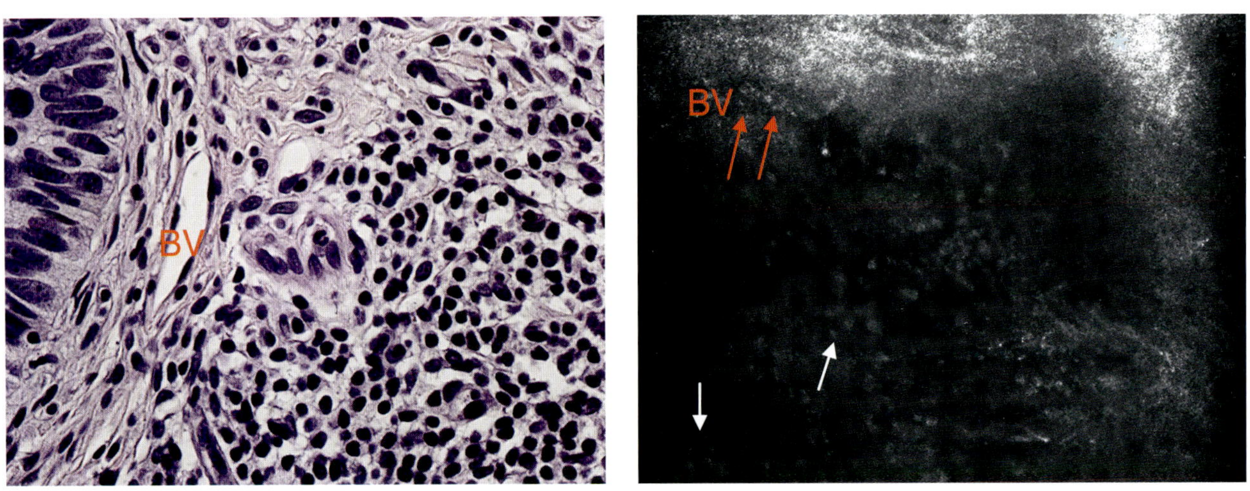

▲ **Figures 3.89, 3.90** Case 2: histology (40×) shows a dilated dermal blood vessel (BV) and dense inflammatory infiltrate adjacent to the tumor in the dermis. RCM (0.45 mm × 0.34 mm) at the level of the superficial dermis demonstrates a dilated, prominent blood vessel (BV), within which refractile round cells can be seen. In areas, an increased number of bright cells can be seen disposed along the endothelium (red arrows). Trafficking of individual leukocytes to endothelial walls was better visualized in real time. Refractile round cells are also seen in the stroma (white arrows).

INFILTRATIVE BASAL CELL CARCINOMA

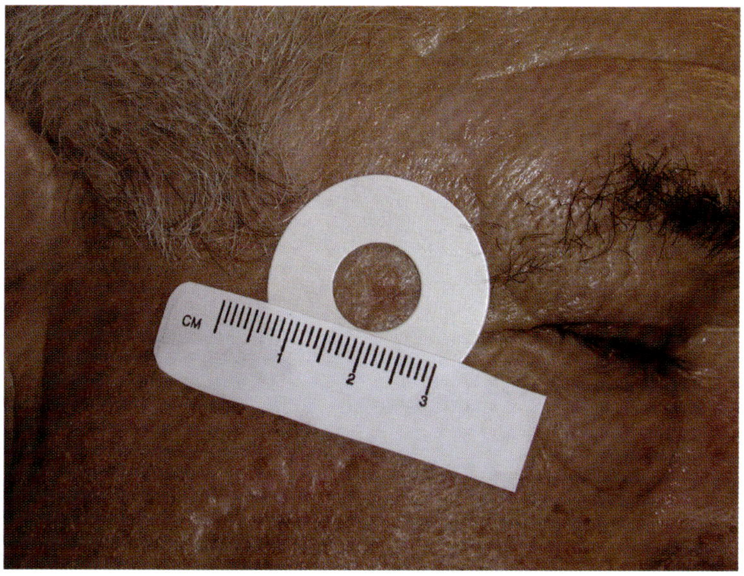

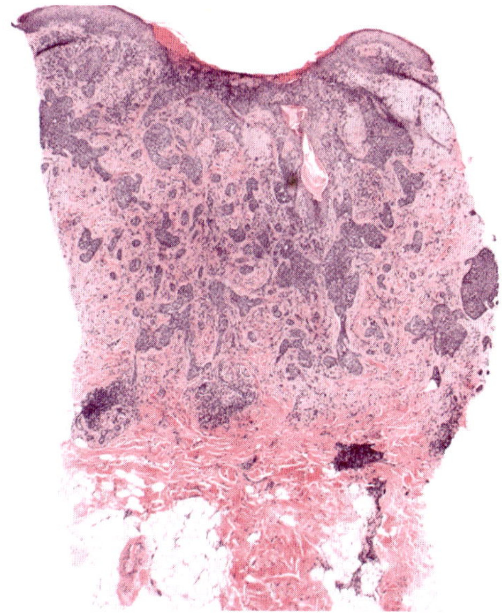

▲ **Figures 3.91, 3.92** Case 3: clinical photograph of a 5 mm depressed erythematous macule on the right temple of a 64-year-old male. Note the scar on the cheek resulting from surgical treatment of a previous BCC. Histology (4×) shows an infiltrative BCC, characterized by jagged, variably sized aggregates of basaloid cells within a fibrotic stroma, which extends into the deep reticular dermis.

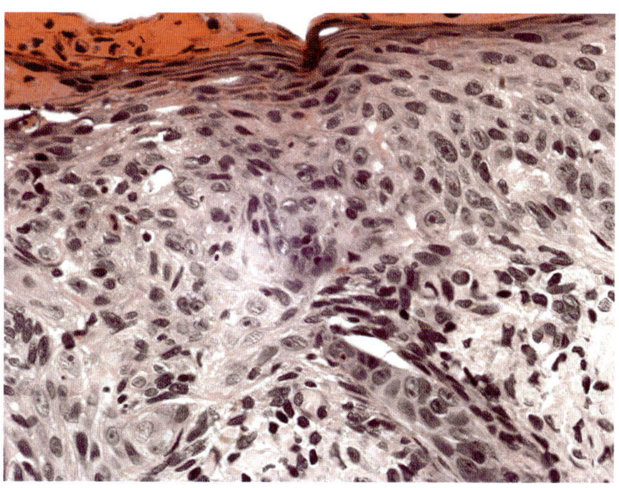

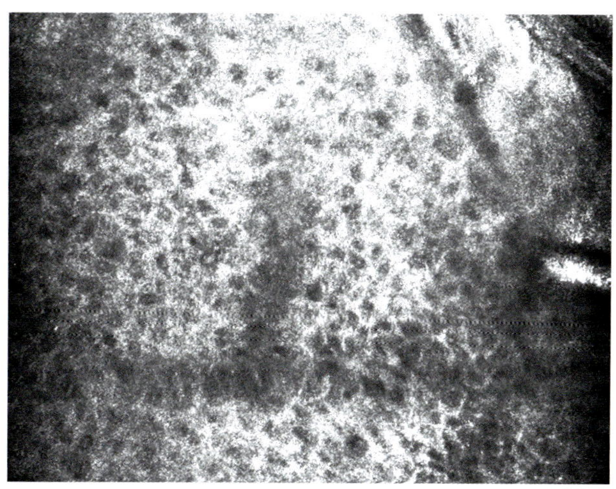

▲ **Figures 3.93, 3.94** Case 3: histology (40×) of epidermis overlying the BCC shows parakeratosis and keratinocytic atypia. RCM (0.45 mm × 0.34 mm) at the level of the stratum granulosum/superficial stratum spinosum reveals an altered honeycomb pattern and keratinocytic pleomorphism.

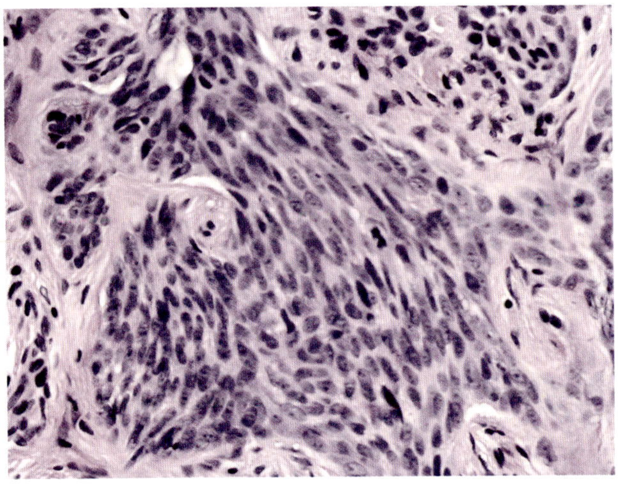

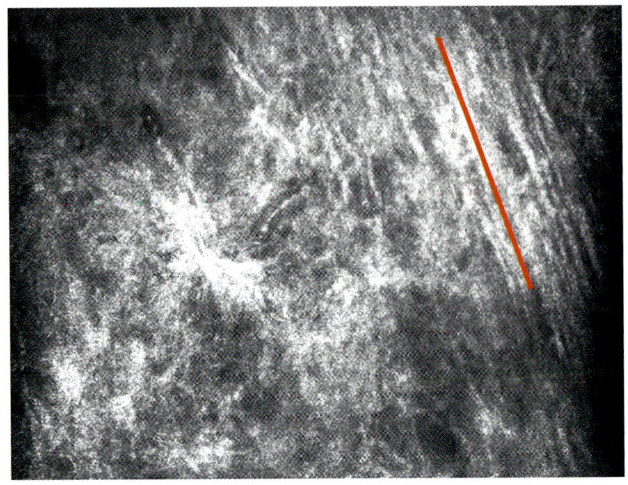

▲ **Figures 3.95, 3.96** Case 3: histology (40×) shows an irregularly shaped tumor cell aggregate with jagged, tapered borders composed of atypical basaloid cells with large oval and elongated nuclei, which are oriented in the same direction, or polarized. Peripheral palisading of nuclei is not seen. RCM (0.45 mm × 0.34 mm) at the level of the superficial dermis reveals, at left, a population of large cells with uniform elongated monomorphic nuclei polarized along the same axis (red line), or streaming. The border between tumor and stroma is difficult to discern.

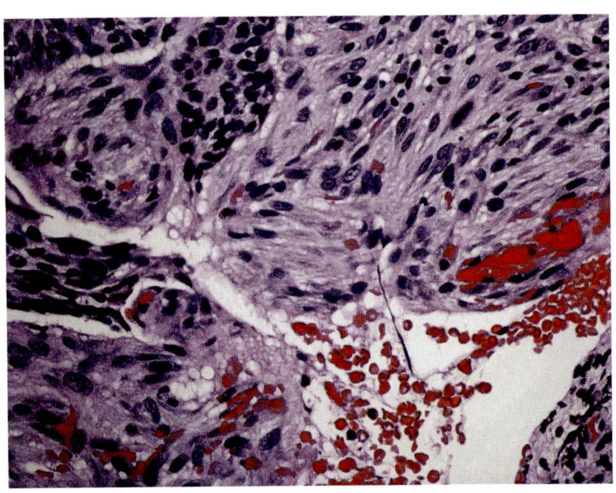

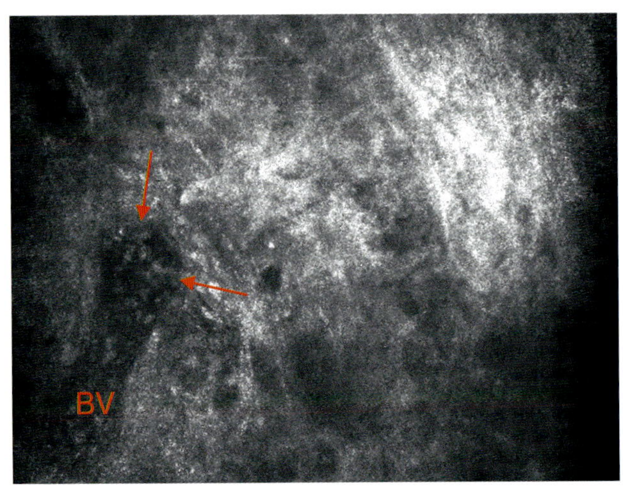

▲ **Figures 3.97, 3.98** Case 3: histology (40×) shows cellular tumoral stroma containing dilated blood vessels. RCM (0.45 mm × 0.34 mm) at the level of the dermis demonstrates dilated blood vessels (BV). Weakly refractile round cells (red arrows) are seen against the luminal blood vessel wall in this still image and were seen undergoing margination and rolling in real time.

PIGMENTED BASAL CELL CARCINOMA

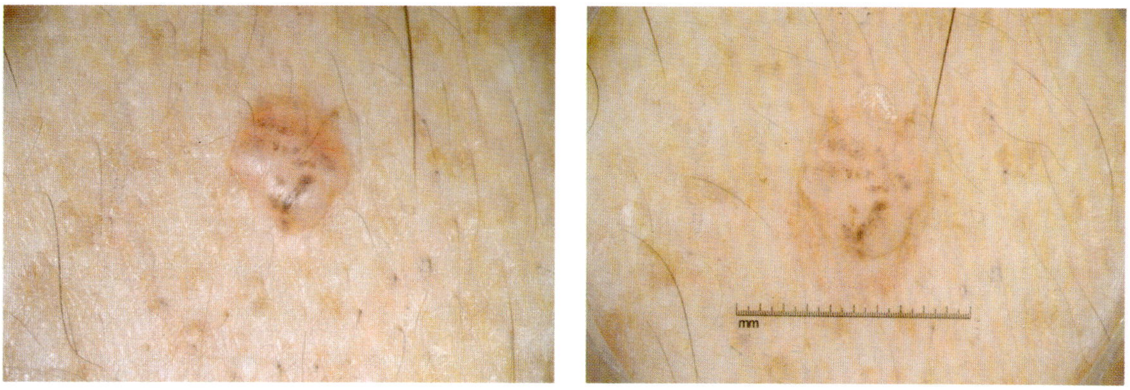

▲ **Figures 3.99, 3.100** Case 4: clinical photograph of a 6 mm papule showing spotty pigmentation and focal telangiectasia on the back of a 46-year-old male. Dermoscopy shows features suggestive of pigmented BCC such as the absence of a pigment network and the presence of structures such as gray-brown ovoid areas, globules, and dots, together with telangiectasia. Reproduced with permission of Elsevier Rights Department from Agero AG, Halpern AC. Reflectance confocal microscopy of pigmented basal cell carcinoma in J Am Acad Dermatol. 2006 Apr: 54(4): 638–43.

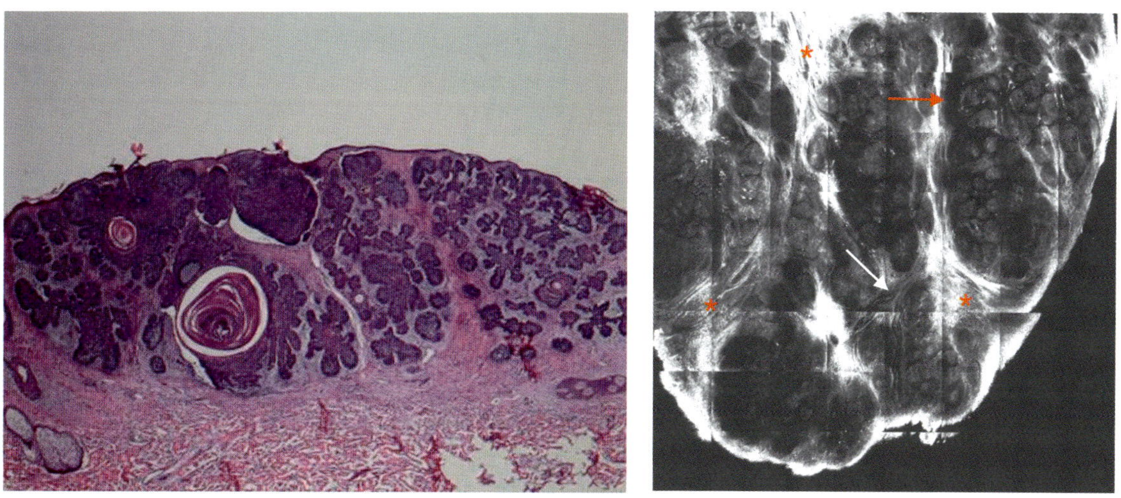

▲ **Figures 3.101, 3.102** Case 4: histology (4×) shows a nodular basal cell carcinoma composed of nodules of lobulated basophilic tumor. Tumor nodules are separated by dense pink fibrous stroma, while, within each tumor nodule, individual tumor lobules are separated by pale blue mucinous stroma. Frank peritumoral clefting is focally seen, but pigment is difficult to discern at this magnification. RCM mosaic (4 mm × 4 mm) at the level of the dermis corresponds nicely to the histology, revealing nodules of weakly to moderately refractile lobulated tumor separated by bright, linear bundles of collagen (asterisks). Within the tumor nodules, dark stroma separates individual tumor lobules; and occasionally peritumoral cleft-like dark spaces are seen (red arrow). An arborizing vessel containing refractile leukocytes (white arrow) is closely apposed to a tumor nodule. Reproduced with permission of Elsevier Rights Department from Agero AG, Halpern AC. Reflectance confocal microscopy of pigmented basal cell carcinoma in J Am Acad Dermatol. 2006 Apr: 54(4): 638–43.

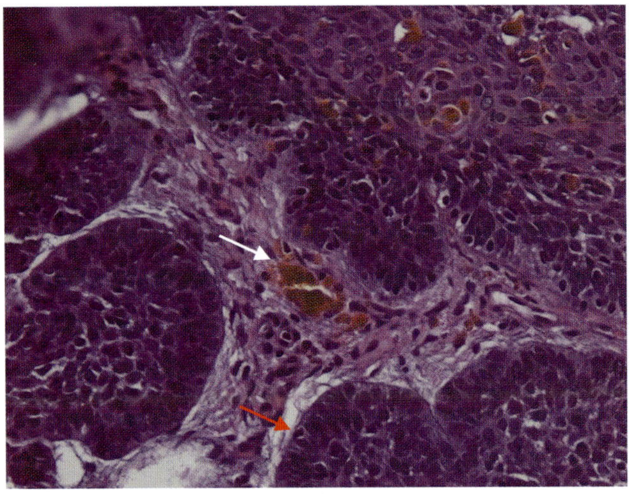

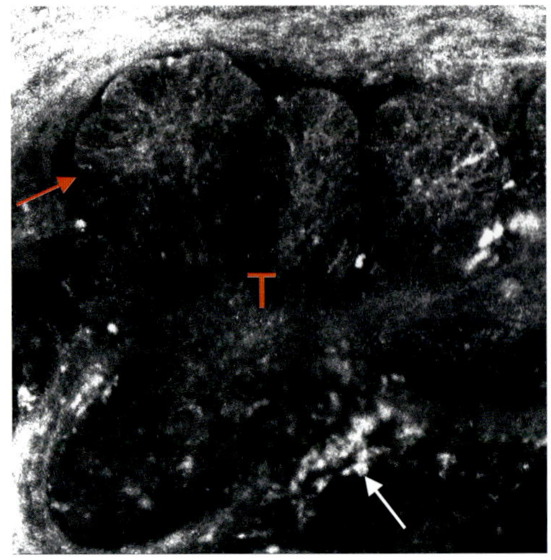

▲ **Figures 3.103, 3.104** Case 4: histology (20×) demonstrates variably pigmented lobulated tumor islands of atypical basaloid cells separated by cellular stroma containing aggregated melanophages (white arrow). Focal peripheral palisading of nuclei (red arrow) and peritumoral mucin are seen. RCM (0.5 mm × 0.5 mm) at the level of the upper dermis demonstrates a lobulated tumor island (T) speckled with brightly refractile dots, dendrites, and granular structures. Subtle peripheral palisading of nuclei (red arrow), extensive peritumoral dark cleft-like spaces, and refractile surrounding stroma containing clusters of plump bright cells (white arrow), corresponding to macrophages, are seen. Reproduced with permission of Elsevier Rights Department from Agero AG, Halpern AC. Reflectance confocal microscopy of pigmented basal cell carcinoma in J Am Acad Dermatol. 2006 Apr: 54(4): 638–43.

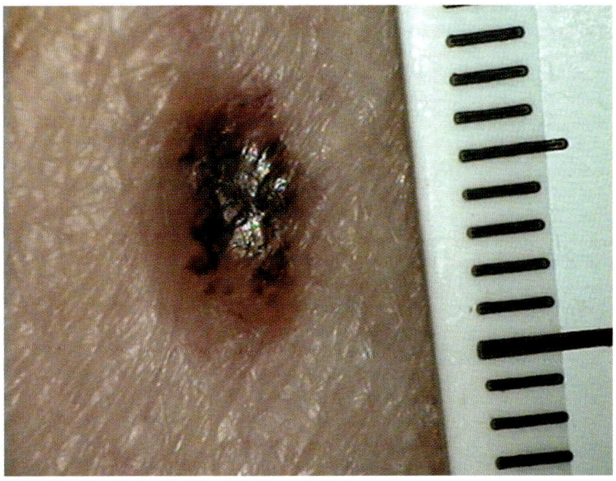

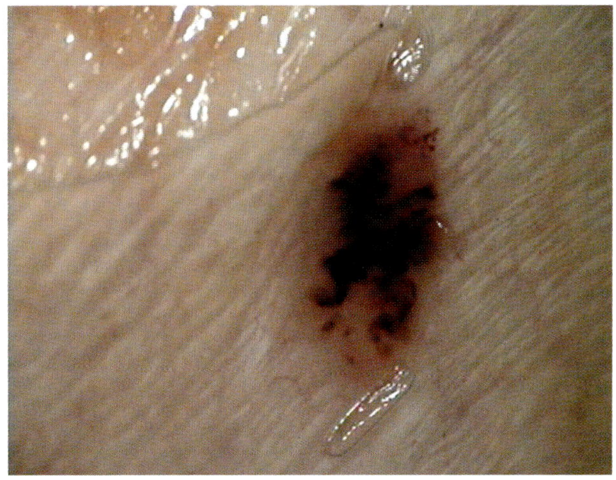

▲ **Figures 3.105, 3.106** Case 5: clinical photograph of a 6 mm irregularly pigmented papule on the chest of a 73-year-old male. Dermoscopy shows features suggestive of pigmented BCC, such as absence of a pigment network and the presence of gray-brown ovoid areas and dots. Reproduced with permission of Elsevier Rights Department from Agero AG, Halpern AC. Reflectance confocal microscopy of pigmented basal cell carcinoma in J Am Acad Dermatol. 2006 Apr: 54(4): 638–43.

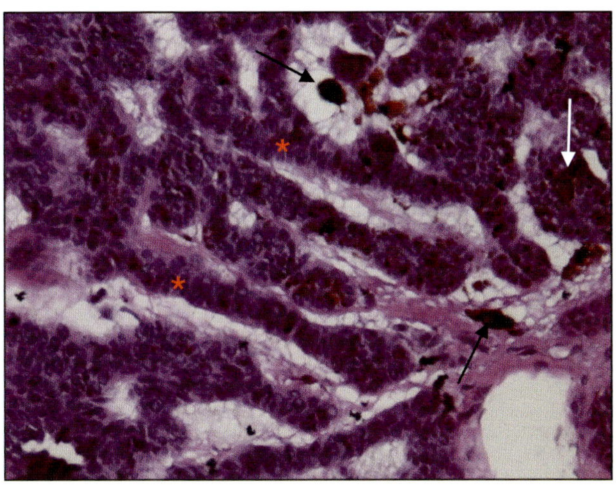

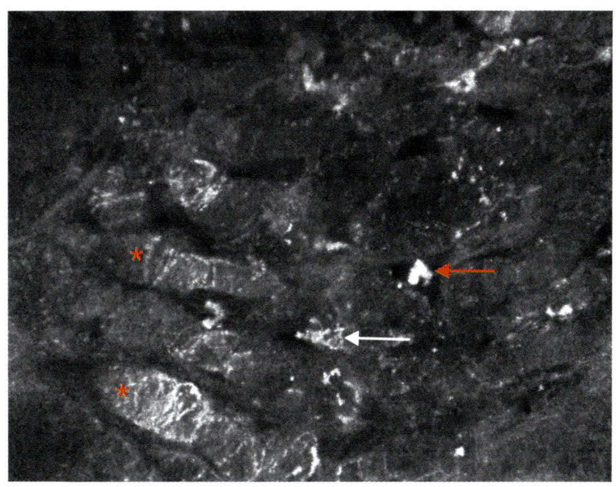

▲ **Figures 3.107, 3.108** Case 5: histology (20×) demonstrates variably pigmented cords of atypical basaloid cells with palisaded nuclei (asterisks) containing rare melanized dendritic melanocytes (white arrow). Peritumoral mucin and stromal melanophages (black arrows) are seen. RCM image (0.45 mm × 0.34 mm) at the level of the dermis reveals cords of tightly packed, variably refractile tumor cells arranged parallel to each other (palisading) (asterisks), surrounded by dark cleft-like spaces. The tumor is speckled with brightly refractile dots and dendrites, and a portion of a brightly refractile, nucleated dendritic cell is seen (white arrow). Within the stroma, plump bright cells (red arrow), corresponding to macrophages, are seen. Reproduced with permission of Elsevier Rights Department from Agero AG, Halpern AC. Reflectance confocal microscopy of pigmented basal cell carcinoma in J Am Acad Dermatol. 2006 Apr: 54(4): 638–43.

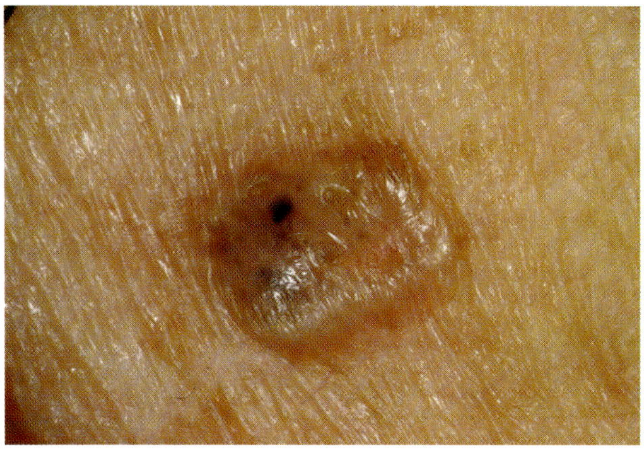

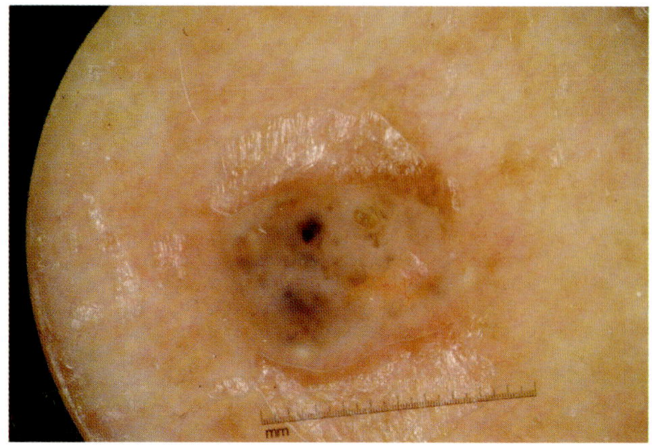

▲ **Figures 3.109, 3.110** Case 6: clinical photograph of a 9 mm erythematous papule with telangiectasia and irregular pigmentation located on the back of a 74-year-old female. Dermoscopy shows absence of a pigment network and presence of gray-brown and blue-gray ovoid areas, blue-gray dots, and arborizing telangiectasia. Reproduced with permission of Elsevier Rights Department from Agero AG, Halpern AC. Reflectance confocal microscopy of pigmented basal cell carcinoma in J Am Acad Dermatol. 2006 Apr: 54(4): 638–43.

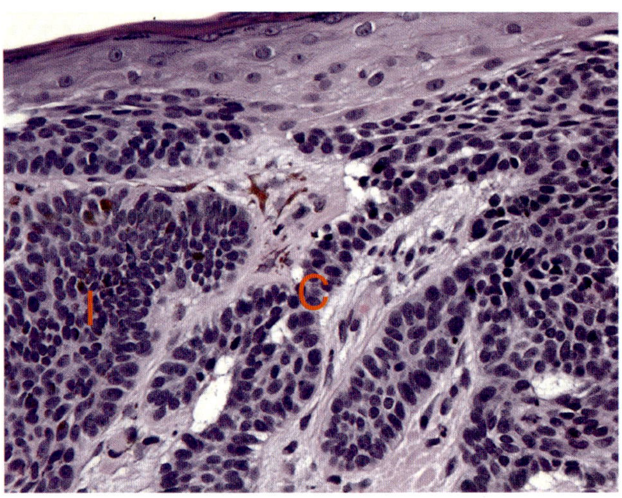

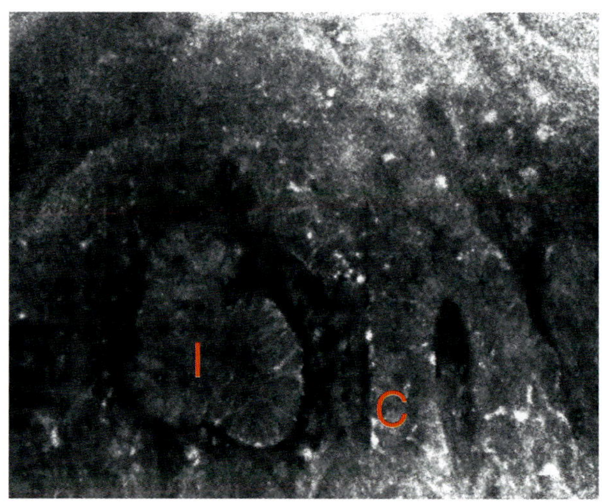

▲ **Figures 3.111, 3.112** Case 6: histology (20×) demonstrates focally pigmented islands and cords of basaloid tumor cells extending from the lower epidermis into the dermis, which show peripheral palisading of nuclei. RCM image (0.45 mm × 0.34 mm) at the level of the dermis reveals islands (I) and cords (C) of tumor composed of tightly packed cells speckled with brightly refractile dots, dendrites, and granular structures. Peripheral palisading of nuclei is somewhat subtle but can be appreciated.

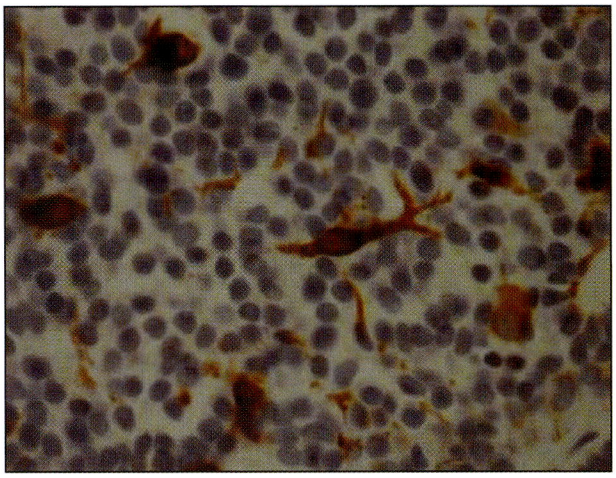

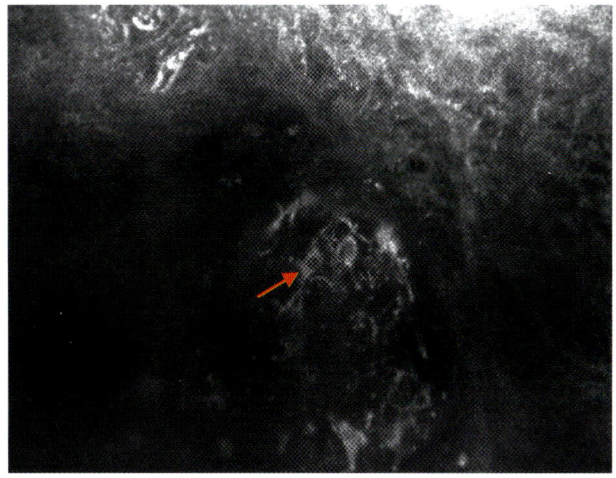

▲ **Figures 3.113, 3.114** Case 7: histology (40×) of Melan-A immunostained section shows colonization of the tumor by dendritic melanocytes. RCM (0.45 mm × 0.34 mm) reveals brightly refractile dendritic cells with round-to-oval nuclei (red arrow) within a tumor island. Reproduced with permission of Elsevier Rights Department from Agero AG, Halpern AC. Reflectance confocal microscopy of pigmented basal cell carcinoma in J Am Acad Dermatol. 2006 Apr: 54(4): 638–43.

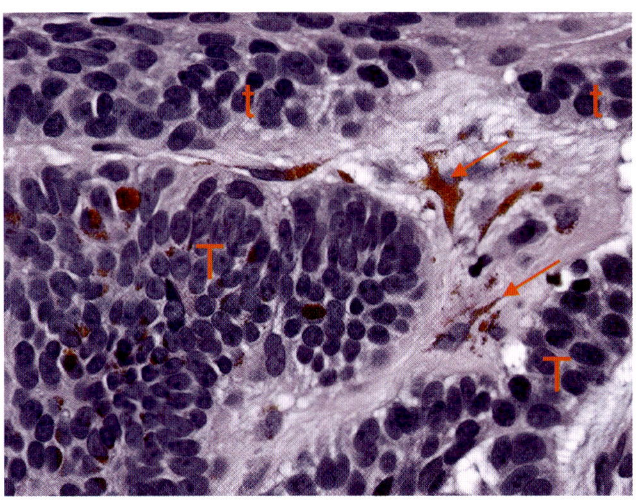

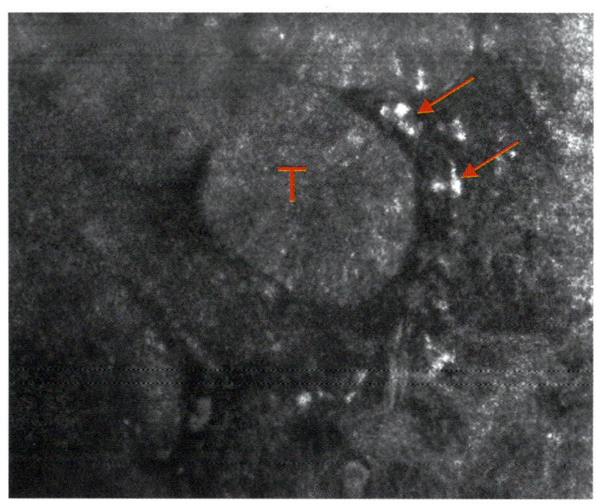

▲ **Figures 3.115, 3.116** Case 7: histology (40×) demonstrates islands of variably pigmented or non-pigmented atypical basaloid cells (T) just below the epidermis, which also contains tumor (t). Within the mucinous stroma are melanophages (red arrows). RCM (0.45 mm × 0.34 mm) at the level of the dermis discloses tumor islands (T) in a variably dark stroma containing plump, bright cells (red arrows), corresponding to melanophages.

CHAPTER 4a

Lentigo

Melissa Gill, Cristiane Benvenuto-Andrade, Marco Ardigo, Juan Luis Santiago Sánchez-Mateos, Lorea Bagazgoitia, Allan C Halpern, and Salvador González

Lentigines are brown or black macules or patches that vary in size, shape, and presentation depending on their etiologic subtype. Clinically, lentigines may be confused with nevi or occasionally melanoma resulting in biopsy.[1–3] Of even more concern is when melanoma is mistaken for lentigo and treated non-invasively for cosmetic purposes, resulting in delay of proper therapy.[4] All lentigo subtypes share basic findings on histology and reflectance confocal microscopy (RCM): hyperpigmentation of and an increased number of uniform, small, regularly spaced melanocytes within the basal layer usually accompanied by elongation of rete ridges, corresponding to a hyperrefractile cobblestone pattern of the basal layer and hyperrefractile dermal papillary rings.[5–7] Melanophages, corresponding to plump bright cells on RCM, may be present on the dermis.[5] Additional RCM features include preservation of the honeycomb pattern of the upper epidermis and an increased number of polymorphous dermal papillae, which assume various geometric shapes ranging from ovoid to annular to polycyclic.[6] The presence of increased numbers of melanocytes in the basal layer may not be appreciated on RCM, as the melanocytes are small, uniform, and evenly distributed, and therefore are difficult to distinguish from hyperpigmented basal keratinocytes on RCM.

Key RCM features of lentigo

- Preserved honeycomb and cobblestone pattern of the epidermis
- Hyperrefractile dermal papillary rings composed of uniform, round cells
- Polymorphous, crowded dermal papillae
- Plump bright cells (melanophages) may be present in the dermis

LENTIGO SIMPLEX

Lentigo simplex is the most common form of lentigo. It usually presents in early childhood, but it can develop at any age. Lentigo simplex can be solitary or multiple, and when multiple may be associated with an inherited syndrome. This type of lentigo is not induced by sun exposure and may occur anywhere on the skin or mucous membranes. Clinically, the lesion is a small, homogeneously pigmented, brown or black, round-to-oval macule with a jagged or smooth margin (Figure 4.1).[3] Lentigo simplex usually has a reticular dermoscopic pattern with a typical and regular light to dark brown pigment network (Figure 4.2).[8] Histologic examination identifies a proliferation of uniform, small melanocytes as solitary units along the sides and tips of elongated, pigmented rete ridges and often finds melanophages in the subjacent dermis (Figures 4.3, 4.5).[5] Reflectance confocal microscopy of lentigo simplex usually reveals the characteristic honeycomb pattern of the stratum granulosum and spinosum, a hyperrefractile basal layer resulting in a pronounced cobblestone pattern at the level of the superficial basal layer (Figure 4.5A) as compared to surrounding non-lesional skin and a very distinctive dermal–epidermal junction (DEJ). Dermal papillary rings form a single layer of bright monomorphic cells around crowded, variably sized dermal papillae, which assume various shapes ranging from round to ovoid to annular (Figure 4.5B).[6] Lentigo simplex may be confused with a lentiginous nevus or small dysplastic nevus clinically. If cell clusters, corresponding to nests of melanocytes on histology, are identified on RCM, the lesion is not a lentigo (Figure 4.5C).

Key RCM features of lentigo simplex

- Preserved honeycomb and cobblestone pattern of the epidermis
- Hyperrefractile dermal papillary rings composed of uniform, round cells
- Polymorphous, crowded dermal papillae with round, ovoid, or annular contours
- Plump bright cells (melanophages) may be present in the dermis

SOLAR LENTIGO

Solar lentigines are benign sharply circumscribed, uniformly pigmented, light brown macules or patches that occur in sun-damaged skin of older adults (Figure 4.6). They are induced by ultraviolet (UV) exposure and are usually located on the shoulders, the scalp, and dorsal hands. Unlike freckles, they persist and do not darken when exposed to sunlight.[3] Dermoscopy shows an irregularly shaped lesion with a 'moth-eaten' border, structureless pigmentation, and occasionally areas with a faint, irregular pigment network or linearly striated pigmentation, creating a 'fingerprint' pattern (Figure 4.7).[9,10] Histologic examination shows a hyperpigmentation of the basal and sometimes suprabasal layers, usually with a more subtle proliferation of melanocytes than seen in lentigo simplex (Figures 4.8, 4.9). The rete ridges range from short and club-shaped to more complex anastomosing finger-like projections creating a reticulated pattern, which overlaps with macular or reticulated seborrheic keratosis, and occasionally are entirely absent, especially in lesions located on the face. Melanophages may be present in the dermis (Figure 4.9).[5]

Reflectance confocal microscopy of solar lentigo usually reveals a normal honeycomb pattern in the upper epidermis, a hyperrefractile cobblestone pattern in the basal layer and sometimes lower stratum spinosum (Figures 4.8A, 4.8B), and hyperrefractile dermal papillary rings composed of a monolayer of uniform cells surrounding crowded round to oval to annular or polycyclic dermal papillae (Figures 4.8B, 4.10, 4.11).[6] Solar lentigo, which overlaps histologically with seborrheic keratosis, not surprisingly, also resembles seborrheic keratosis on RCM, showing cerebriform architecture of the epidermis, as described previously in Chapter 3a.[6] In this setting, the dermal papillae have such complex polycyclic shapes that they appear more like dark sulci and the dermal papillary rings have no resemblance to ring shapes; thus, the general RCM features of lentigo are less prominent. Solar lentigo with a loss of rete ridges on histology is best visualized at the level of the superficial basal layer on RCM, where it appears as a well-demarcated area showing a hyperrefractile cobblestone pattern as compared to surrounding non-lesional skin (see Figure 6.119 in Chapter 6d).[7] Dermal plump bright cells, corresponding to melanophages, may be present (Figure 4.11), but there is no evidence of a melanocytic proliferation in the dermis (Figures 4.12, 4.13).

Solar lentigo may be difficult to differentiate from lentigo maligna (LM)/lentigo maligna melanoma (LMM) clinically. Both can be large and occur on the face, making excisional biopsy cosmetically and often functionally challenging. Furthermore, small biopsies risk underdiagnosis of LM/LMM, as LM/LMM often contains areas resembling solar lentigo histologically.[11] In this setting, RCM provides a potential advantage, as the whole lesion can be analyzed in vivo. If features of melanoma, such as loss of the honeycomb or cobblestone pattern of the epidermis, effacement of the DEJ with loss of defined dermal papillae, presence of numerous, coarse or branching dendritic structures, pleomorphic bright cells, and/or 'pagetoid' nucleated cells, are identified, a diagnosis of lentigo should not be rendered, but rather a diagnosis of LM/LMM should be considered.[6]

Key RCM features of solar lentigo

- Preserved honeycomb and cobblestone pattern of the epidermis
- Hyperrefractile dermal papillary rings composed of uniform, round cells
- Polymorphous, crowded dermal papillae with ovoid to annular or polycyclic contours
- or cerebriform architecture of the epidermis
- or well-demarcated hyperrefractile cobblestone pattern of the epidermis
- Plump bright cells (melanophages) may be present in the dermis

INK SPOT LENTIGO

Ink spot lentigo, also known as reticulated black solar lentigo, is an uncommon variant of solar lentigo that typically occurs in phototype I or II individuals of Celtic origin. It presents in adulthood in a background of solar damage as a dark brown or black, reticuted macule with an extremely irregular wiry or beaded border, reminiscent of an ink spot (Figure 4.14).[1] Dermoscopy shows a well-demarcated lesion with an irregular border and a broadened dark brown or black, pigmented network occasionally with a central homogeneous area (Figure 4.15).[12] Histologic examination shows prominent hyperpigmentation, often of several entire rete ridges, with or without extension of pigmentation throughout all levels of the epidermis (Figures 4.16, 4.18). Suprapapillary plates may be relatively spared. Melanocytes may be near normal or slightly increased in number, but are small and uniform in size and shape. Melanophages are often present in the subjacent dermis.[1,2,13]

Reflectance confocal microscopy finds features which correlate nicely with dermoscopic and histologic features. RCM mosaics from the lower epidermis and DEJ illustrate a well-demarcated lesion with an irregular border, composed of hyperrefractile small round cells with a similar architecture to the surrounding epidermis, giving the impression that a bright carpet has been placed on the epidermis: thus, the term carpet-like distribution (Figure 4.17). The stratum corneum may show hyperrefractile particles or globules. The stratum granulosum and upper spinosum show a preserved honeycomb pattern and may show admixed refractile particles, refractile globules, or cobblestone cells (Figure 4.18A). The lower stratum spinosum and basal layer show a hyperrefractile cobblestone pattern, which may be most pronounced over the rete ridges. RCM at the level of the DEJ reveals hyperrefractile dermal papillary rings, composed of uniform, round cells, and often a cobblestone pattern of the rete ridges (Figure 4.18B). The dermal papillae are crowded and range from round to oval to annular or polycyclic in shape.[6] Dermal plump bright cells, corresponding to melanophages, may be present, but there is no evidence of a melanocytic proliferation in the dermis.

Ink spot lentigo may be confused with melanoma clinically due to its dark color and irregular border.[1] Melanocyte cytomorphology, melanocyte architecture, and keratinocyte cell borders are the main factors to be used in differentiating ink spot lentigines from melanomas under RCM;[14] i.e. melanocytes, if distinguishable, are small, uniform and evenly distributed along the basal layer. The honeycomb and cobblestone patterns of the epidermis are preserved. There is no effacement of the DEJ architecture, although the junction between statum basalis and stratum spinosum may be less pronounced when rete are hyperpigmented and show a cobblestone pattern. Refractile particles and globules may be present in the superficial epidermis, but no prominent, complex dendritic strucures are seen. 'Pagetoid' cells and cell clusters are absent.

Key RCM features of ink spot lentigo

- Preserved honeycomb and cobblestone pattern of the epidermis
- Variable presence of brightly refractile particles/globules within the superficial epidermis
- Carpet-like distribution of uniform, small round bright cells in the lower epidermis, or a diffuse cobblestone pattern (if present, dermal papillary rings often blend into the stratum spinosum)
- Hyperrefractile dermal papillary rings composed of uniform, round cells
- Polymorphous, crowded dermal papillae with round, ovoid, annular, or polycyclic contours

REFERENCES

1. Bolognia JL. Reticulated black solar lentigo ('ink spot' lentigo). Arch Dermatol 1992; 128:934–40.
2. Kaddu S, Soyer HP, Wolf IH et al. [Reticular lentigo]. Der Hautarzt; Zeitschrift fur Dermatologie, Venerologie, und verwandte Gebiete 1997; 48:181–5.

3. Trout CR, Levine NS, Chang MW. Disorders of hyperpigmentation: lentigo. In: Bolognia JL, Jorizzo JL, Rapini RP, eds. Dermatology, 1st edn, Vol. 1. New York: Mosby, Elsevier; 2003: 981–7.

4. Lee PK, Rosenberg CN, Tsao H et al. Failure of Q-switched ruby laser to eradicate atypical-appearing solar lentigo: report of two cases. J Am Acad Dermatol 1998; 38:314–7.

5. Weedon D. Lentigines, nevi and melanomas. In: Skin Pathology, 2nd edn. New York: Churchill Livingstone; 2002: 803–58.

6. Langley RG, Burton E, Walsh N et al. In vivo confocal scanning laser microscopy of benign lentigines: comparison to conventional histology and in vivo characteristics of lentigo maligna. J Am Acad Dermatol 2006; 55:88–97.

7. Yamashita T, Negishi K, Hariya T et al. Intense pulsed light therapy for superficial pigmented lesions evaluated by reflectance-mode confocal microscopy and optical coherence tomography. J Invest Dermatol 2006; 126:2281–6.

8. Pehamberger H, Steiner A, Wolff K. In vivo epiluminescence microscopy of pigmented skin lesions. I. Pattern analysis of pigmented skin lesions. J Am Acad Dermatol 1987; 17:571–83.

9. Elgart GW. Seborrheic keratoses, solar lentigines, and lichenoid keratoses. Dermatoscopic features and correlation to histology and clinical signs. Dermatol Clin 2001; 19:347–57.

10. Sahin MT, Ozturkcan S, Ermertcan AT et al. A comparison of dermoscopic features among lentigo senilis/initial seborrheic keratosis, seborrheic keratosis, lentigo maligna and lentigo maligna melanoma on the face. J Dermatol 2004; 31:884–9.

11. Dalton SR, Gardner TL, Libow LF et al. Contiguous lesions in lentigo maligna. J Am Acad Dermatol 2005; 52:859–62.

12. Wang SQ, Rabinovitz H, Oliviero MC. Dermoscopic patterns of solar lentigines and seborrheic keratoses. In: Marghoob AA, Braun RP, Kopf AW, eds. Atlas of Dermoscopy. Abingdon, UK: Taylor & Francis; 2005: 60–6.

13. Haas N, Hermes B, Henz BM. Detection of a novel pigment network feature in reticulated black solar lentigo by high-resolution epiluminescence microscopy. Am J Dermatopathol 2002; 24:213–7.

14. Gerger A, Koller S, Kern T et al. Diagnostic applicability of in vivo confocal laser scanning microscopy in melanocytic skin tumors. J Invest Dermatol 2005; 124:493–8.

LENTIGO SIMPLEX

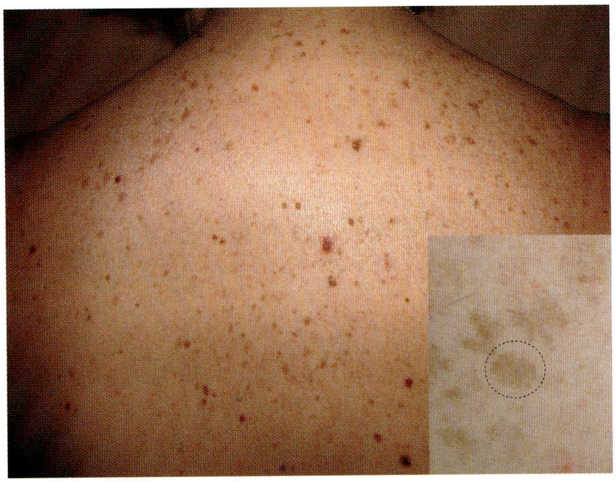

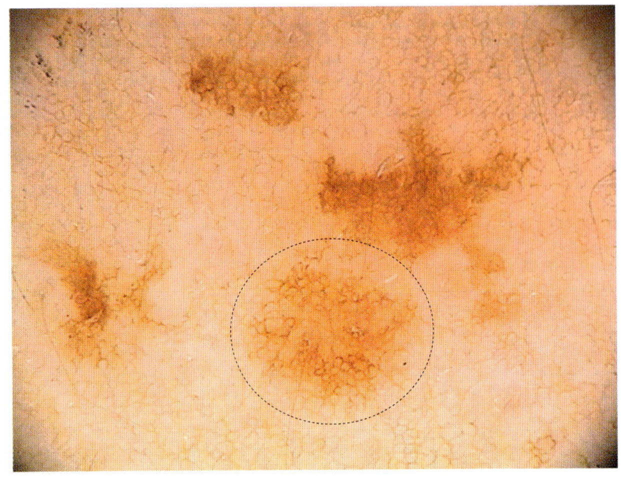

▲ **Figures 4.1, 4.2** Clinical photograph of the upper back of a 45-year-old woman showing multiple pigmented lesions. Inset close-up photograph shows a 4 mm, oval, evenly pigmented, light brown macule (circled) surrounded by similarly colored macules and patches with irregular borders. Dermoscopic image reveals a symmetrical reticular lesion (circled) with a typical and regular light brown pigment network, compatible with lentigo simplex. Note by contrast, the irregular 'moth-eaten' borders of the surrounding pigmented macules, suggestive of solar lentigo.

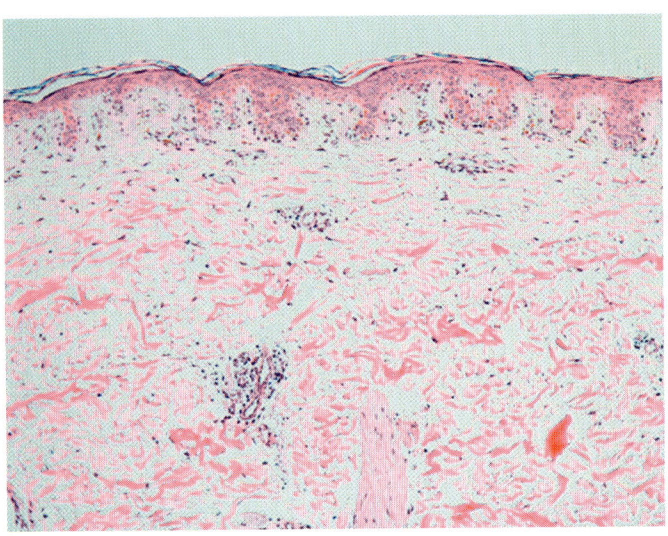

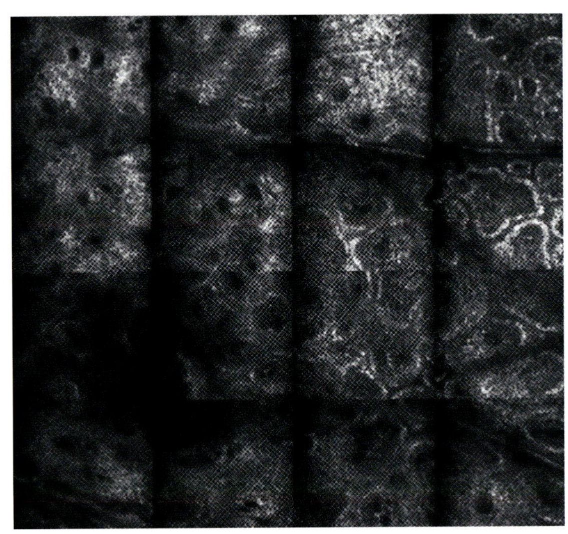

▲ **Figures 4.3, 4.4** Histology (10×) shows features of lentigo simplex, including hyperpigmentation of the basal layer and an increased number of small, uniform melanocytes along the sides and tips of bulbous rete ridges. Notably, the lesion does not otherwise disturb the architecture of the epidermis. RCM mosaic (2 mm × 2 mm) at the level of the DEJ reveals variably sized and shaped hyperrefractile dermal papillary rings.

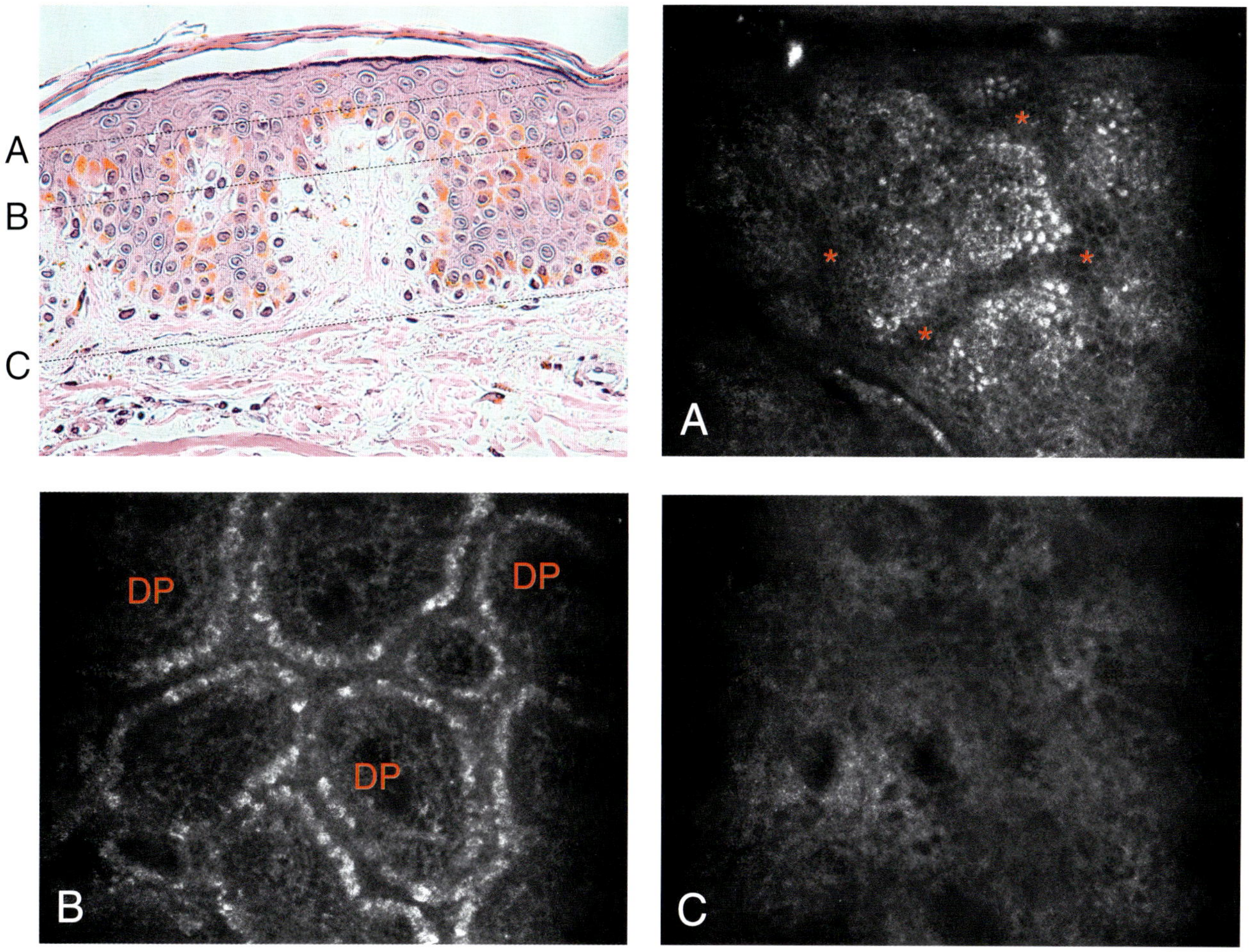

▲ **Figure 4.5** Histology (20×) shows hyperpigmentation of the basal layer and an increased number of small, uniform melanocytes along the sides and tips of bulbous rete ridges. A few melanophages, but not melanocytes, are seen in the subjacent dermis. Horizontal lines labeled A, B, and C indicate from where each RCM image (0.475 mm × 0.340 mm) is captured. At level A, islands of small, round, uniform cells forming a hyperrefractile cobblestone pattern are seen at the level of the superficial basal layer in suprapapillary plates, surrounded by rete ridges showing a normal honeycomb pattern of the stratum spinosum (asterisks). At the level of the DEJ (B), bright dermal papillary rings composed of a layer of monomorphic bright cells surround crowded variably sized and shaped dermal papillae (DP). There is no evidence of a melanocytic proliferation, such as cell clusters, or individual nucleated refractile cells, in the superficial dermis (C).

SOLAR LENTIGO

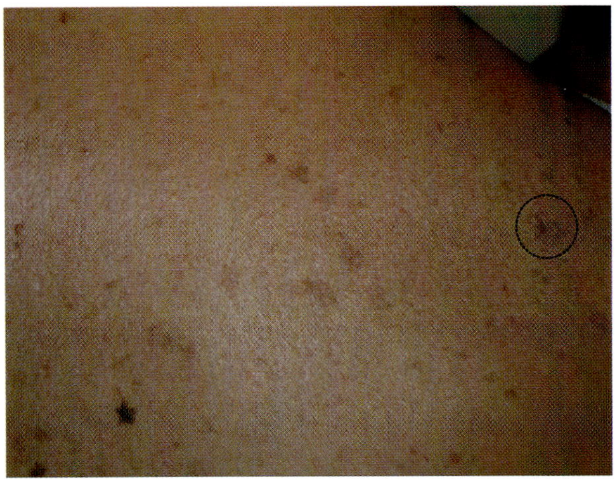

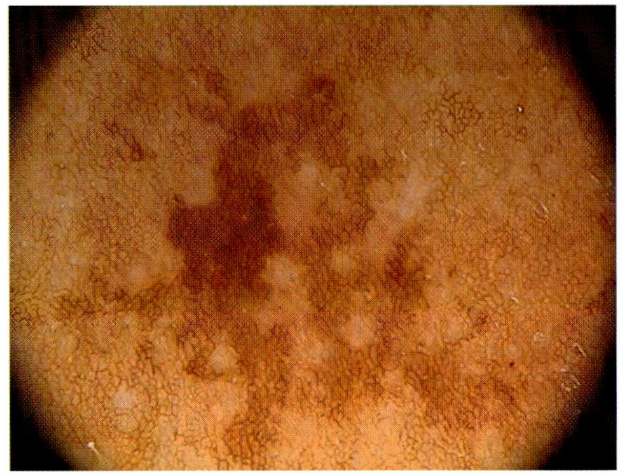

▲ **Figures 4.6, 4.7** Clinical photograph of a 9 mm asymptomatic, irregular brown macule (circled) on the back of a 36-year-old man. Note the background of actinic damage. Dermoscopy reveals an irregularly shaped lesion with a 'moth-eaten' border showing areas with structureless pigmentation and areas with a faint, irregular pigment network.

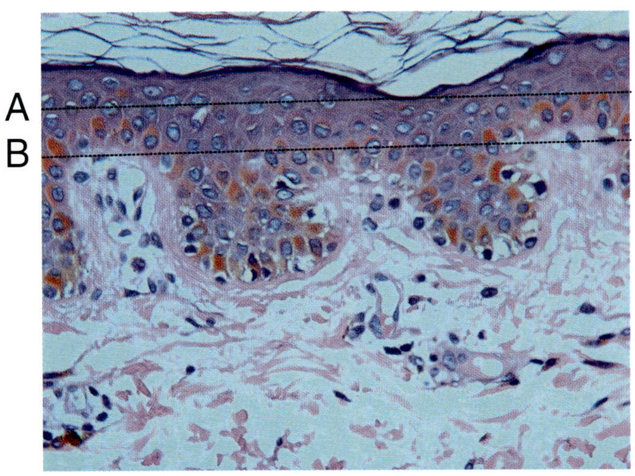

▲ **Figure 4.8** Histology (20×) shows diffuse hyperpigmentation of the basal layer and patchy hyperpigmentation of the stratum spinosum. A slightly increased number of uniform small melanocytes are also seen along the sides and tips of rete ridges. Horizontal lines labeled A and B indicate from where each RCM image (0.475 mm × 0.340 mm) is captured. An expanded cobblestone pattern, formed by small round bright cells, corresponding to supranuclear melanin caps, is seen in the lower stratum spinosum/superficial basal layer (A) and in the superficial DEJ (B), where uniformly hyperrefractile, variably sized and shaped dermal papillary rings are also identified.

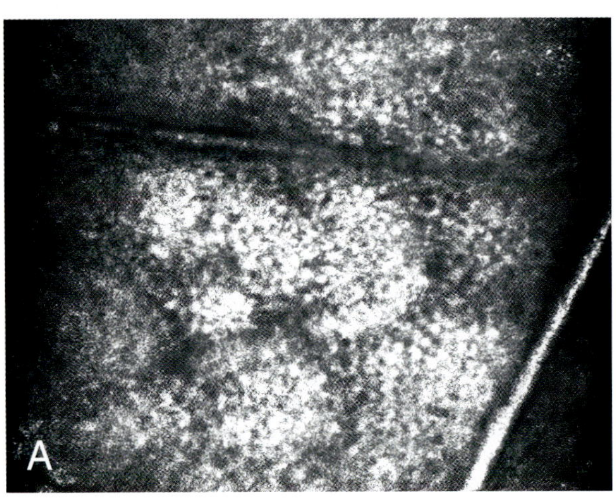

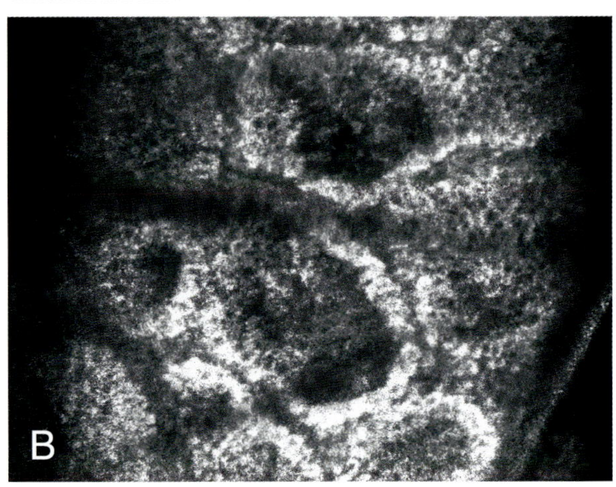

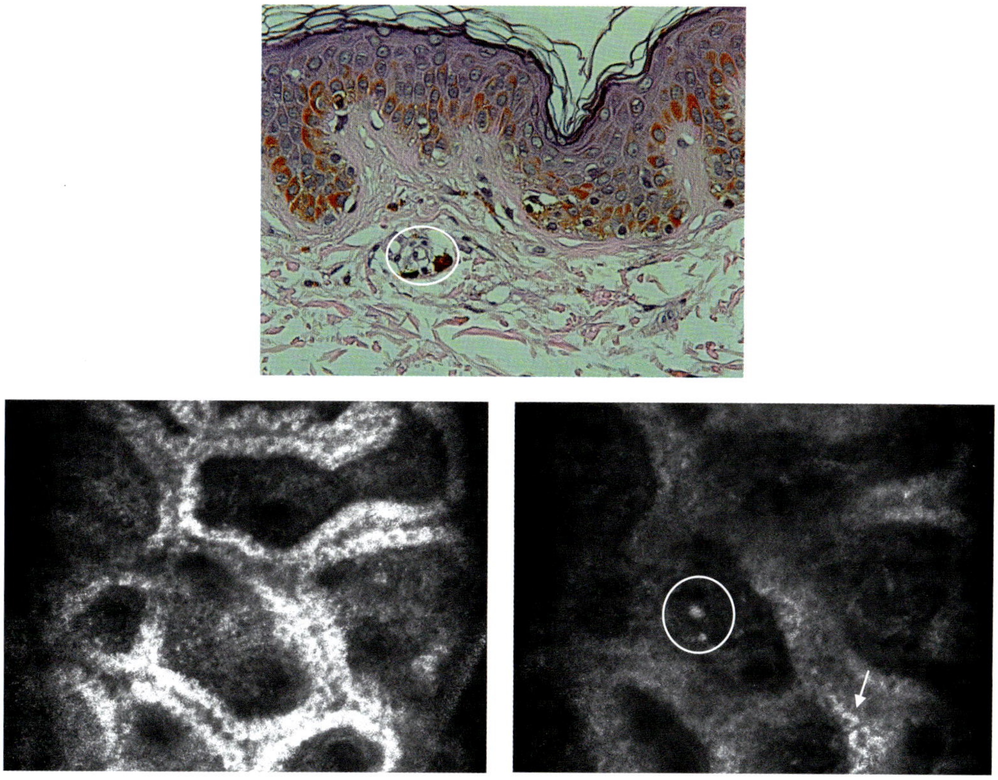

▲ **Figures 4.9–4.11** Histology (20×) from another area shows similar features and an even more subtle proliferation of melanocytes. A few melanophages (circled) are noted in the papillary dermis. RCM (0.475 mm × 0.340 mm) at the level of the mid DEJ (left) shows hyperrefractile dermal papillary rings, composed of uniform, round bright cells, surrounding crowded, variably sized dermal papillae, which range from round to annular to polycyclic in shape. Dermal papillary rings at the level of the deep DEJ (right) are less bright, due to decreased light penetration, allowing for easy visualization of individual pigmented basal keratinocytes (white arrow), which have a central round nucleus and abundant bright cytoplasm. Plump bright cells (circled) are seen in the papillary dermis.

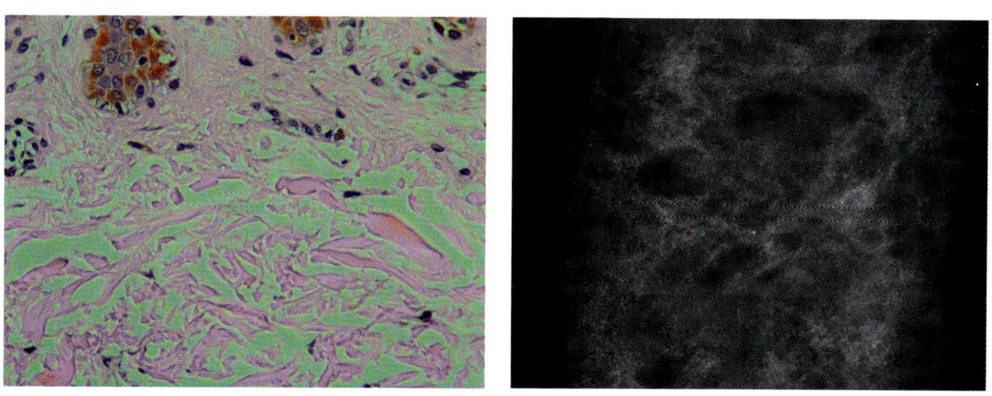

▲ **Figures 4.12, 4.13** There is no evidence of a melanocytic proliferation in the superficial reticular dermis on histology (20×) or on RCM (0.475 mm × 0.340 mm).

INK SPOT LENTIGO

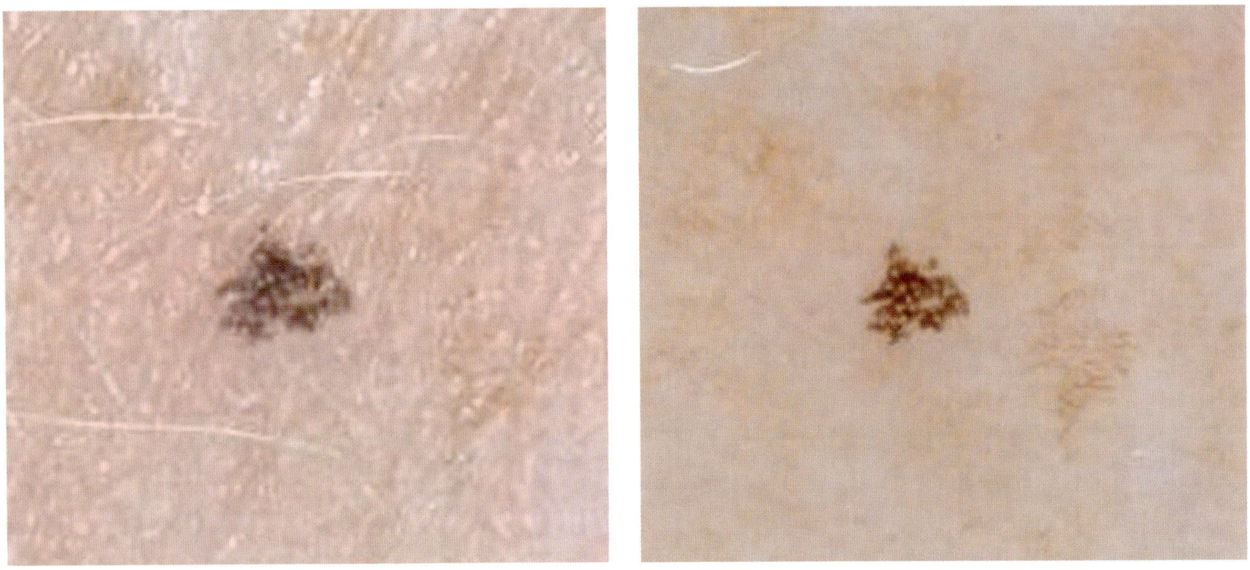

▲ **Figures 4.14, 4.15** Clinical photograph of a 1 mm asymptomatic brown macule on the right arm of a 32-year-old woman with extensive actinic damage. Dermoscopic photograph reveals a well-demarcated lesion with an irregular border and broadened dark brown pigmented network.

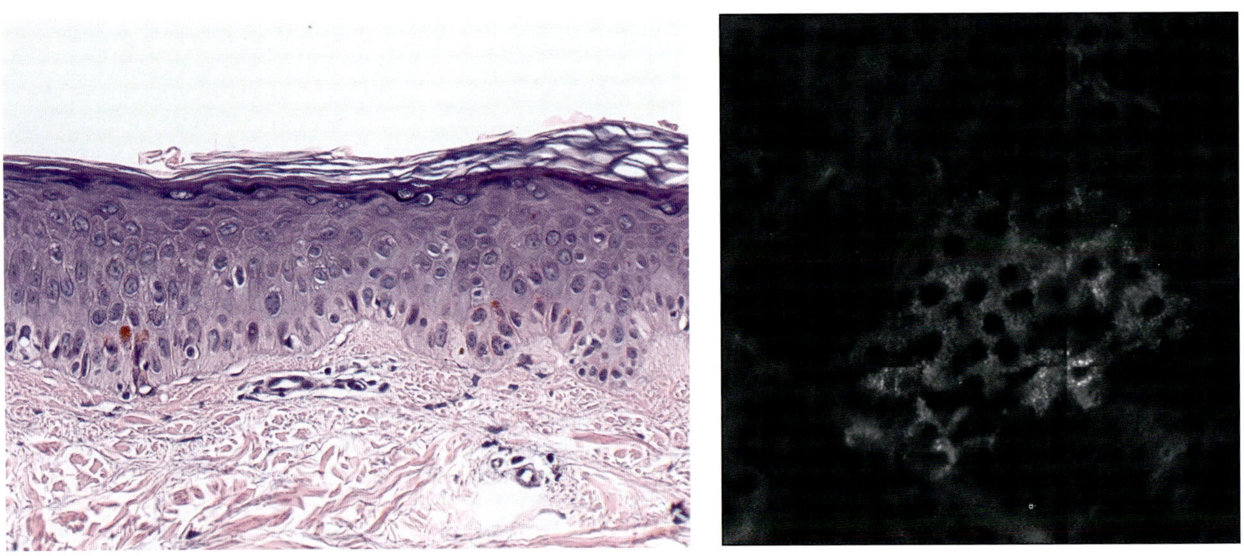

▲ **Figures 4.16, 4.17** Histology (20×) shows background actinic damage and the characteristic hyperpigmentation of the basal layer found in lentigines. RCM mosaic (1.5 mm × 1.5 mm) at the level of the DEJ, like dermoscopy, shows an easily visualized lesion with an irregular border and sharp lateral circumscription. The lesion is composed of uniform, bright cells and has an architecture similar to surrounding non-lesional skin, giving the impression that a bright carpet has merely been placed over the skin: thus, the origin of the term 'carpet-like distribution'.

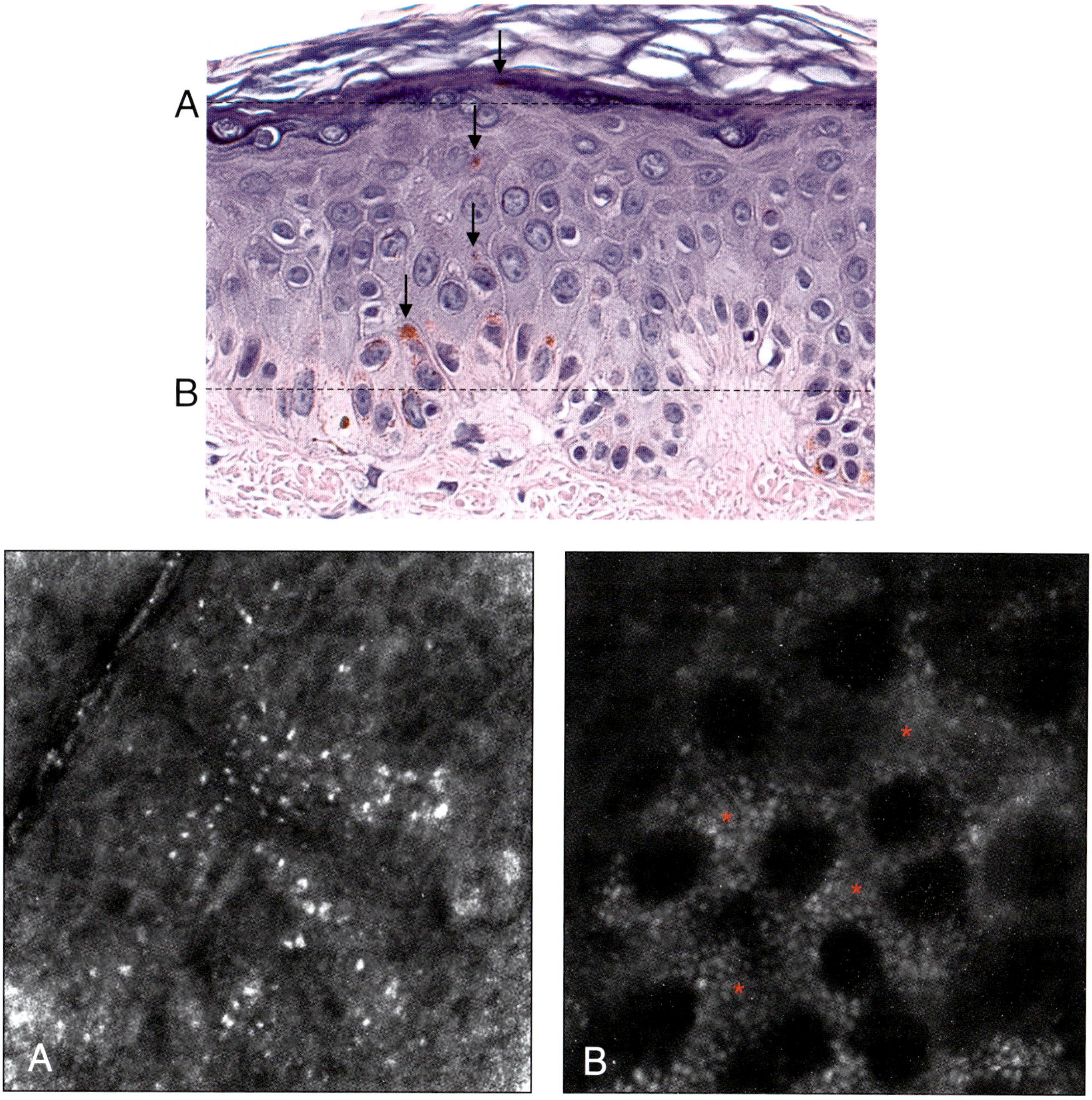

▲ **Figure 4.18** At higher magnification, histology (40×) shows that pigmentation is most pronounced in the rete ridges, but can be seen at all levels of epidermis (arrows); horizontal lines labeled A and B indicate from where each confocal image (0.5 mm × 0.5 mm) is captured. RCM at the level of the stratum granulosum (A) identifies several small brightly refractile particles and a few larger brightly refractile globules within keratinocytes; the background honeycomb pattern can still be appreciated. RCM at the level of the upper DEJ (B) shows a diffuse cobblestone pattern, or a 'carpet-like' distribution of homogeneous, round, bright cells not only in the stratum basalis but also throughout the stratum spinosum of the rete (asterisks).

CHAPTER 4b

Congenital and common acquired melanocytic nevi

Melissa Gill, Jocelyn A Lieb, and Cristiane Benvenuto-Andrade

Melanocytic nevi are benign neoplasms composed of melanocytes. They can be present at birth or acquired at any age. Depending on subtype and melanin content, nevi can range in size, shape (macule, plaque, papule, polyp, or papilloma), and color (flesh-tone, pink, tan, brown, or black). Dermoscopic and histologic features also vary depending on subtype. In general, however, all characteristically show symmetry and homogeneity on dermoscopy and circumscription, symmetry, an absence of cytologic atypia, and maturation (decrease in nest size, cell size, and melanization with progressive descent into the dermis) on histology.

The melanin present in melanocytic neoplasms provides contrast, making them ideal for evaluation by reflectance confocal microscopy (RCM).[1] On RCM, individual nevocytes generally appear as round or oval cells with central round nuclei surrounded by refractile cytoplasm; their brightness depends on the quantity and possibly the quality of cytoplasmic melanin (Figure 4.23C).[2] Careful examination of both the attributes of the melanocytic proliferation and its surrounding epidermis allows for in-vivo categorization of superficial melanocytic neoplasms with surprising sensitivity and specificity.[3–5] The limited imaging depth of currently available RCM imaging devices, however, prevents the adequate evaluation of some compound nevi and most intradermal nevi. Furthermore, malignant intradermal features may be difficult to discern. For this reason, in its present configuration, RCM is most useful for the evaluation of flat benign or malignant pigmented lesions or raised malignant pigmented lesions (melanomas) with a prominent in-situ component.

Reflectance confocal microscopic examination of a benign nevus begins with mosaics, which characteristically reveal a well-circumscribed and symmetrical lesion (Figures 4.31, 4.38). Benign nevi tend to show preservation of the skin's architecture, such that keratinocyte cell borders are easily visualized within the normal honeycomb and cobblestone patterns of the epidermis (Figures 4.23A, 4.32A, 4.39B).[3–8] Some nevi may show an expanded cobblestone pattern of the epidermis (Figure 4.39A–C) and/or edged papillae (Figures 4.38, 4.39C, 4.39D, 4.41), secondary to hypermelanization of keratinocytes and, in the case of edged papillae, pigmented keratinocytes and melanocytes along the sides of rete ridges, resulting in hyperrefractile dermal papillary rings.[4,5,9] The rete may be elongated, but dermal papillary rings tend to be regular in size, shape and distribution (Figures 4.22, 4.31, 4.38).[9]

Nests of melanocytes appear on RCM as refractile, round to oval, cellular aggregates, termed cell clusters. Cell cluster brightness depends on the extent of melanization. Individual melanocytes within a cell cluster may be easy to distinguish or blend in with surrounding cells. In benign nevi, RCM mosaics reveal cell clusters that are uniform in size and shape and evenly distributed at the dermal–epidermal junction (junctional cell clusters) and/or in the dermis (dermal cell clusters) (Figures 4.22, 4.31, 4.38, 4.41). Cell clusters are characteristically dense and homogeneous (Figures 4.32C, 4.34, 4.39C, 4.39D, 4.41), corresponding to cohesive nests of uniform melanocytes on histology (Figures 4.32, 4.33, 4.39, 4.40). Moreover, loose and/or dishomogeneous cell clusters, corresponding to discohesive and/or internally pleomorphic melanocytic nests on histology, are uncommon.[3–7,10,11] Cerebriform cell clusters have as yet generally not been identified in benign nevi and are considered specific for melanoma.[4,5,10,11] Decreasing cell cluster brightness with increasing depth is a feature of maturation (Figures 4.23C, 4.23D), which corresponds to decreasing melanization with increasing depth on histology (Figure 4.23). In addition to nested melanocytes, some benign nevi show an increased number of solitary melanocytes along the sides and tips of rete ridges (Figures 4.37, 4.39, 4.40). As these are (by definition) small, uniform, round, and lack cytologic atypia, they can be difficult to distinguish from pigmented basal keratinocytes on RCM (Figures 4.39C, 4.39D, 4.41).[4–7] In general, 'pagetoid' melanocytosis should not be observed in benign nevi.[4,5,8] Likewise, some reports suggest individual nucleated refractile cells in the papillary dermis are a feature of concern on RCM,[4,5] but they have also been reported in congenital nevi[12] and melanocytes arranged as solitary units can certainly be found in the papillary dermis of benign nevi on histology. Further studies are needed to determine the significance of these cells.

As described above, several RCM features are more frequently attributed to benign nevi, but, like histology, no one feature alone is diagnostic of nevus vs melanoma. Under special circumstances, such as acute ultraviolet (UV) exposure or trauma, melanocytes can be seen above the basal layer in benign nevi.[13] Moreover, activated intraepidermal Langerhans cells in inflamed nevi appear as dendritic cells in the mid and upper epidermis and may be difficult to distinguish from dendritic melanocytes.[14] Some studies report that if dendritic structures are present in benign nevi, they are thin and without complex branching.[3,6,7] In summary, when evaluating a pigmented lesion using RCM, as with histology, all features must be taken together in the global context of the lesion with incorporation of clinical findings to avoid misclassification.

Key RCM features of benign melanocytic nevi

- Well circumscribed and symmetrical
- Preservation of the normal honeycomb and cobblestone patterns of the epidermis
- Uniformly sized and shaped dermal papillary rings
- +/– Edged papillae
- Dense, homogeneous cell clusters, uniform in size and shape, and distributed evenly

CONGENITAL MELANOCYTIC NEVUS

By definition, congenital melanocytic nevi (CMN) are present at birth or soon thereafter. They tend to be uniformly pigmented papules or plaques and range in color from tan to black (Figure 4.19). They are commonly classified by size as small (<1.5 cm), medium (1.5–19.9 cm), or large (≥20 cm). Melanoma may develop in association with CMN and the relative risk seems to be greater with increasing size.[15,16] CMN show a variety of global patterns on dermoscopy, including globular, reticular, reticuloglobular, and diffuse brown pigmentation with or without remnant globules or network fragments. Regardless of pattern, however, they are overall homogeneous and symmetrical (Figure 4.20).[17] On histologic examination, congenital melanocytic nevi have cytologic features similar to those found in common acquired melanocytic nevi (CAMN), but differ architecturally. CMN are usually compound or intradermal. The junctional component may be nested or lentiginous (see below). Dermal melanocytes tend to be distributed in more diffuse aggregate and cords, which splay individually between collagen bundles and extend as aggregates and nests around adnexal structures, blood vessels, and nerves (Figures 4.21, 4.23, 4.24, 4.26). Nevus usually involves the reticular dermis and occasionally extends into the subcutis.[18] Lesions with clinical hypertrichosis show an increased number and size of hair follicles.

Congenital nevi may be indistinguishable from common acquired nevi on RCM, as the diagnostic features allowing for a histologic designation of congenital pattern nevus are based on the dermal architecture, which is only superficially visualized using RCM. CMN may simply show generic benign nevus features on RCM, as described above

(Figures 4.22, 4.23A–D, 4.27). Occasionally, cell clusters or aggregates extending along adnexal or vascular structures may be visualized, suggesting congenital patterning (Figure 4.25). Additional features that may be encountered in congenital nevi include slightly loose cell clusters, corresponding to discohesive nests at the dermal-epidermal junction and aggregates and cords of melanocytes in the dermis (Figure 4.23A–D), and individual nucleated refractile cells in the papillary dermis.[12] It would be unexpected, however, to find associated cellular atypia or pleomorphism.

As patients grow, their congenital nevi may develop and undergo subtle changes in size, color, and texture, raising concern for melanoma development. Although most biopsy specimens from these changing lesions show histologic features of CMN without any evidence of melanoma, many patients are left with disfiguring scars. Therefore, RCM may become an interesting additional tool for the non-invasive quasi-histologic study of changing CMN, helping to detect early superficial melanomas. According to a published series of cases,[12] RCM allows for the identification of features characteristic of melanoma development in CMN, although future studies are needed to determine the sensitivity and specificity of such an approach. Owing to the limited imaging depth of currently available devices, RCM is as yet not helpful for the evaluation of deeper dermal changes, such as distinguishing between a proliferative nodule and nodular melanoma arising in a congenital nevus.

Key RCM features of congenital melanocytic nevi

- Well circumscribed and symmetrical
- Preservation of the normal honeycomb and cobblestone patterns of the epidermis
- Uniformly sized and shaped dermal papillary rings
- +/– Edged papillae
- Dense or slightly loose, homogeneous cell clusters, uniform in size and shape, and distributed evenly
- Cell clusters or aggregates in a periadnexal and/or perivascular distribution

COMMON ACQUIRED MELANOCYTIC NEVUS

Common acquired melanocytic nevi, also called banal nevi, are not present at birth. They usually develop during the first three decades of life, but can occur at any age. Most acquired nevi are <5 mm in diameter. Many clinical and histologic subtypes of CAMN have been described. These benign melanocytic neoplasms range in shape (macular, papular, papillomatous, or polypoid) and color (flesh-tone, pink, tan, brown, or near black) depending on subtype, but all are symmetrical with even pigmentation and regular borders (Figure 4.28). Similarly, CAMN can show a variety of patterns on dermoscopy, depending on the anatomic location of the melanocytic proliferation and the amount and distribution of melanin pigment. Patterns include a regular pigment network, regular globules, regularly distributed dots, and homogeneous areas; regardless of pattern, the lesion shows symmetrical distribution of pigmentation and pattern (Figure 4.29).[19] On histology, CAMN are generally grouped according to the anatomic location of the melanocytic proliferation within the skin and correspondingly termed junctional (tips of rete ridges), compound (tips of rete ridges and dermis), or intradermal (dermis only). All are well circumscribed, symmetric, and composed of nested melanocytes without cytologic atypia (Figures 4.30, 4.32, 4.33). If there is a dermal component, maturation is present (Figure 4.32). CAMN show the features generally attributed to benign nevi on both histology and RCM, but periadnexal and perivascular nests are usually not seen (Figures 4.31, 4.32A–D, 4.34).[18]

Lentiginous nevus is a histologic subtype of CAMN with distinctive clinical, dermoscopic, and histologic features that are well appreciated on RCM. These nevi may be junctional or compound. As they usually do not extend beyond the papillary or superficial reticular dermis, these nevi are generally quite flat (Figures 4.35, 4.37). As indicated by the name, these nevi show features of lentigo in addition to melanocytic nests. As such, they are characterized by a proliferation of solitary and nested melanocytes along the sides and tips of elongated, pigmented rete ridges (Figures 4.37, 4.39, 4.40). Hyperpigmentation of keratinocytes may extend throughout all layers of the epidermis, resulting in a near black color clinically and homogeneous pigmentation in the otherwise regular reticular pigment network on dermoscopy (Figures 4.36, 4.39).[18,19] Not surprisingly, these lesions also show features of lentigo on RCM, including an expanded cobblestone pattern, hyperpigmented dermal papillary rings, or edged dermal papillae, in addition to the presence of small, dense, homogeneous cell clusters distributed evenly throughout the lesion (Figures 4.38, 4.39A–D, 4.41).

Key RCM features of common acquired melanocytic nevi

- Well circumscribed and symmetrical
- Preservation of the normal honeycomb and cobblestone patterns of the epidermis
- Uniformly sized and shaped dermal papillary rings
- +/– Edged papillae
- Dense, homogeneous cell clusters, uniform in size and shape, and distributed evenly
- **Lentiginous nevi:** expanded cobblestone pattern and edged papillae are typical

REFERENCES

1. Rajadhyaksha M, Grossman M, Esterowitz D et al. In vivo confocal scanning laser microscopy of human skin: melanin provides strong contrast. J Invest Dermatol 1995; 104:946–52.
2. Busam KJ, Charles C, Lee G et al. Morphologic features of melanocytes, pigmented keratinocytes, and melanophages by in vivo confocal scanning laser microscopy. Mod Pathol 2001; 14:862–8.
3. Gerger A, Koller S, Weger W et al. Sensitivity and specificity of confocal laser-scanning microscopy for in vivo diagnosis of malignant skin tumors. Cancer 2006; 107:193–200.
4. Pellacani G, Cesinaro AM, Seidenari S. Reflectance-mode confocal microscopy of pigmented skin lesions – improvement in melanoma diagnostic specificity. J Am Acad Dermatol 2005; 53:979–85.
5. Pellacani G, Guitera P, Longo C et al. The impact of in vivo reflectance confocal microscopy for the diagnostic accuracy of melanoma and equivocal melanocytic lesions. J Invest Dermatol 2007; Jul 26: [Epub ahead of print].
6. Langley RG, Rajadhyaksha M, Dwyer PJ et al. Confocal scanning laser microscopy of benign and malignant melanocytic skin lesions in vivo. J Am Acad Dermatol 2001; 45:365–76.
7. Gerger A, Koller S, Kern T et al. Diagnostic applicability of in vivo confocal laser scanning microscopy in melanocytic skin tumors. J Invest Dermatol 2005; 124:493–8.
8. Pellacani G, Cesinaro AM, Seidenari S. Reflectance-mode confocal microscopy for the in vivo characterization of pagetoid melanocytosis in melanomas and nevi. J Invest Dermatol 2005; 125:532–7.
9. Pellacani G, Cesinaro AM, Longo C et al. Microscopic in vivo description of cellular architecture of dermoscopic pigment network in nevi and melanomas. Arch Dermatol 2005; 141:147–54.
10. Pellacani G, Cesinaro AM, Seidenari S. In vivo assessment of melanocytic nests in nevi and melanomas by reflectance confocal microscopy. Mod Pathol 2005; 18:469–74.
11. Pellacani G, Cesinaro AM, Seidenari S. In vivo confocal reflectance microscopy for the characterization of melanocytic nests and correlation with dermoscopy and histology. Br J Dermatol 2005; 152:384–6.
12. Marghoob AA, Charles CA, Busam KJ et al. In vivo confocal scanning laser microscopy of a series of congenital melanocytic nevi suggestive of having developed malignant melanoma. Arch Dermatol 2005; 141:1401–12.
13. Petronic-Rosic V, Shea CR, Krausz T. Pagetoid melanocytosis: when is it significant? Pathology 2004; 36:435–44.
14. Busam KJ, Marghoob AA, Halpern A. Melanoma diagnosis by confocal microscopy: promise and pitfalls. J Invest Dermatol 2005; 125:vii.
15. Krengel S, Hauschild A, Schafer T. Melanoma risk in congenital melanocytic naevi: a systematic review. Br J Dermatol 2006; 155:1–8.
16. Zaal LH, Mooi WJ, Klip H et al. Risk of malignant transformation of congenital melanocytic nevi: a retrospective nationwide study from The Netherlands. Plast Reconstr Surg 2005; 116:1902–9.
17. Marghoob AA, Fu JM, Sachs D. Dermoscopic features of congenital melanocytic nevi. In: Marghoob AA, Braun RP, Kopf AW, eds. Atlas of Dermoscopy. Abingdon, UK: Taylor & Francis; 2005: 141–59.
18. McKee P, Calonje E, Granter S. Melanocytic nevi. In: McKee PH, Calonje E, Granter SR, eds. Pathology of the Skin with Clinical Correlations, Vol. 2. Philadelphia: Elsevier Mosby; 2005: 1242–94.
19. Bauer J, Blum A. Dermoscopic features of common melanocytic nevi of the junctional compound and dermal type. In: Marghoob AA, Braun RP, Kopf AW, eds. Atlas of Dermoscopy. Abingdon, UK: Taylor & Francis; 2005: 181–7.

CONGENITAL MELANOCYTIC NEVUS

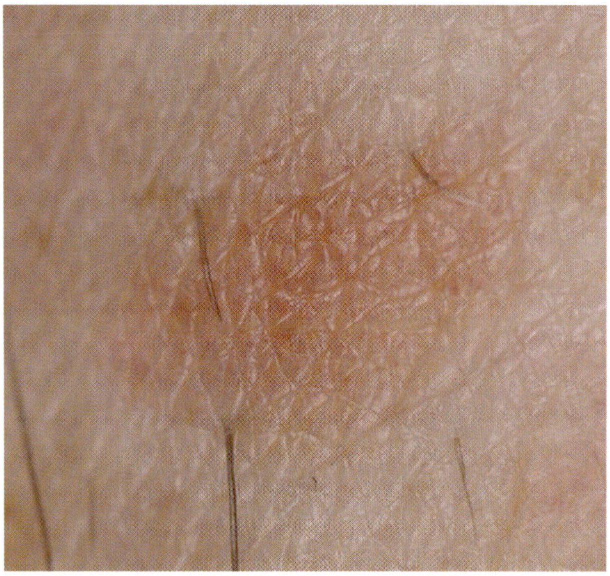

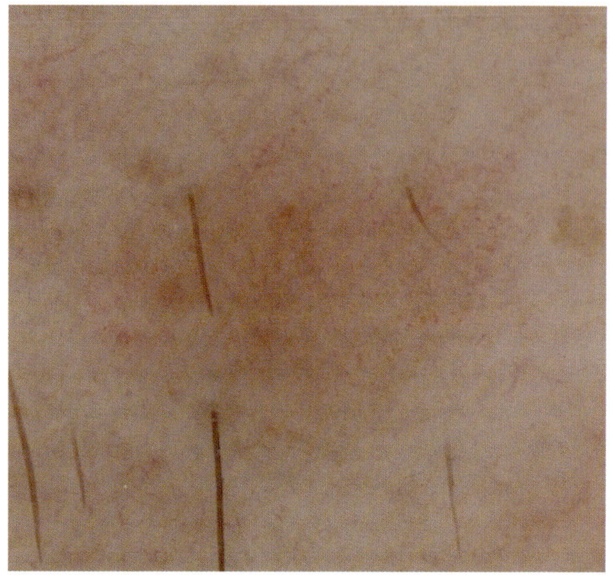

▲ **Figures 4.19, 4.20** Clinical photograph of a 6 mm tan plaque on the left anterior forearm of a 48-year-old man, which has been present since birth. Dermoscopic photograph reveals a tan homogeneous lesion with scattered light brown globules.

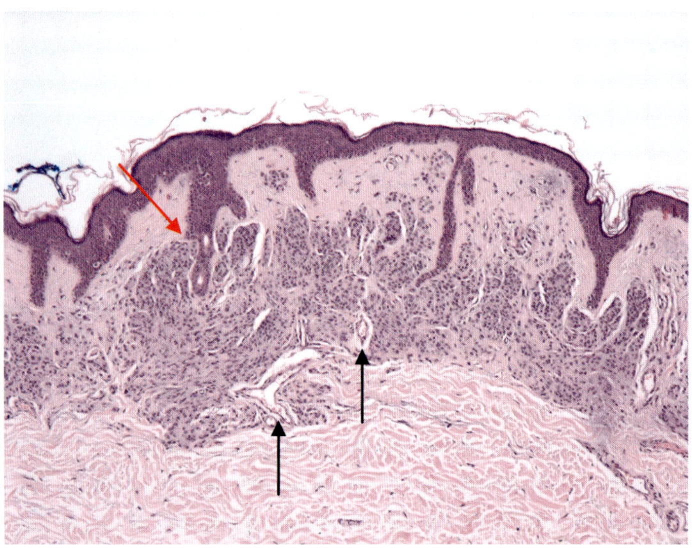

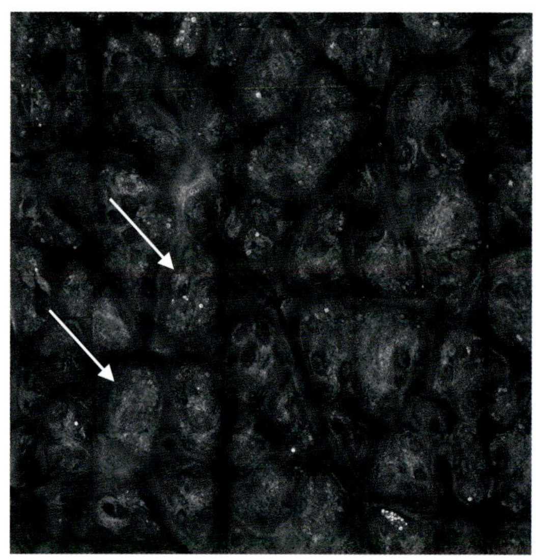

▲ **Figures 4.21, 4.22** Histology (10×) shows nests of melanocytes within the dermis, which mature with descent and show extension along an eccrine duct (red arrow) and close association with the superficial vascular plexus (black arrows). RCM mosaic (2.0 mm × 2.0 mm) at the level of the deep DEJ shows diffuse distribution of refractile, medium-sized, dense cell clusters within the papillary dermis (white arrows).

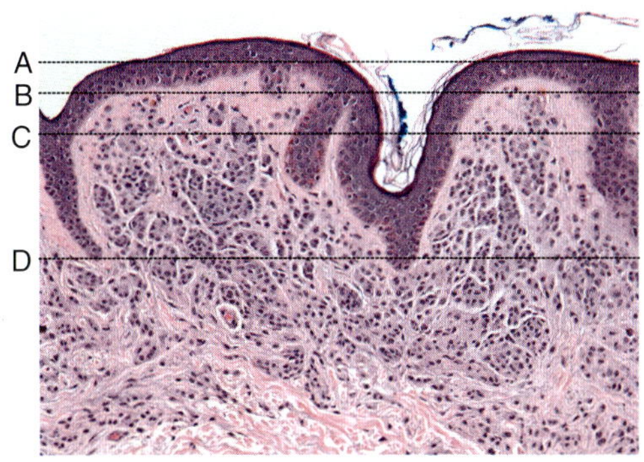

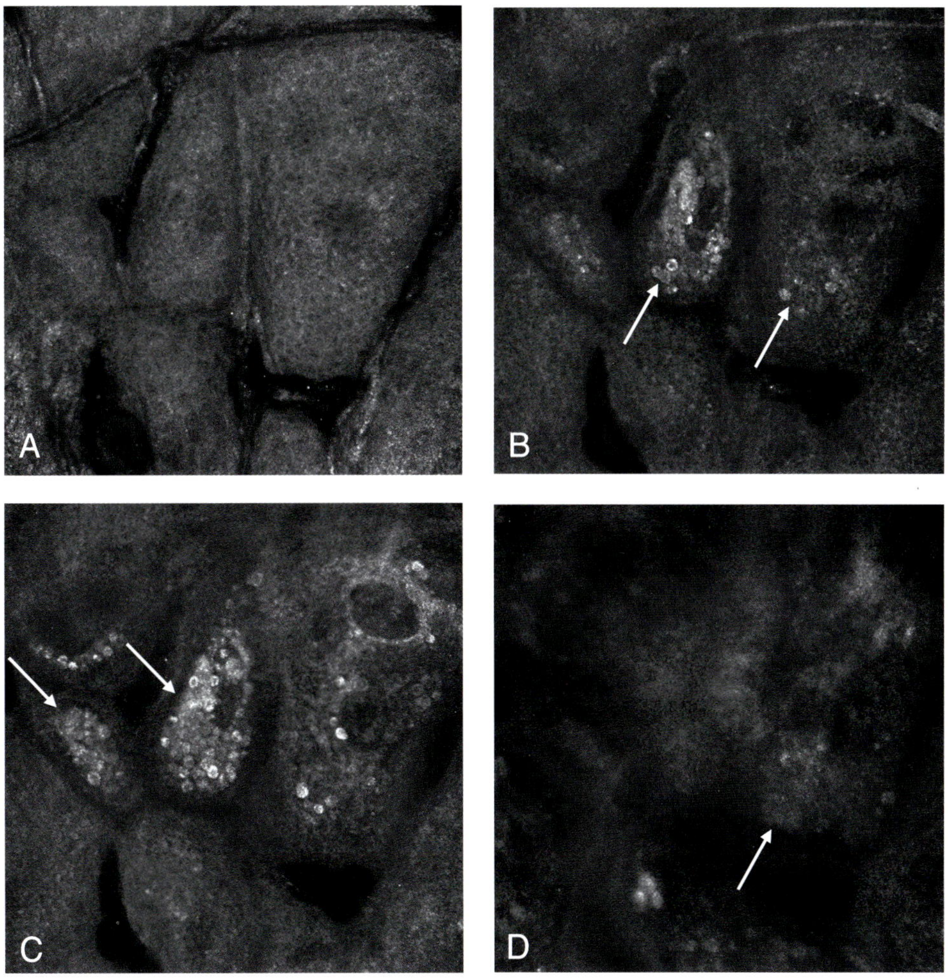

▲ **Figure 4.23** Histology (20×) shows solitary and nested small, bland, melanocytes in the dermis. Horizontal lines labeled A–D indicate from where each confocal image is captured. RCM (0.5 mm × 0.5 mm) at the level of the stratum spinosum (A) shows a normal honeycomb pattern. At the upper DEJ (B), the surface of bright cell clusters (arrows) are seen just below the epidermis. At the lower DEJ (C), slightly loose cell clusters (arrows), composed of uniform round cells with bright cytoplasm and central small round dark nucleus, fill the dermal papillae. At the level of the dermis (D), clusters of less bright nucleated cells (arrow) are seen, but there is loss of detail and contrast.

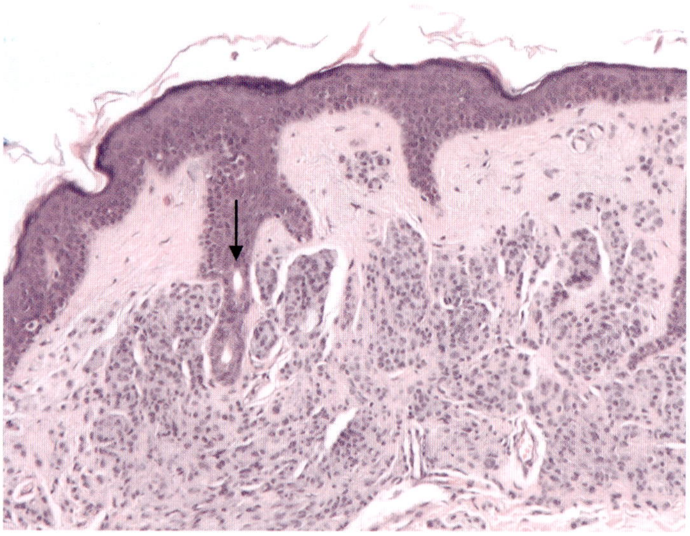

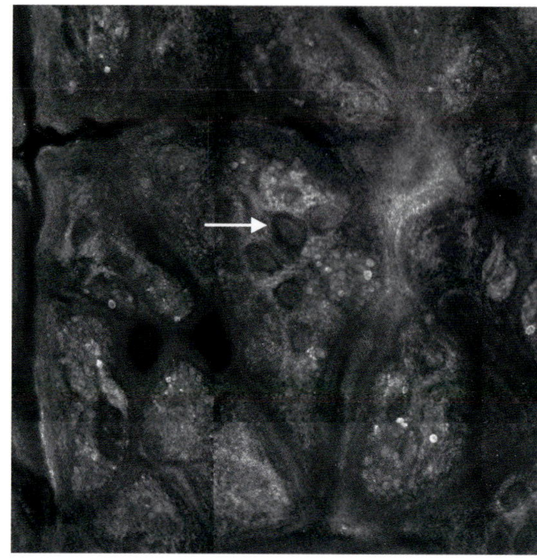

▲ **Figures 4.24, 4.25** The nevus cells seen aggregated around an eccrine duct (black arrow) on histology (20×) can also be seen on RCM mosaic (1.0 mm × 1.0 mm) as homogeneous, round, variably refractile, nucleated cells surrounding a group of round, weakly refractile donut-shaped structures (white arrow). These grouped donut-shaped structures represent the coiling eccrine duct; one can appreciate the darker outer ring with an internal weakly refractile 'donut shape' and a central, small dark lumen, which correspond to the bilayer of ductular cells and the duct lumen.

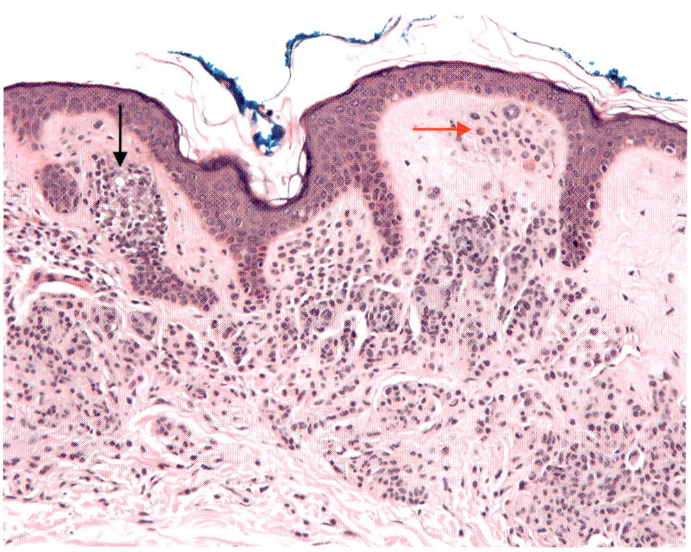

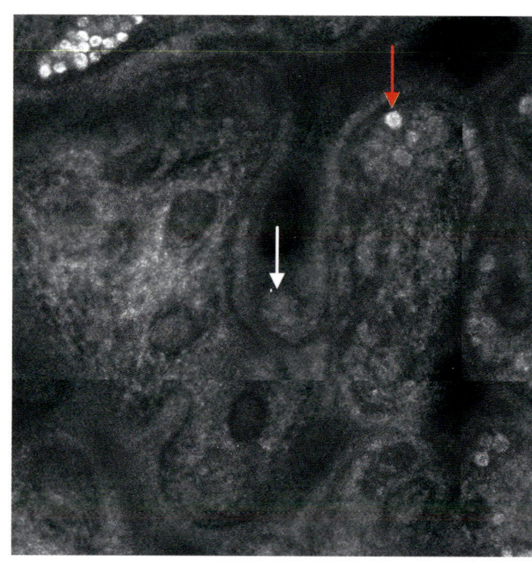

▲ **Figures 4.26, 4.27** Histology (20×) shows a junctional melanocytic nest (black arrow) and a few superficial nevus cells which are more heavily pigmented (red arrow) than most. Corresponding RCM at the level of the DEJ reveals a small dense cell cluster connected to a rete ridge (white arrow) and scattered nucleated round cells in the papillary dermis which have much brighter cytoplasm than most (red arrow).

COMMON ACQUIRED MELANOCYTIC NEVUS

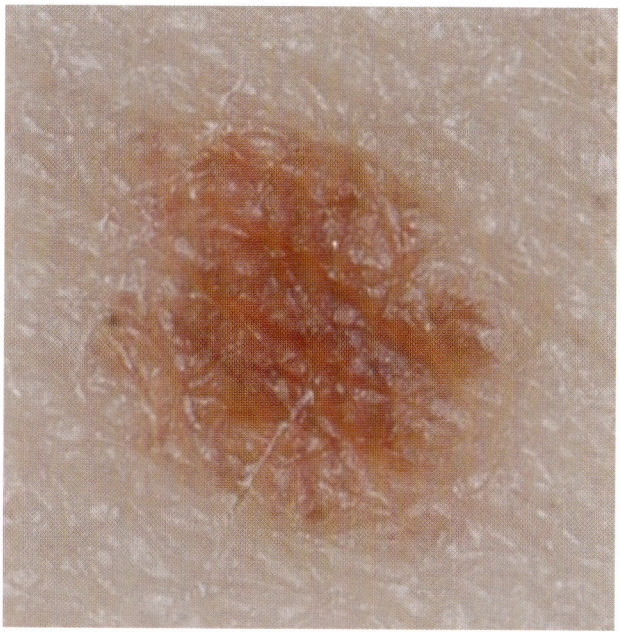
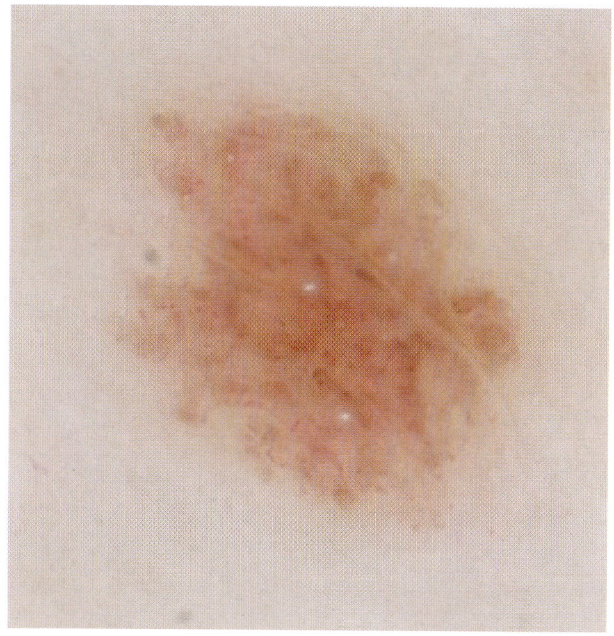

▲ **Figures 4.28, 4.29** Clinical photograph of a 3 mm brown macule near the right axilla of a 32-year-old woman. Dermoscopic photograph reveals a brown lesion with a regular globular pattern.

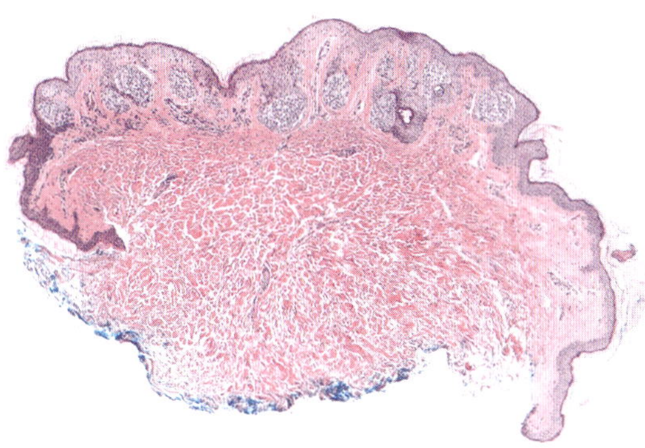
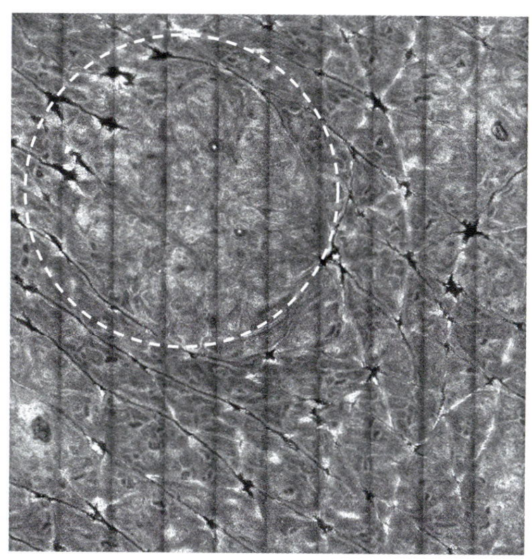

▲ **Figures 4.30, 4.31** Histology (4×) shows a well-circumscribed, symmetrical proliferation of nested melanocytes at the DEJ and in the superficial dermis. Corresponding RCM mosaic (5.0 mm × 5.0 mm) at the level of the superficial DEJ shows a symmetrical, well-circumscribed lesion (circled).

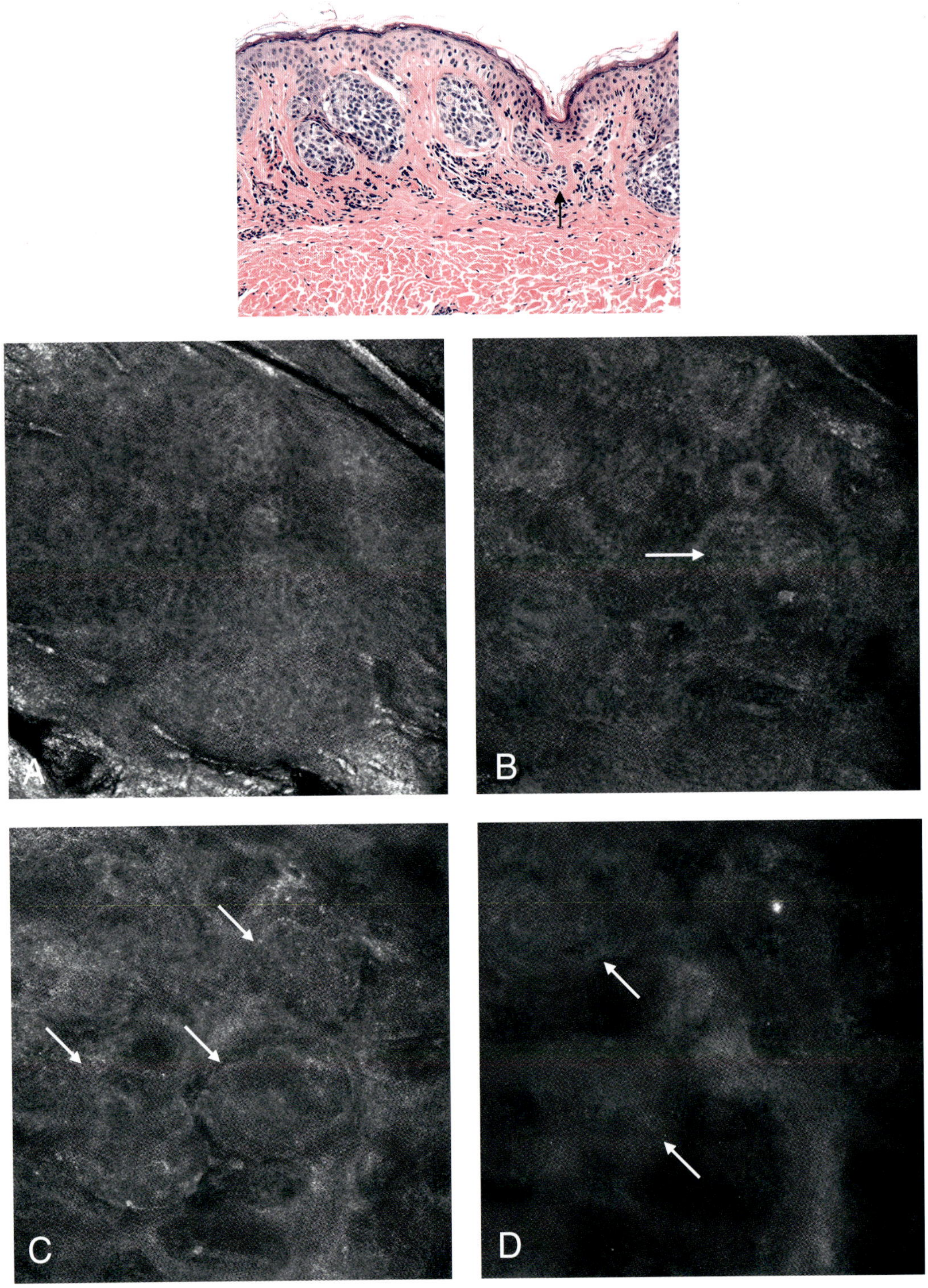

▲ **Figure 4.32** Histology (20×) shows melanocytic nests at the tips of rete ridges and a few small nests (arrow) in the dermis. Corresponding RCM (0.5 mm × 0.5 mm) at the level of the stratum granulosum/spinosum (A) and the deep stratum spinosum (B) show a normal honeycomb pattern. In (B), the tips of a few dermal papillae can be seen; one is expanded by a dense cell cluster (white arrow). At the deep DEJ (C) and in the dermis (D) several similarly sized small dense cell clusters (white arrows) composed of weakly refractile cells are seen.

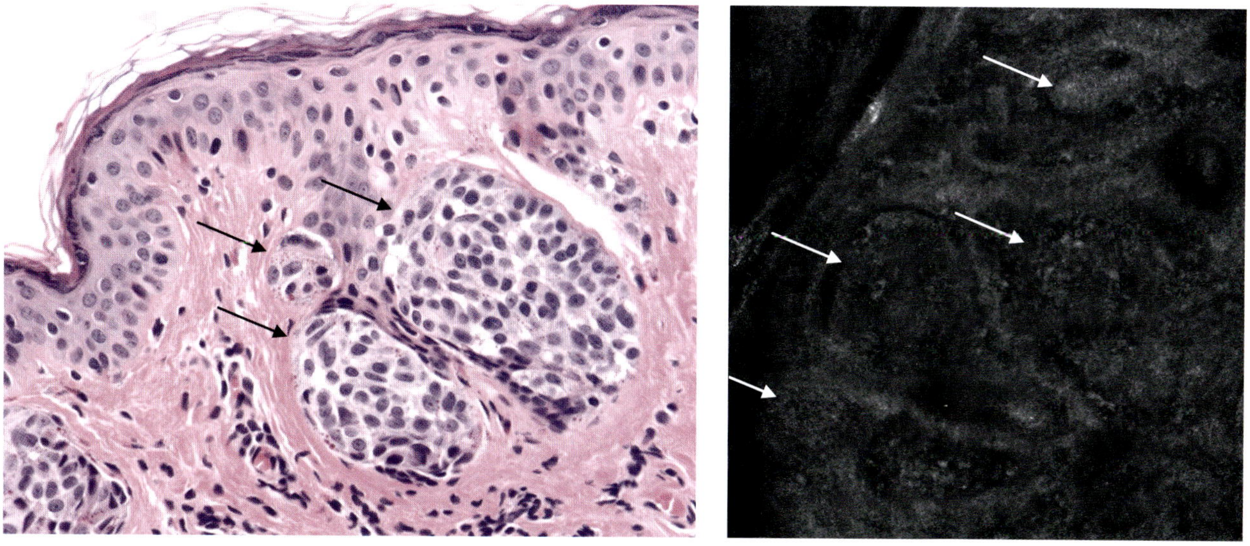

▲ **Figures 4.33, 4.34** On high power, histology (40×) shows bland, uniform melanocytes forming nests along a rete ridge (black arrows). On corresponding RCM, dense cell clusters (white arrows) can be seen connected to rete ridges.

COMMON AQUIRED MELANOCYTIC NEVUS, LENTIGINOUS TYPE

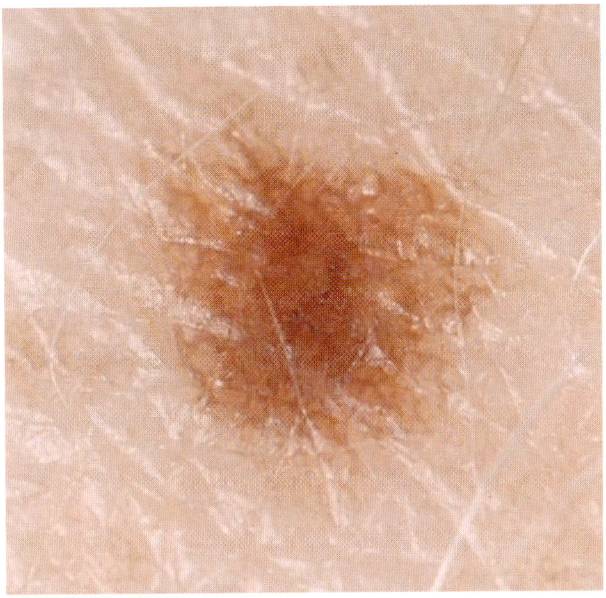

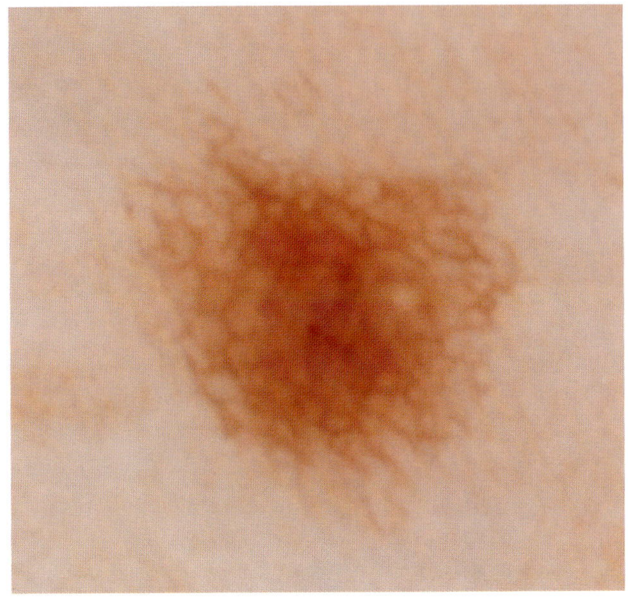

▲ **Figures 4.35, 4.36** Clinical photograph of a 2 mm brown macule on the right posterior shoulder of a 33-year-old man. Dermoscopic photograph reveals a symmetric lesion with a regular brown reticular pigment network showing central homogeneous pigmentation.

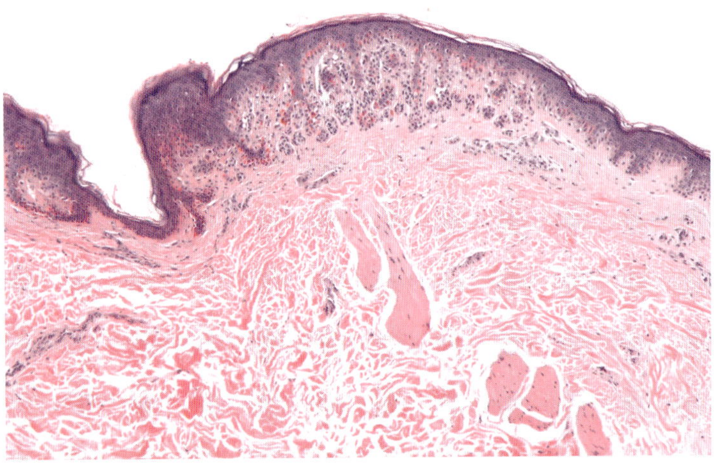

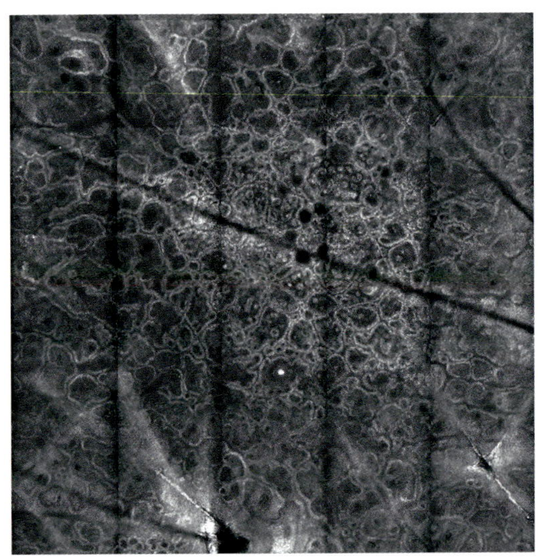

▲ **Figures 4.37, 4.38** Histology (4×) shows a symmetrical proliferation of solitary and nested melanocytes along the sides and tips of elongated, pigmented rete ridges and within the superficial dermis. The hyperpigmentation of the basal layer is limited to the lesion. RCM mosaic (2.5 mm × 2.5 mm) at the level of the DEJ shows a well-demarcated lesion characterized by hyperrefractile dermal papillary rings and variably bright, diffusely distributed, small cell clusters. Dermal papillae are notably edged and quite uniform in size and shape.

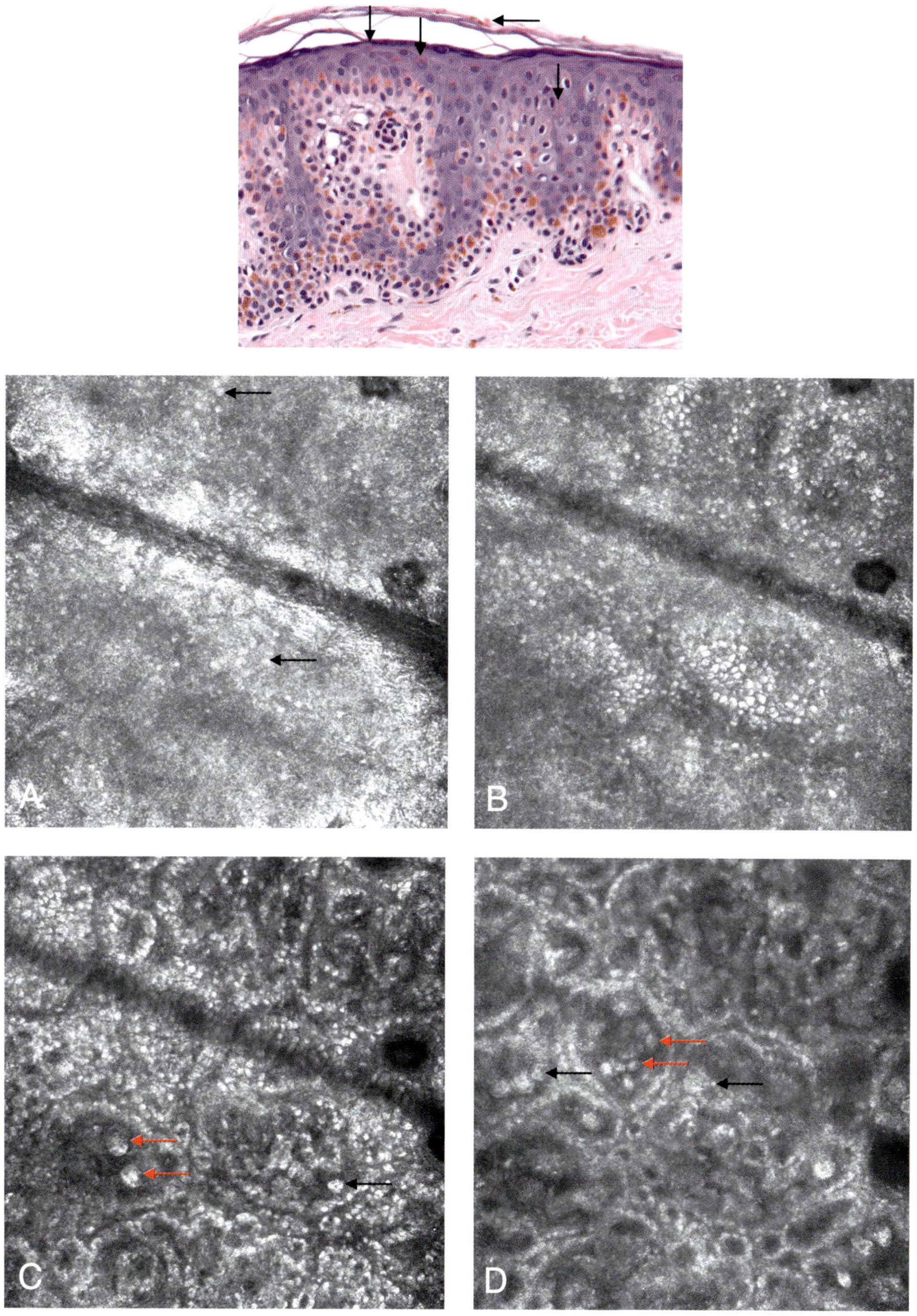

▲ **Figure 4.39** Histology (40×) shows small, uniform melanocytes singly and as small nests along the sides and tips of rete ridges and within the superficial dermis. Hypermelanization is seen at the basal layer and scattered at all levels of the epidermis (arrows). Corresponding RCM (0.5 mm × 0.5 mm) at the stratum corneum/stratum granulosum (A) shows a honeycomb pattern with focal cobblestoning (black arrows). At the surface of the basal layer (B), a more diffuse cobblestone pattern is seen. Bright, small, dense cell clusters are seen attached to rete ridges (black arrows) and within the papillary dermis (red arrows) at the superficial (C) and deep DEJ (D). Differentiation between basal keratinocytes and melanocytes is difficult.

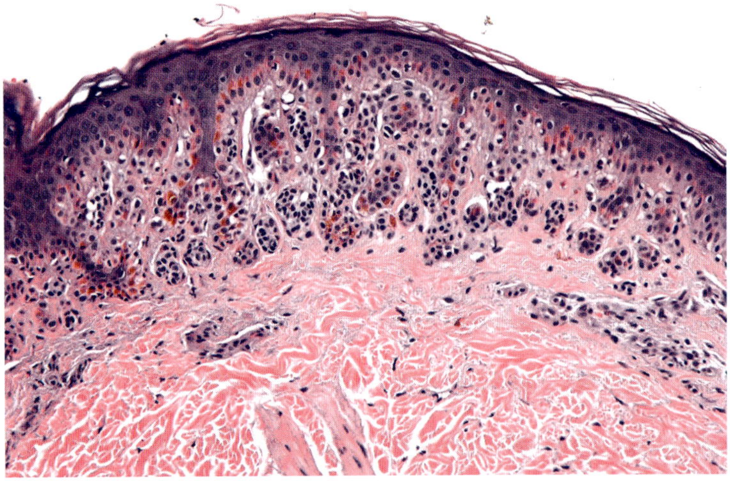

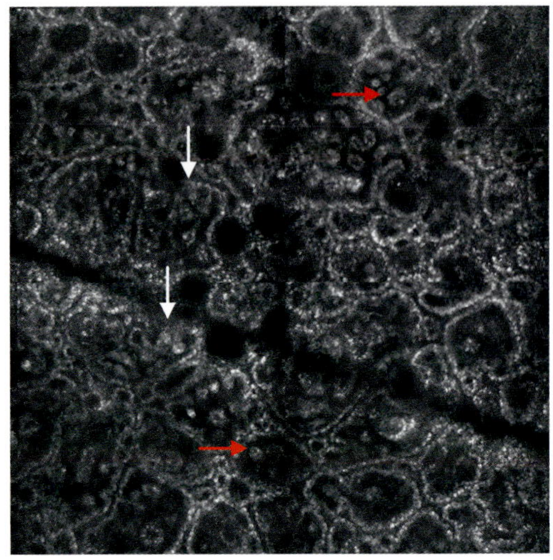

▲ **Figures 4.40, 4.41** Histology (20×) shows regular elongation and hyperpigmentation of the rete ridges. Nevus cells and nests are small and uniform in size throughout the lesion. RCM mosaic (1 mm × 1 mm) at the level of the DEJ demonstrates edged papillae, or a central dermal papilla rimmed by melanocytes and basal keratinocytes which are uniform in size, shape, and refractility. Also present are several small dense cell clusters, which are uniform in size and shape and distributed evenly at DEJ (white arrows) and within the papillary dermis (red arrows).

CHAPTER 4c

Dysplastic nevi

Alon Scope, Ashfaq A Marghoob, Allan C Halpern, and Ruby Delgado

Dysplastic nevi (DN, atypical moles) are acquired melanocytic nevi significant for being markers for increased melanoma risk and possible precursors of melanoma, occurring in both familial and sporadic forms.[1–4] Epidemiologic, morphologic, and genetic studies have placed DN as intermediate lesions in the hierarchy of melanocytic neoplasia between ordinary common nevi and cutaneous melanoma.[5,6]

There exists an enormous clinical variability in the morphology of DN. However, most DN are macular or maculopapular lesions, at least 5 mm in diameter, with an irregular asymmetric outline, indistinct borders, and variable pigmentation. DN can be clinically challenging to differentiate from melanoma in that they share some of the features of the ABCD acronym used to clinically identify melanoma.[7] It is not uncommon to see only one DN on an individual; however, the numbers can range from <10 to >100 per patient. Although DN may occur anywhere on the skin, they are most frequently observed on the trunk, particularly the upper back of adolescents and adults.[8] In addition, similar to the distribution of melanoma, DN can often be seen on the legs of women. In familial cases, DN may first appear on the scalp of children.[8,9]

The heterogeneous dermoscopic appearance of dysplastic nevi has been incorporated into a classification that characterizes them based on structural features into reticular, globular, or homogeneous patterns (or a combination of these); and further classifies them by pigment distribution: namely, central hypo- or hyperpigmented, eccentric peripheral hypo- or hyperpigmented, and multifocal hypo- or hyperpigmented.[10,11] On dermoscopy, the morphologic overlap between DN and melanoma can be again observed, even when dermoscopic scoring algorithms are applied.[12,13]

Histologically, dysplastic nevi are characterized by a disordered intraepidermal nevomelanocytic proliferation, mostly positioned at the dermal–epidermal junction (DEJ), which may extend into the papillary dermis. Foremost criteria in the diagnosis of a DN are a discontinuous lentiginous melanocytic proliferation (confined to the sides and tips of elongated rete ridges), junctional nest disarray manifested by variation in size, shape, and location of nests and fusion of adjacent nests (with an accompanying distortion of the rete ridges), and, in the case of compound DN, a junctional melanocytic component which extends beyond the dermal component creating a 'shoulder'. Other histologic features include stromal changes, such as concentric and lamellar fibroplasia, neovascularization, and a dermal inflammatory response.[14–16] It is recognized that DN represent a histologic spectrum, ranging from lesions that deviate slightly from common nevi to lesions that may be interpreted as bordering on early or radial-growth phase melanoma. For this reason, it has been proposed that an attempt should be made to grade their degree of atypia (dysplasia) into slight, moderate, and severe, according to a combination of architectural and cytologic features.[17,18]

Because most DN are clinically flat and are histologically superficial melanocytic lesions, the major histologic architectural features characterizing DN are apparent by reflectance confocal microscopy (RCM). RCM analysis of DN also shows a spectrum of findings intermediary between common nevi and melanoma (Figures 4.42–4.102, Cases 1–8: spectrum of DN from slight to severe atypia). Some of the RCM features of DN that may be distinctive from common nevi are an irregular epidermal rete meshwork with variation in size and shape of dermal papillae (Figures 4.51, 4.53, 4.67, 4.69); a greater variation in the size, shape, and location of cell clusters (nests), including the presence of cell clusters in suprapapillary plates (Figures 4.45, 4.59, 4.61, 4.63, 4.77, 4.79); fusion of epidermal rete by confluent junctional cell clusters (Figures 4.71, 4.77, 4.85, 4.86); enlarged misshapen cell clusters (Figures 4.59, 4.61, 4.63); an increased number of solitary medium to large nucleated cells with refractile cytoplasms, compatible with melanocytes, at the DEJ (Figures 4.91, 4.93, 4.100).[19–22]

As with dermoscopy and histology, there is some overlap in RCM features of DN and melanoma. Nonetheless, the degree and frequency of atypical features help to distinguish DN from melanoma, as do some fairly sensitive and specific findings. While DN may have an atypical honeycomb or cobblestone pattern of the epidermis, a frank disarranged epidermal pattern (effacement of the normal upper epidermal architecture by unevenly distributed bright, pleomorphic granular particles and cells) is much more common in melanoma.[23–26] Moreover, 'pagetoid' melanocytes are infrequently observed in DN, and when seen, are focal and few (Figure 4.102).[24–26] Edged papillae (Figures 4.51, 4.53) are more frequent in DN than in melanoma, whereas non-edged papillae, in which delineated bright dermal papillary rings are not seen due to a less orderly melanocytic proliferation often involving suprabasal layers, are more frequently seen in melanoma than DN.[25–27] Cell clusters in DN are mostly dense (Figures 4.45, 4.47, 4.61, 4.63, 4.77, 4.85, 4.87), while in melanoma loose, sparse, and cerebriform cell clusters may be observed.[24–26,28] While sporadic atypical cells can be seen in both melanoma and DN (Figures 4.91, 4.100), numerous markedly atypical cells (i.e. cells irregular in size, shape, and reflectivity), distributed throughout the lesion, are seen only in melanoma (Figures 4.91, 4.100).[23,25–27] Isolated refractile cells containing an eccentric nucleus located in the dermal papillae are rarely observed in DN compared with melanoma.[25–27] Preliminary studies demonstrate that combinations of the above noted features have high sensitivity and specificity for differentiating melanoma from nevi, including DN.[23,25,26]

Key RCM features of dysplastic nevi

- Variable distortion of normal epidermal honeycomb and cobblestone patterns
- Slight-to-complex distortion of the DEJ architecture:
  - Variation in size and shape of dermal papillae
  - Altered contour of the rete ridges
- Junctional cell cluster disarray:
  - Variation in size, shape, and location of cell clusters
  - Enlarged, misshapen cell clusters
  - Presence of cell clusters in suprapapillary plates
- Variable cellular atypia
- Dense cell clusters predominate

Reflectance confocal microscopy holds opportunities for the study of dysplastic nevi. First, RCM may help in better defining salient features that distinguish DN from melanoma and further classify the degree of disorder seen in DN. Furthermore, in some cases, RCM taken together with histopathology provides an almost three-dimensional view of the growth pattern of DN (Figures 4.70, 4.71, 4.76, 4.77, 4.84, 4.85). An added benefit of RCM is that it affords the unique ability to monitor the growth patterns of DN in vivo at a quasi-histologic level over time. Thus, for the first time, the opportunity exists to view nevus cells in a dynamic instead of static mode, which may in turn add to the understanding of DN and melanoma development and progression. On the other hand, although RCM may capture general cytologic contours, such as nuclear size and cell size and shape (i.e. epithelioid, spindled, etc.), of the atypical melanocytic proliferation, evaluation of cytoplasmic and nuclear detail, needed for grading of cytologic atypia, must await further sophistication of RCM instruments.

REFERENCES

1. Clark WH Jr, Reimer RR, Greene M et al. Origin of familial malignant melanomas from heritable

melanocytic lesions. 'The B-K mole syndrome'. Arch Dermatol 1978; 114:732–8.

2. Elder DE, Goldman LI, Goldman SC et al. Dysplastic nevus syndrome: a phenotypic association of sporadic cutaneous melanoma. Cancer 1980; 46:1787–94.
3. Greene MH, Clark WH Jr, Tucker MA et al. Acquired precursors of cutaneous malignant melanoma. The familial dysplastic nevus syndrome. N Engl J Med 1985; 312:91–7.
4. Halpern AC, Guerry D 4th, Elder DE et al. Dysplastic nevi as risk markers of sporadic (nonfamilial) melanoma. A case–control study. Arch Dermatol 1991; 127: 995–9.
5. Elder DE, Clark WH Jr, Elenitsas R et al. The early and intermediate precursor lesions of tumor progression in the melanocytic system: common acquired nevi and atypical (dysplastic) nevi. Semin Diagn Pathol 1993; 10:18–35.
6. Hussein MR. Melanocytic dysplastic naevi occupy the middle ground between benign melanocytic naevi and cutaneous malignant melanomas: emerging clues. J Clin Pathol 2005; 58:453–6.
7. Friedman RJ, Rigel DS, Kopf AW. Early detection of malignant melanoma: the role of physician examination and self-examination of the skin. CA Cancer J Clin 1985; 35:130–51.
8. Naeyaert JM, Brochez L. Clinical practice. Dysplastic nevi. N Engl J Med 2003; 349:2233–40.
9. Tucker MA, Greene MH, Clark WH Jr et al. Dysplastic nevi on the scalp of prepubertal children from melanoma-prone families. J Pediatr 1983; 103:65–9.
10. Hofmann-Wellenhof R, Blum A, Wolf IH et al. Dermoscopic classification of atypical melanocytic nevi (Clark nevi). Arch Dermatol 2001; 137: 1575–80.
11. Blum A, Soyer HP, Garbe C et al. The dermoscopic classification of atypical melanocytic naevi (Clark naevi) is useful to discriminate benign from malignant melanocytic lesions. Br J Dermatol 2003; 149:1159–64.
12. Henning JS, Dusza SW, Wang SQ et al. The CASH (color, architecture, symmetry, and homogeneity) algorithm for dermoscopy. J Am Acad Dermatol 2007; 56:45–52.
13. Nachbar F, Stolz W, Merkle T et al. The ABCD rule of dermatoscopy. High prospective value in the diagnosis of doubtful melanocytic skin lesions. J Am Acad Dermatol 1994; 30:551–9.
14. Elder DE, Green MH, Guerry DT et al. The dysplastic nevus syndrome: our definition. Am J Dermatopathol 1982; 4:455–60.
15. Rhodes AR, Mihm MC Jr, Weinstock MA. Dysplastic melanocytic nevi: a reproducible histologic definition emphasizing cellular morphology. Mod Pathol 1989; 2:306–19.
16. Clemente C, Cochran AJ, Elder DE et al. Histopathologic diagnosis of dysplastic nevi: concordance among pathologists convened by the World Health Organization Melanoma Programme. Hum Pathol 1991; 22:313–9.
17. Duncan LM, Berwick M, Bruijn JA et al. Histopathologic recognition and grading of dysplastic melanocytic nevi: an interobserver agreement study. J Invest Dermatol 1993; 100:318S–21S.
18. Arumi-Uria M, McNutt NS, Finnerty B. Grading of atypia in nevi: correlation with melanoma risk. Mod Pathol 2003; 16:764–71.
19. Busam KJ, Charles C, Lee G et al. Morphologic features of melanocytes, pigmented keratinocytes, and melanophages by in vivo confocal scanning laser microscopy. Mod Pathol 2001; 14:862–8.
20. Scope A, Benvenuto-Andrade C, Agero AL et al. Correlation of dermoscopic structures of melanocytic lesions to reflectance confocal microscopy. Arch Dermatol 2007; 143:176–85.
21. Pellacani G, Cesinaro AM, Seidenari S. In vivo assessment of melanocytic nests in nevi and melanomas by reflectance confocal microscopy. Mod Pathol 2005; 18:469–74.
22. Langley RG, Rajadhyaksha M, Dwyer PJ et al. Confocal scanning laser microscopy of benign and malignant melanocytic skin lesions in vivo. J Am Acad Dermatol 2001; 45:365–76.
23. Gerger A, Koller S, Weger W et al. Sensitivity and specificity of confocal laser-scanning microscopy for in vivo diagnosis of malignant skin tumors. Cancer 2006; 107:193–200.
24. Pellacani G, Cesinaro AM, Seidenari S. Reflectance-mode confocal microscopy for the in vivo characterization of pagetoid melanocytosis in melanomas and nevi. J Invest Dermatol 2005; 125:532–7.
25. Pellacani G, Cesinaro AM, Seidenari S. Reflectance-mode confocal microscopy of pigmented skin lesions – improvement in melanoma diagnostic specificity. J Am Acad Dermatol 2005; 53:979–85.
26. Pellacani G, Guitera P, Longo C et al. The impact of in vivo reflectance confocal microscopy for the

diagnostic accuracy of melanoma and equivocal melanocytic lesions. J Invest Dermatol 2007; Jul 26: (Epub ahead of print).

27. Pellacani G, Cesinaro AM, Longo C et al. Microscopic in vivo description of cellular architecture of dermoscopic pigment network in nevi and melanomas. Arch Dermatol 2005; 141:147–54.

28. Pellacani G, Cesinaro AM, Seidenari S. In vivo confocal reflectance microscopy for the characterization of melanocytic nests and correlation with dermoscopy and histology. Br J Dermatol 2005; 152:384–6.

DYSPLASTIC NEVI

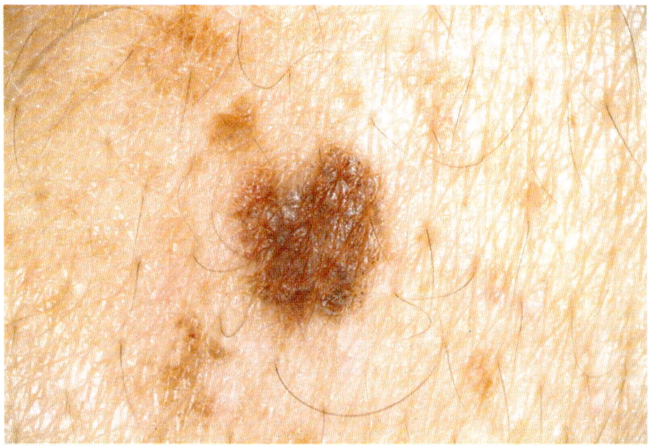

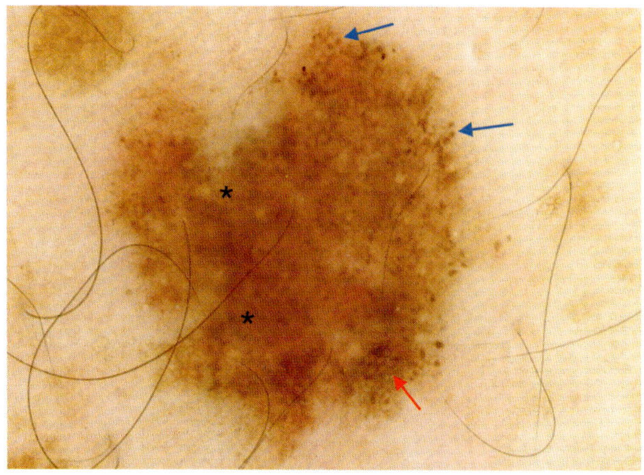

▲ **Figures 4.42, 4.43** Case 1: clinical photograph of a 7 mm, irregular brown-gray papule on the mid back of a 48-year-old male patient. Dermoscopic photograph reveals a multicomponent pattern with peripheral globules (blue arrows), atypical network (red arrow), and regression structures (asterisks).

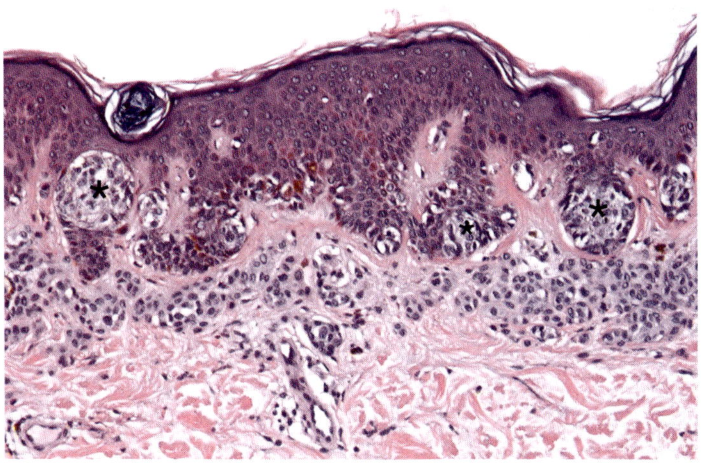

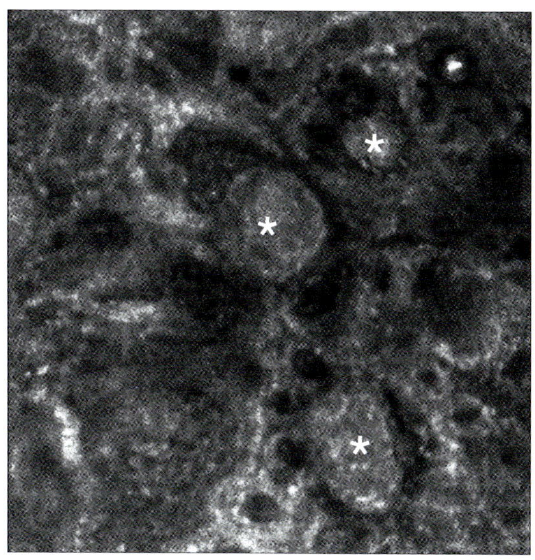

▲ **Figures 4.44, 4.45** Case 1: histology (10×) of DN characterized by variation in size and location of junctional nests (asterisks). Junctional architectural disorder is seen on RCM (0.5 mm × 0.5 mm) as discrete dense junctional clusters (nests) (asterisks) interrupting the dermal papillae pattern of the DEJ.

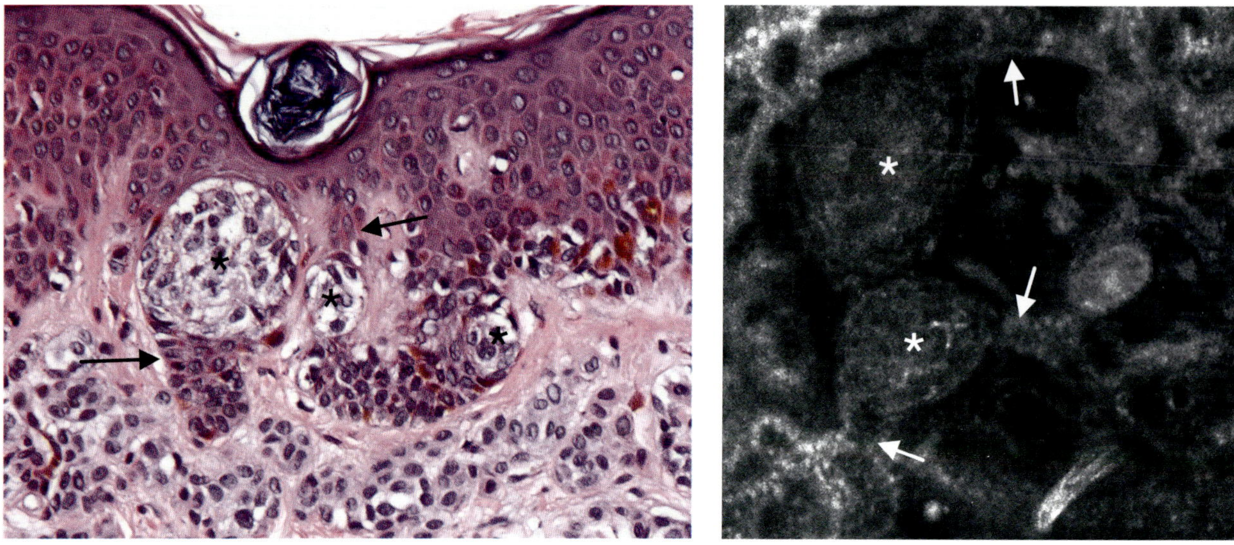

▲ **Figures 4.46, 4.47** Case 1: on histology (20×) and RCM (0.5 mm × 0.5 mm), oval-shaped junctional dense cell clusters (asterisks) protrude from elongated rete ridges (black arrows on histology, white arrows on RCM).

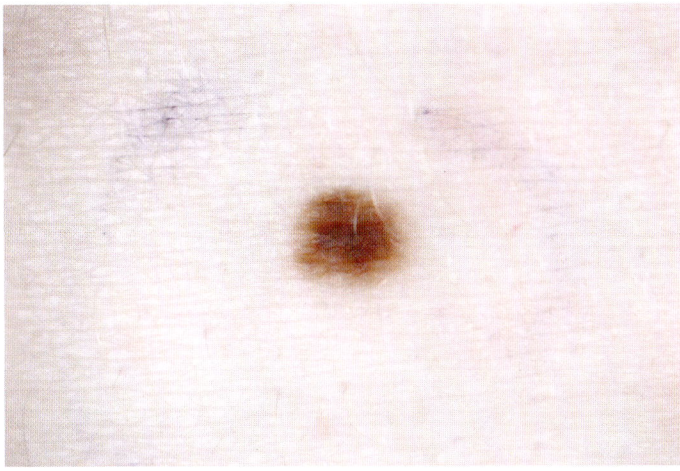

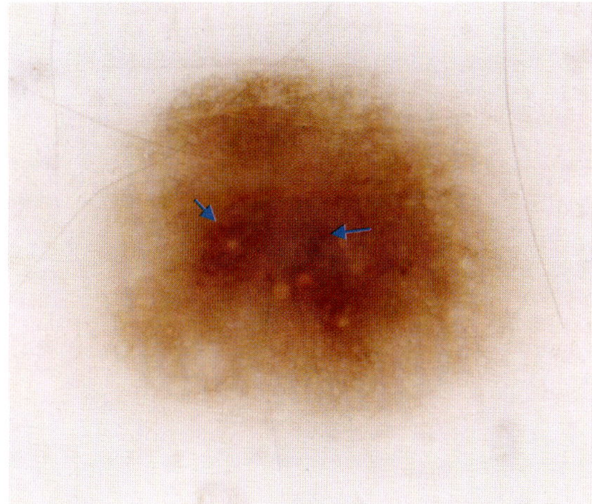

▲ **Figures 4.48, 4.49** Case 2: clinical photograph of a 4 mm, brown lesion on the lower back of a 40-year-old male patient with a history of melanoma. Dermoscopic photograph reveals a reticular pattern with central globules (blue arrows).

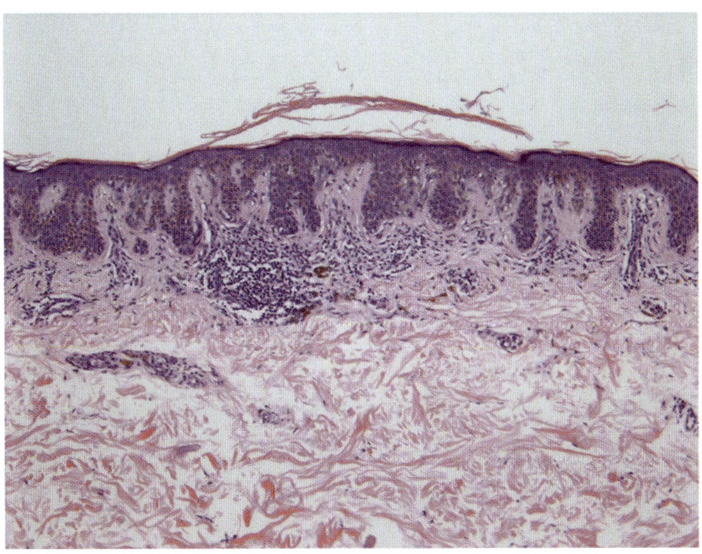

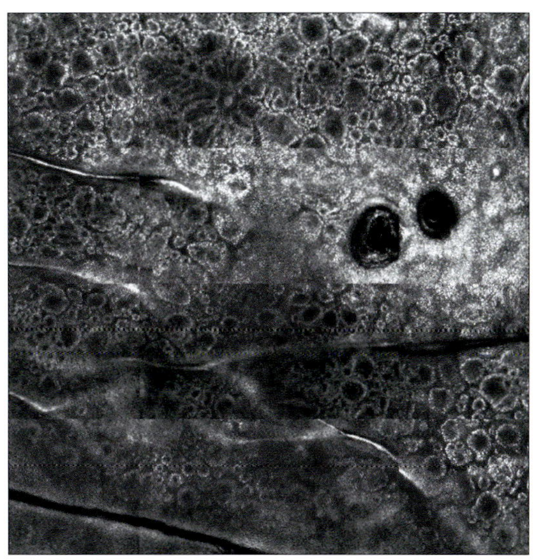

▲ **Figures 4.50, 4.51** Case 2: histology (10×) of DN showing irregular elongation and fusion of the rete ridges. Corresponding RCM mosaic (2 mm × 2 mm) at the level of the DEJ shows a meshwork pattern with edged dermal papillae of variable size, shape, and brightness.

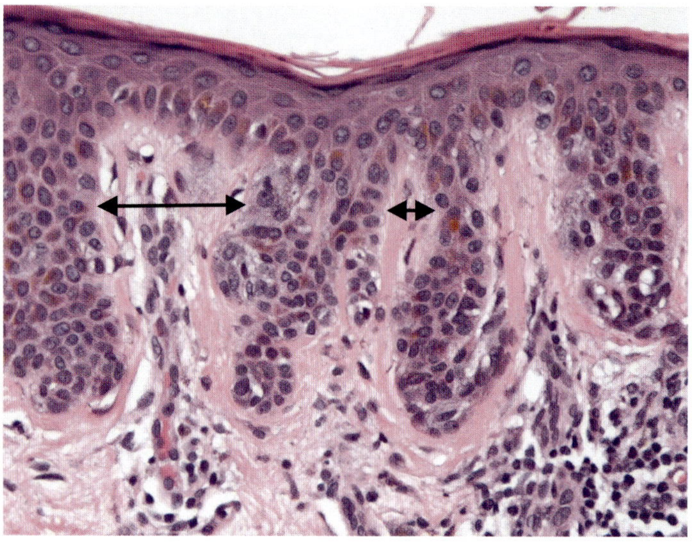

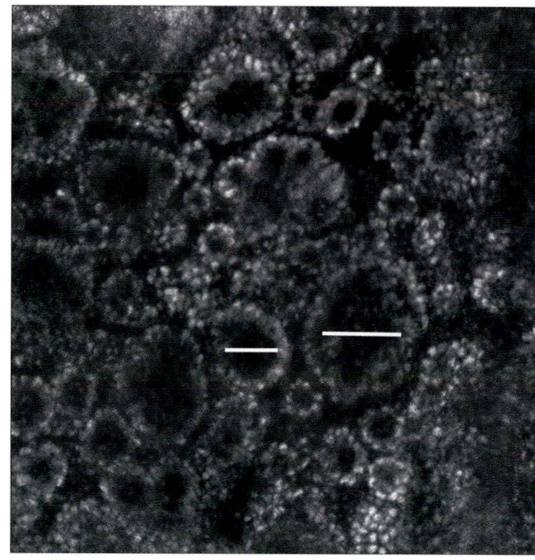

▲ **Figures 4.52, 4.53** Case 2: histology (20×) of DN showing a lentiginous proliferation of melanocytes along asymmetrical, irregularly spaced (black arrows) rete ridges, corresponding on RCM (0.5 mm × 0.5 mm) to variation in size (white bars) and shape of edged papillae.

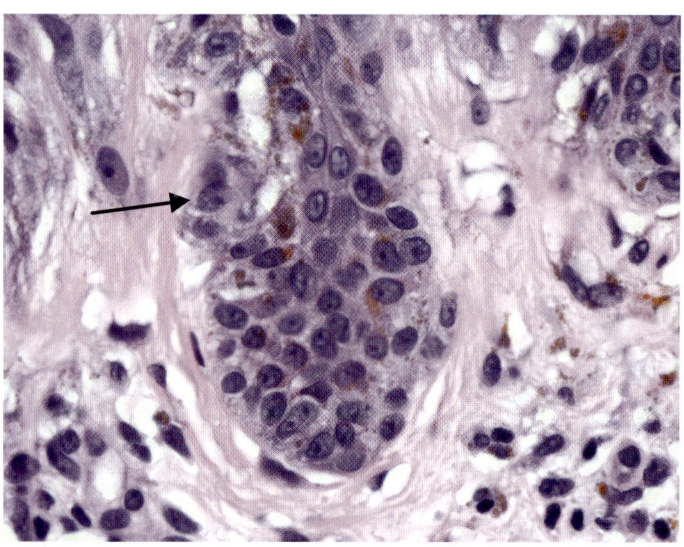

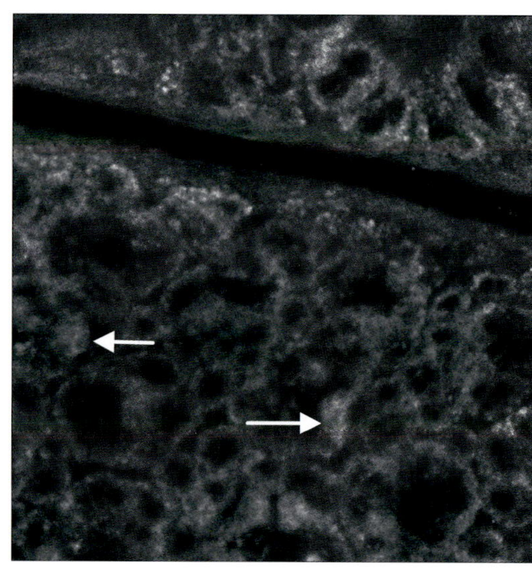

▲ **Figures 4.54, 4.55** Case 2: clusters of epithelioid melanocytes (black arrow), growing along the sides of rete ridges on histology (40×), appear on RCM (0.5 mm × 0.5 mm) at the level of the DEJ as bright junctional dense cell clusters that bulge into the dermal papillae (white arrows).

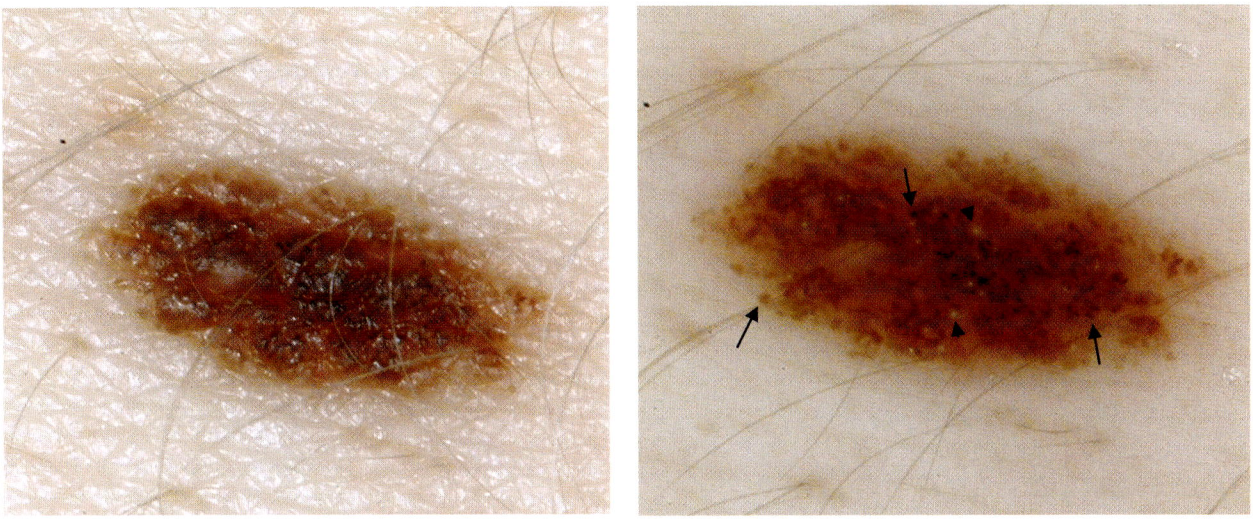

▲ **Figures 4.56, 4.57** Case 3: clinical photograph of a 5.5 mm brown papule on the back of a 29-year-old male patient. Dermoscopic photograph reveals an irregular globular pattern composed of globules of variable size and color (arrows) and multiple milia-like cysts (arrowheads).

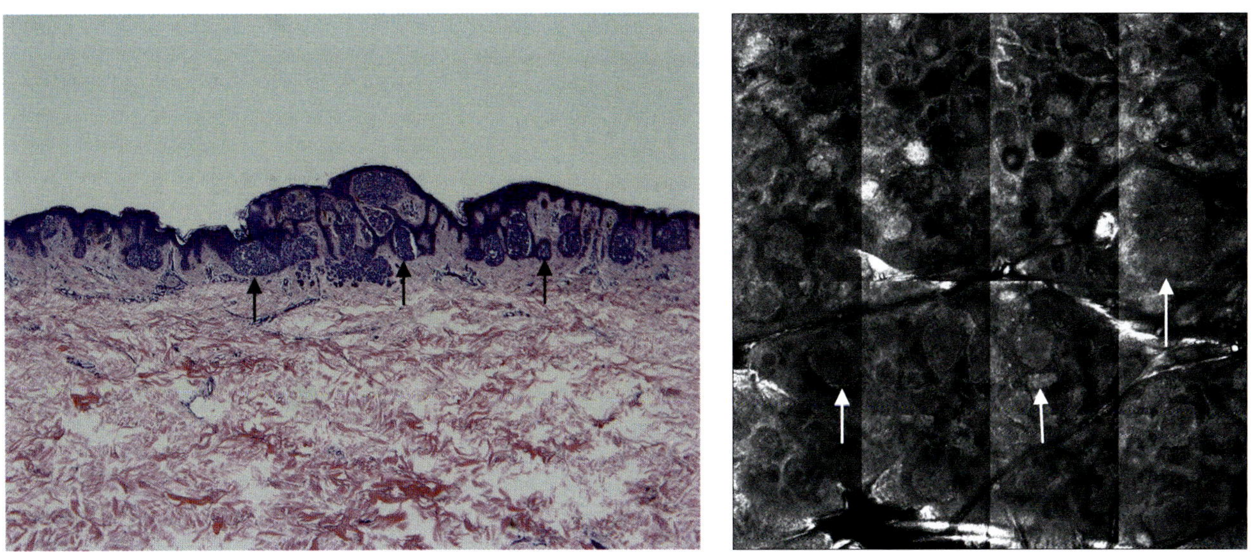

▲ **Figures 4.58, 4.59** Case 3: histology (4×) of DN showing junctional nests of variable size (black arrows) distending the rete ridges. Corresponding RCM mosaic (2 mm × 2 mm) at the level of the DEJ shows dense cell clusters (nests) of variable size (white arrows).

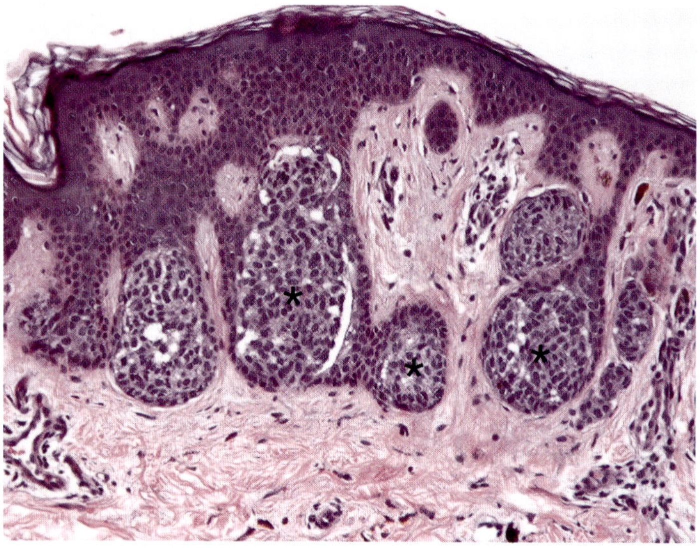

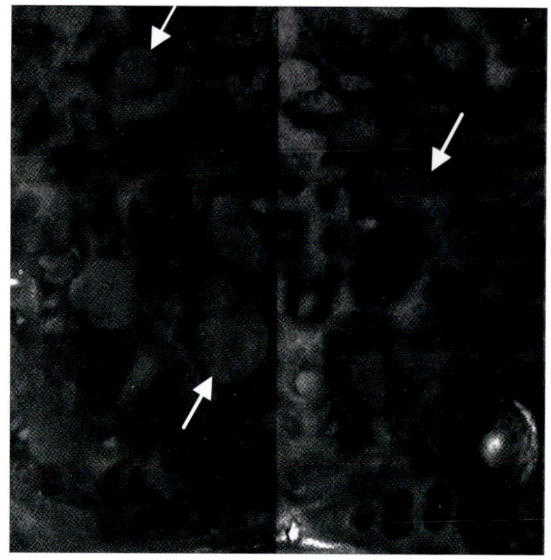

▲ **Figures 4.60, 4.61** Case 3: histology (20×) shows junctional nests (asterisks) of variable size distending the rete ridges. Corresponding RCM mosaic (1 mm × 1 mm) at the level of the deep DEJ shows dense junctional clusters (white arrows) of variable size bulging into the dermal papillae.

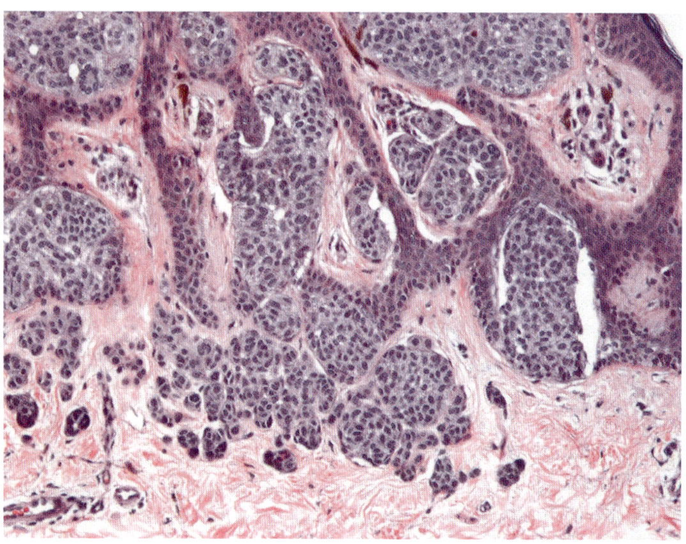

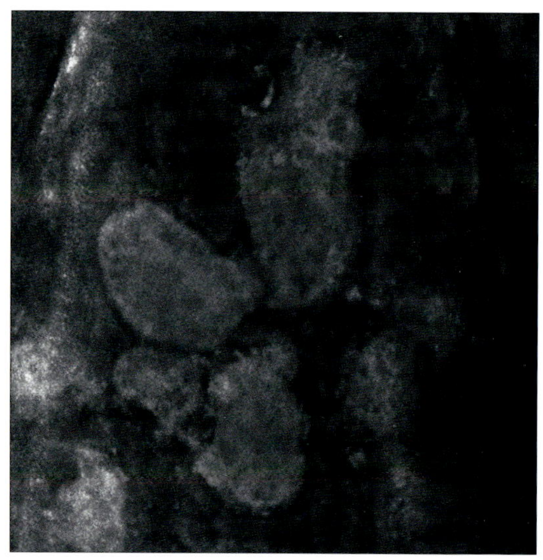

▲ **Figures 4.62, 4.63** Case 3: in this DN, expansive junctional nests distending the rete ridges on histology (20×) translate into misshapen dense cell clusters on RCM (0.5 mm × 0.5 mm).

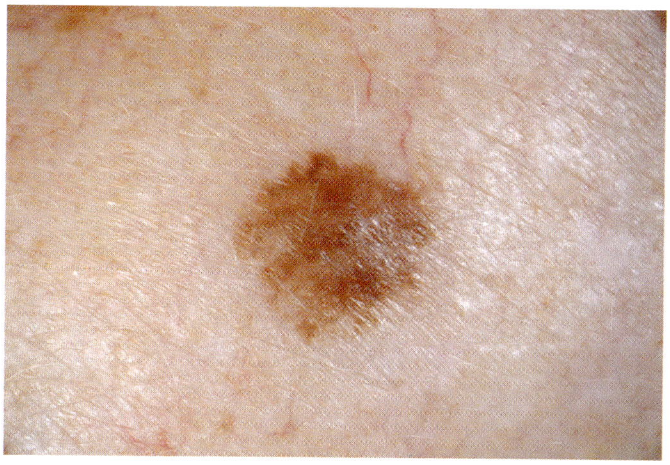

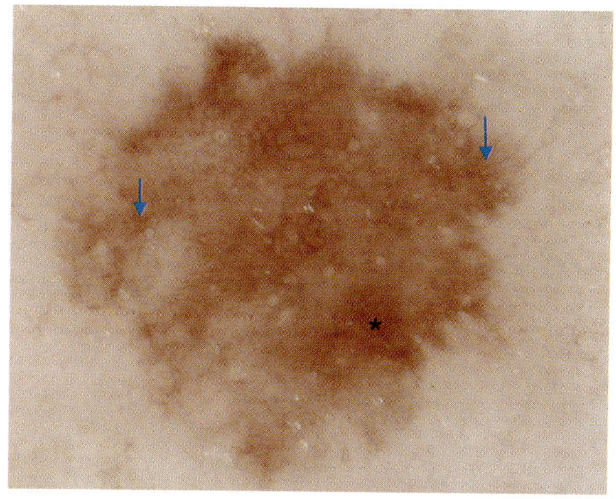

▲ **Figures 4.64, 4.65** Case 4: clinical photograph of a 6 mm irregular brown papule on the shoulder of a 78-year-old female patient. Dermoscopic photograph reveals a reticular pattern with areas of atypical network (asterisk) and branched streaks (blue arrows).

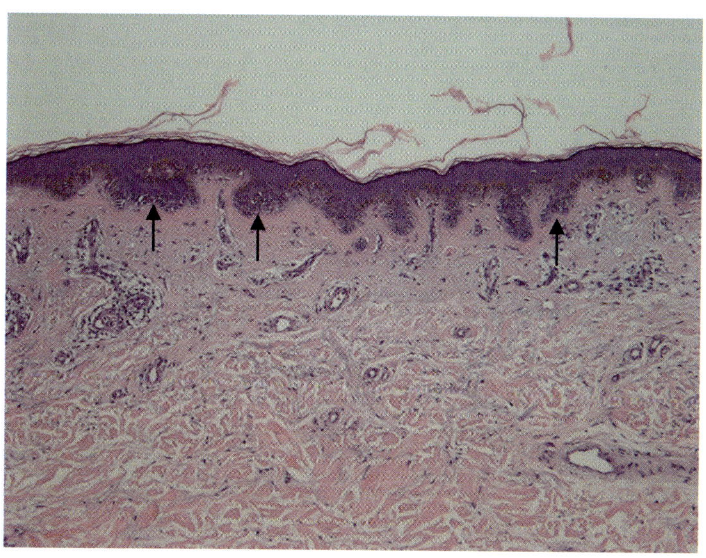

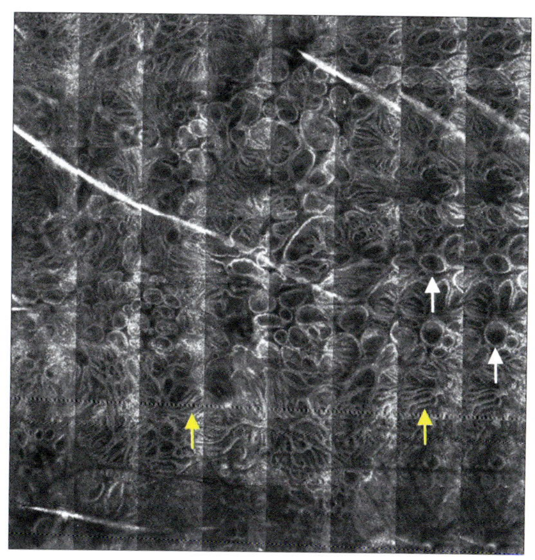

▲ **Figures 4.66, 4.67** Case 4: histology (10×) of DN showing rete ridges that are angulated, irregularly spaced, and focally fused (black arrows). On corresponding RCM mosaic (4 mm × 4 mm) at the level of the DEJ, this translates to an irregular rete meshwork with variation in size and shape of the dermal papillae, from round-oval (white arrows) to elongated, slit-like (yellow arrows).

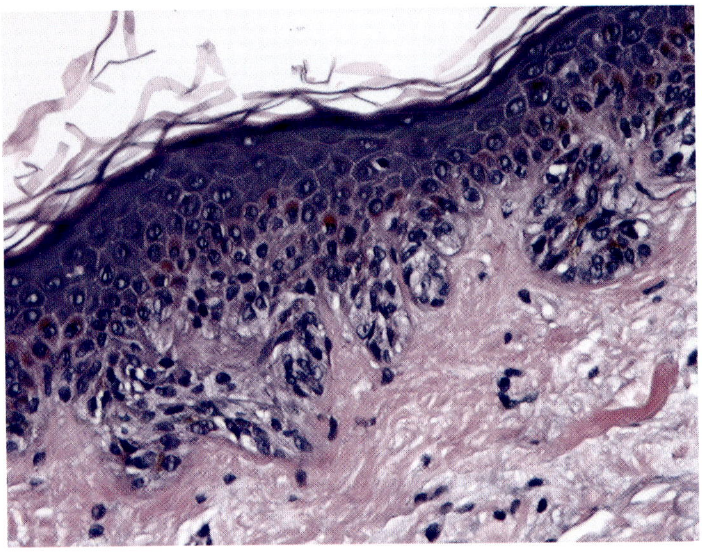

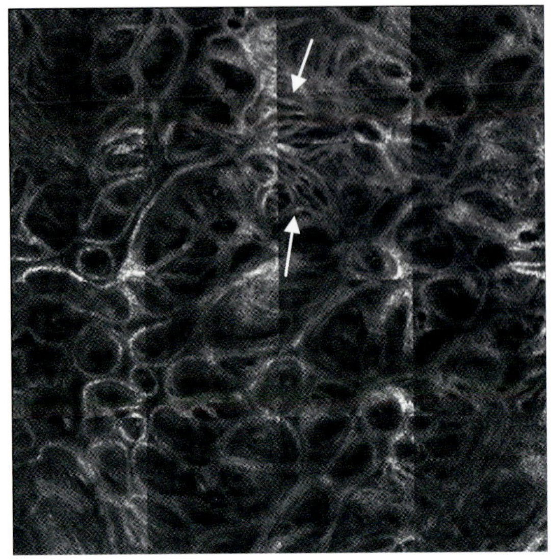

▲ **Figures 4.68, 4.69** Case 4: histology (10×) of DN shows elongated angulated rete ridges harboring a junctional melanocytic proliferation, corresponding to a complex rete meshwork with bright branching cords (white arrows) on RCM mosaic (2 mm × 2 mm) at the level of the DEJ.

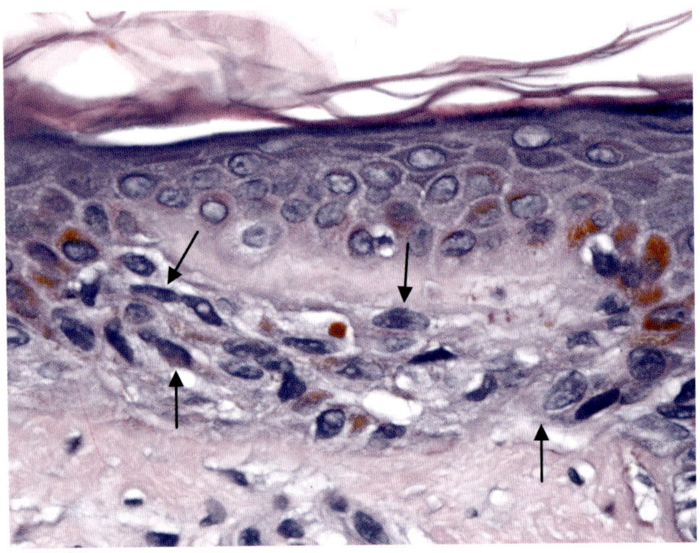

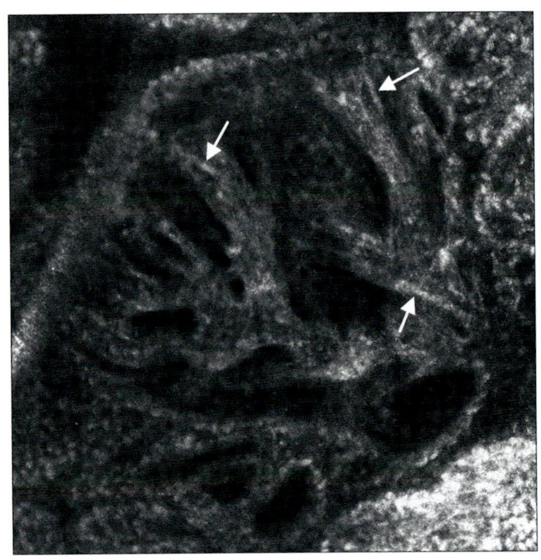

▲ **Figures 4.70, 4.71** Case 4: on higher magnification histology (40×), fusion of rete ridges by spindle cell aggregates can be seen (black arrows); corresponding RCM (0.5 mm × 0.5 mm) shows elongated and branching cord-like aggregates in which ill-defined fusiform elements can be seen (white arrows).

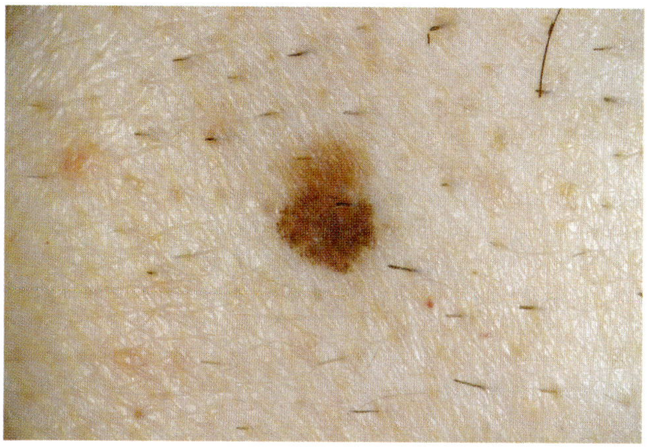

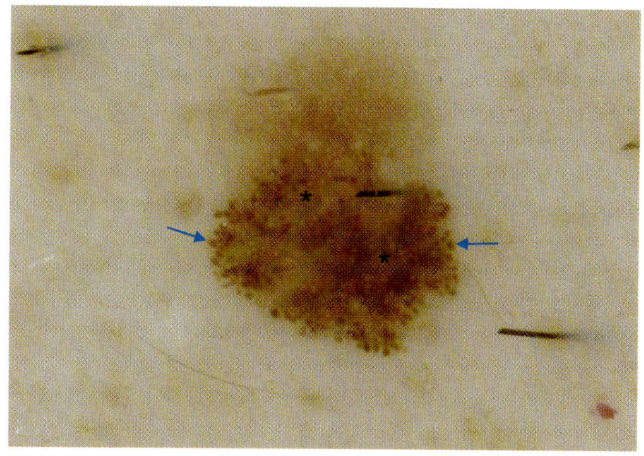

▲ **Figures 4.72, 4.73** Case 5: clinical photograph of a 5 mm irregular brown lesion on the chest of a 37-year-old male patient with a history of melanoma. Dermoscopic photograph reveals a reticular-globular pattern with peripheral globules (blue arrows) and central network (asterisks), a pattern that can be seen in growing melanocytic lesions.

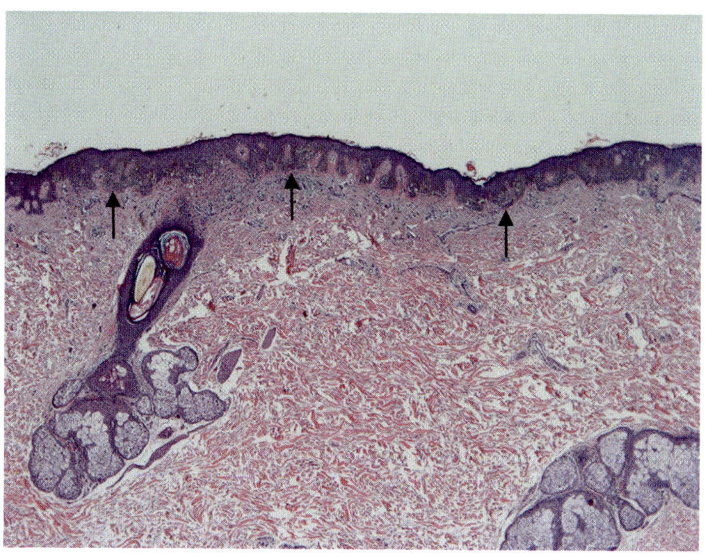

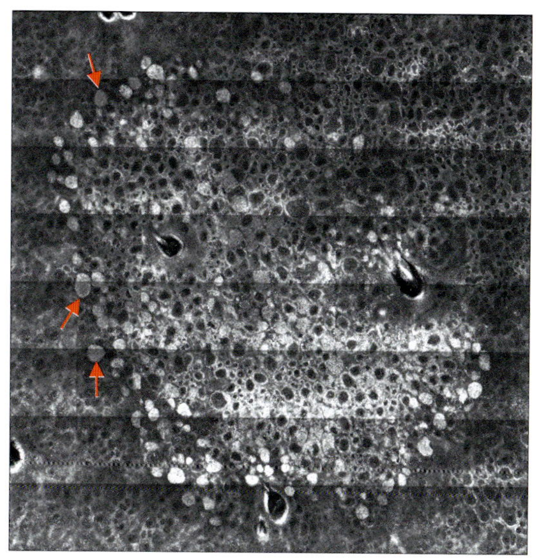

▲ **Figures 4.74, 4.75** Case 5: histology (4×) shows fusion of the rete ridges by junctional nests (black arrows). Corresponding RCM mosaic (4 mm × 4 mm) shows large junctional dense cell clusters that protrude into dermal papillae while still connected to the basal cell layer that rims the papillae (red arrows). The pattern of peripheral dense cell clusters and a central bright rete meshwork with interspersed dense cell clusters seen on the RCM mosaic nicely mirrors the pattern seen on dermoscopy above.

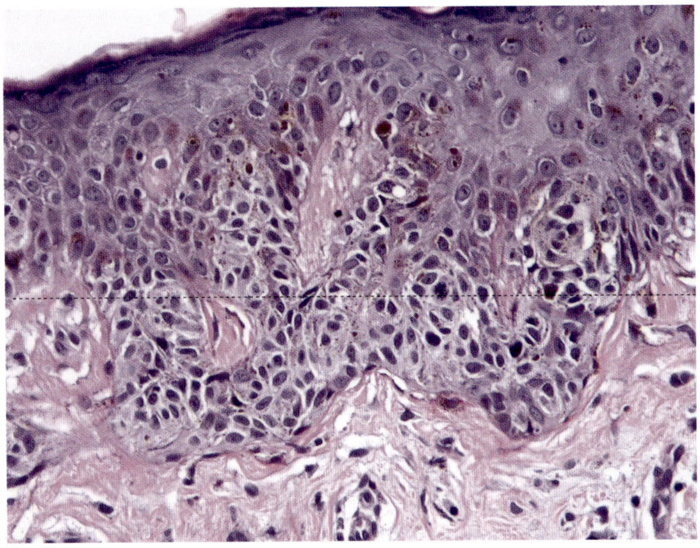

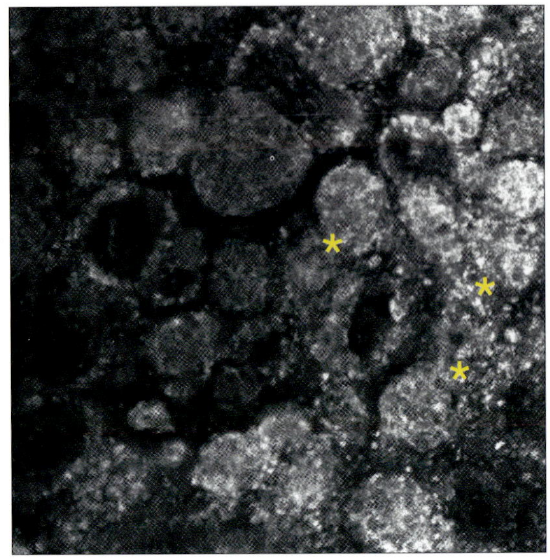

▲ **Figures 4.76, 4.77** Case 5: architectural disarray of the DN is seen on histology (10×) as a confluent nevomelanocytic proliferation at the DEJ; dashed line indicates from where the corresponding RCM image was obtained. RCM (0.5 mm × 0.5 mm) at the level of the DEJ discloses a mostly nested growth pattern seen as dense cell clusters, with confluence between some of the clusters (asterisks).

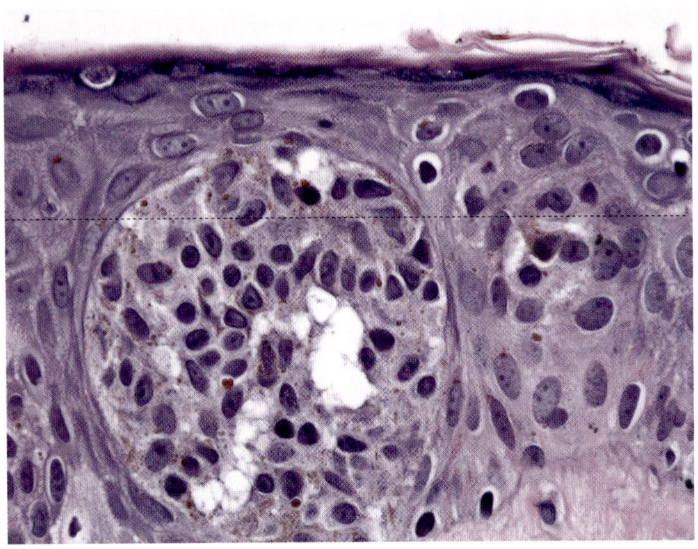

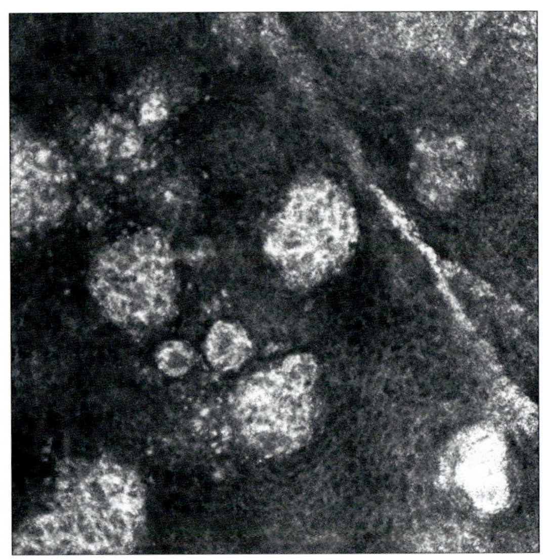

▲ **Figures 4.78, 4.79** Case 5: in other areas of the DN, large pigmented epithelioid melanocytic nests nearly filling the entire thickness of the epidermis can be seen on histology (40×); dashed line indicates from where the corresponding RCM image was obtained. This correlates on RCM (0.5 mm × 0.5 mm) to the unusual finding of bright oval to polygonal dense cell clusters appearing at the level of the upper stratum spinosum.

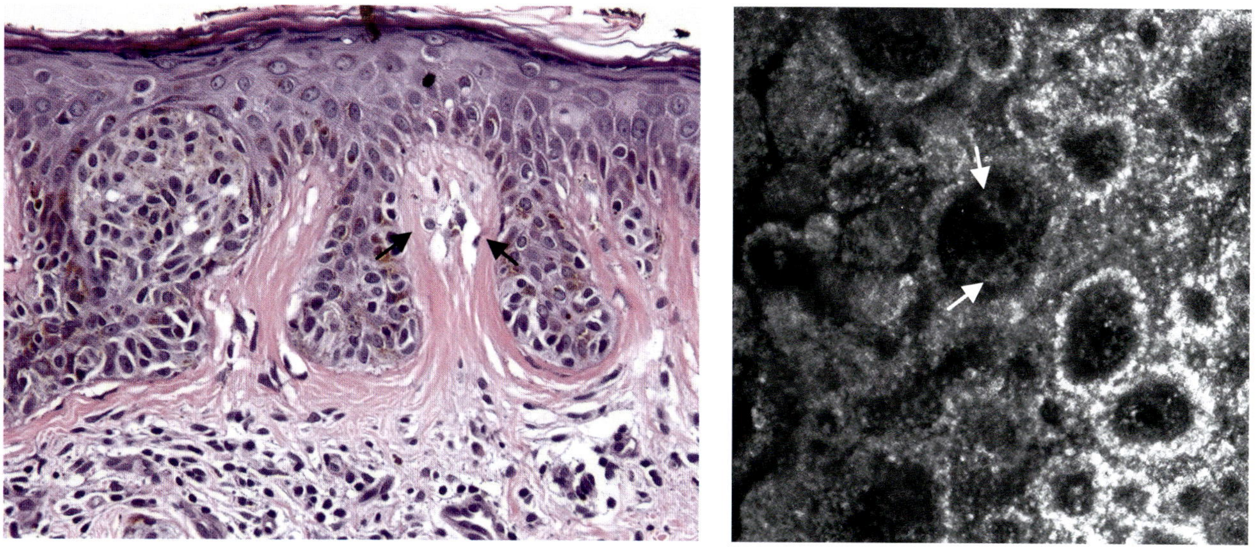

▲ **Figures 4.80, 4.81** Case 5: sheaths of condensed collagen (concentric eosinophilic fibroplasia) surrounding rete ridges (black arrows) can be seen on histology (20×), corresponding to prominent bright fibrillar elements (white arrows) compatible with collagen within the dermal papillae on RCM (0.5 mm × 0.5 mm).

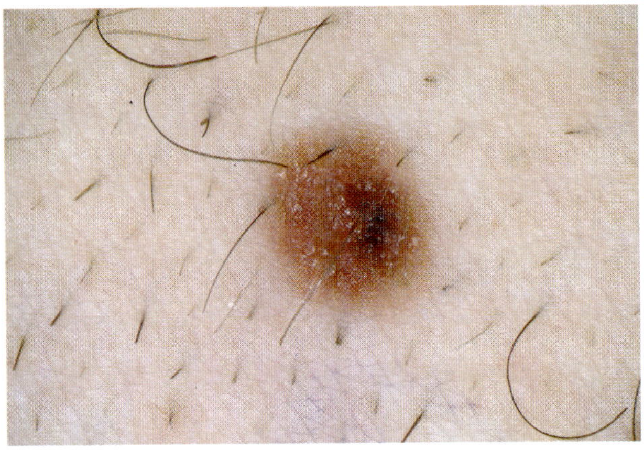

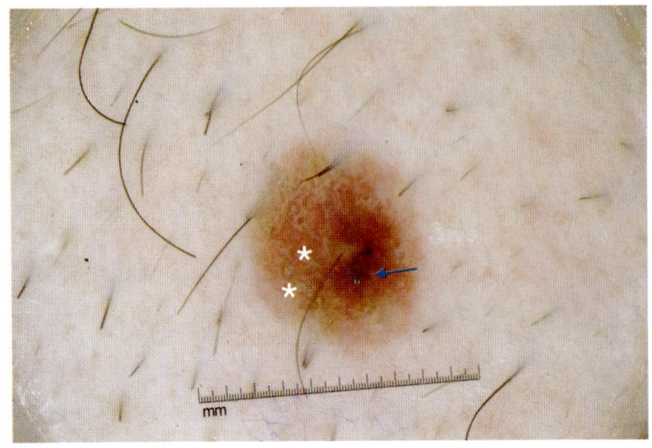

▲ **Figures 4.82, 4.83** Case 6: clinical photograph of a 6 mm, pink-tan papule on the chest of a 33-year-old male patient with history of melanoma. Dermoscopic photograph reveals a complex pattern with a negative network area (asterisks) and eccentric blue-brown blotch (blue arrow).

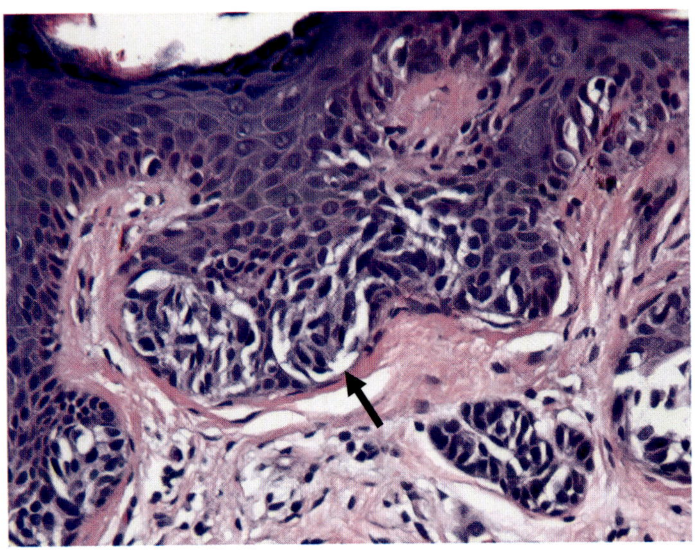

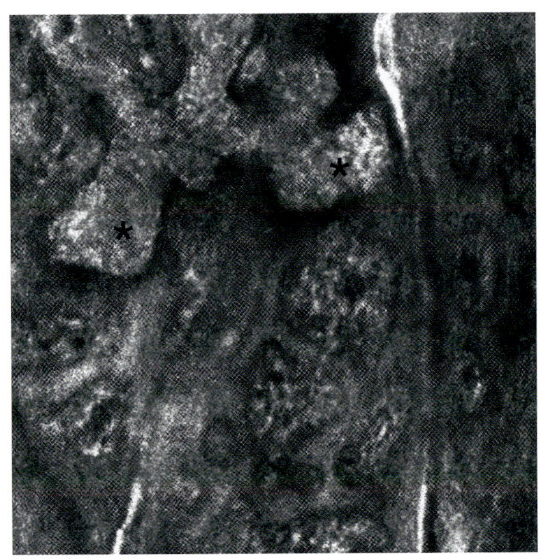

▲ **Figures 4.84, 4.85** Case 6: DN with abnormally shaped, confluent junctional nests (black arrow) seen on histology (20×). RCM (0.5 mm × 0.5 mm) at the DEJ level reveals an elaborate, bright, junctional dense cell cluster (asterisks) with a pseudopod-like configuration.

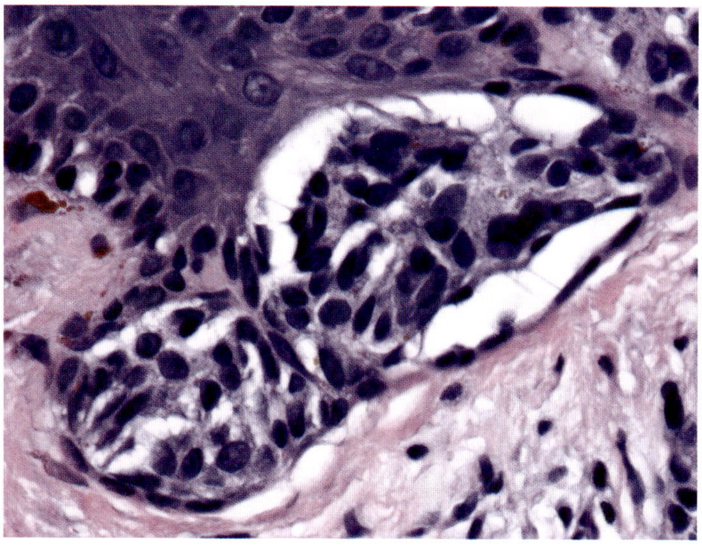

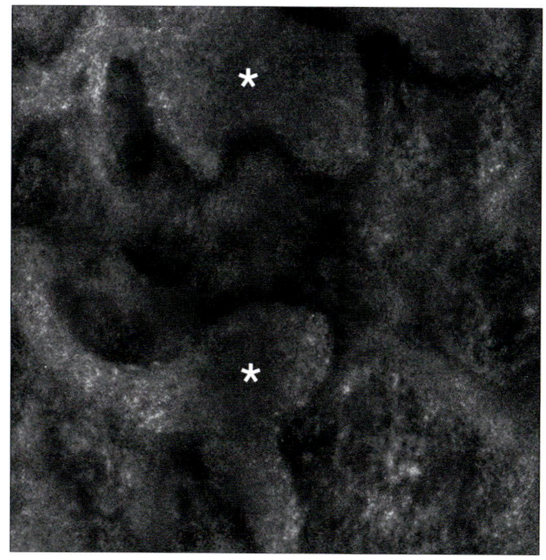

▲ **Figures 4.86, 4.87** Case 6: contrary to the clear cellular composition of the junctional nest seen on histology (40×), the RCM image (0.5 mm × 0.5 mm) does not disclose clear cellular outlines within the junctional dense cell clusters (asterisks).

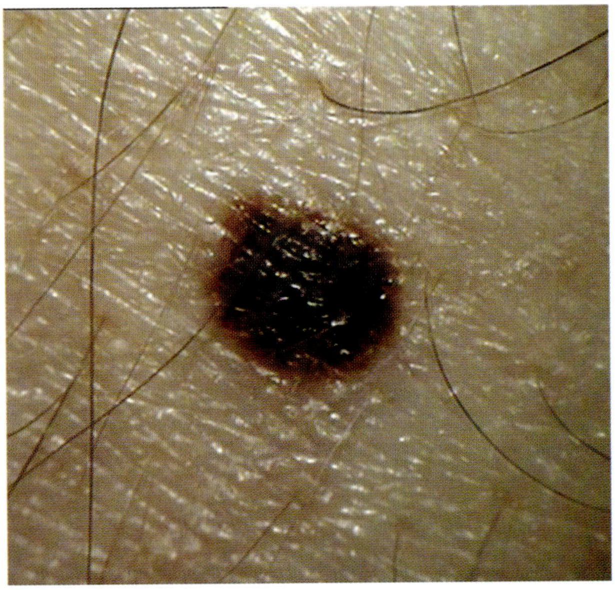

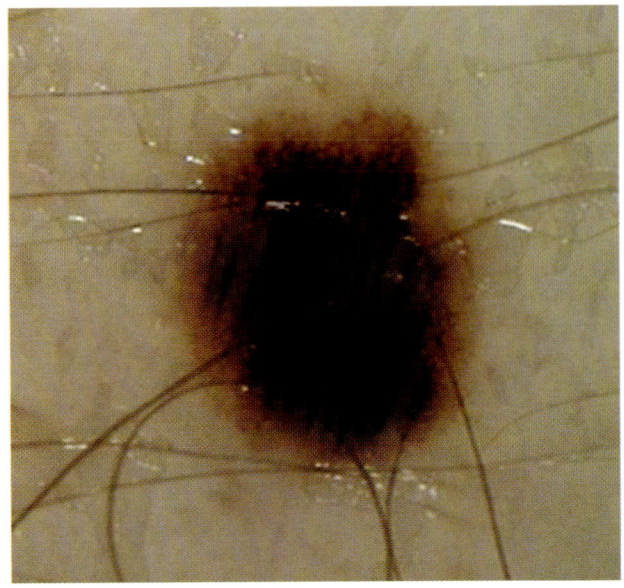

▲ **Figures 4.88, 4.89** Case 7: clinical photograph of a 7 mm dark brown papule on the back of a 27-year-old male patient with a history of melanoma. This lesion has become larger and darker compared with baseline photography. Dermoscopic photograph reveals a reticular pattern with a central hyperpigmented blotch.

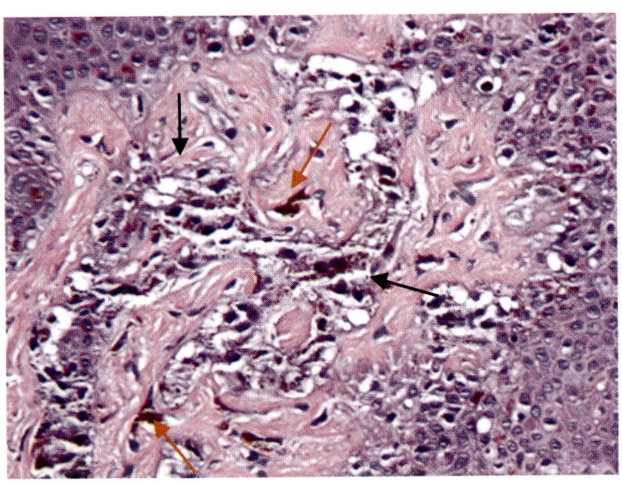

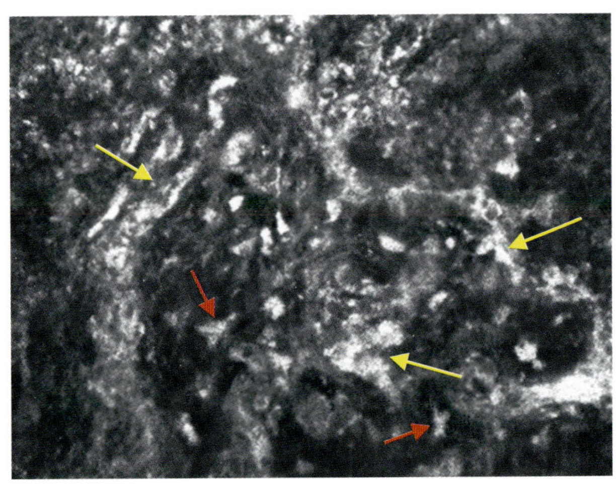

▲ **Figures 4.90, 4.91** Case 7: histology of DN (20×, horizontal section) shows a junctional melanocytic proliferation (black arrows) with marked architectural disarray. This pattern is reproduced on RCM (0.475 mm × 0.340 mm) at the level of the DEJ as junctional thickenings (yellow arrows). Melanophages seen within the dermis on histology appear as fuzzy bright dermal cells (red arrows in both) on RCM.

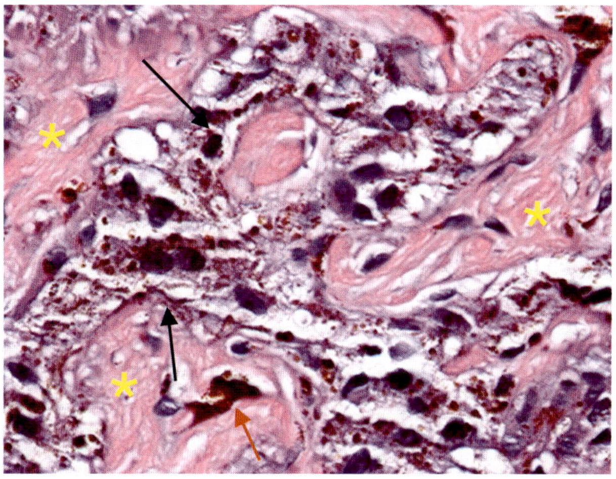

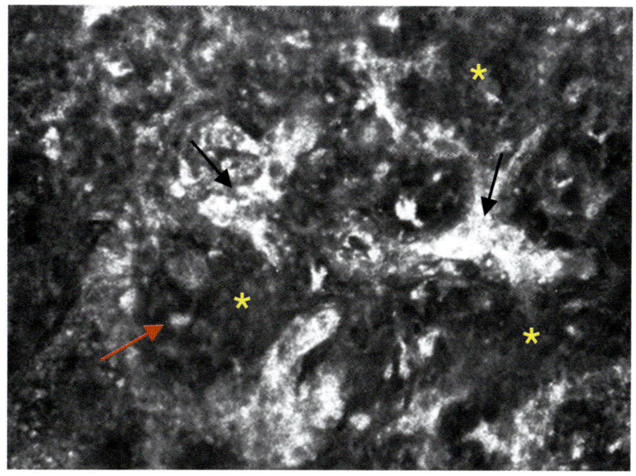

▲ **Figures 4.92, 4.93** Case 7: histology (40×, horizontal section) and corresponding RCM (0.475 mm × 0.340 mm) show junctional melanocytic aggregates (black arrows in both) and melanophages in the papillary dermis (red arrows in both). The prominent collagenous stroma (asterisks) on histology is recapitulated as low-refractility fibrillar dermal elements on RCM (in both).

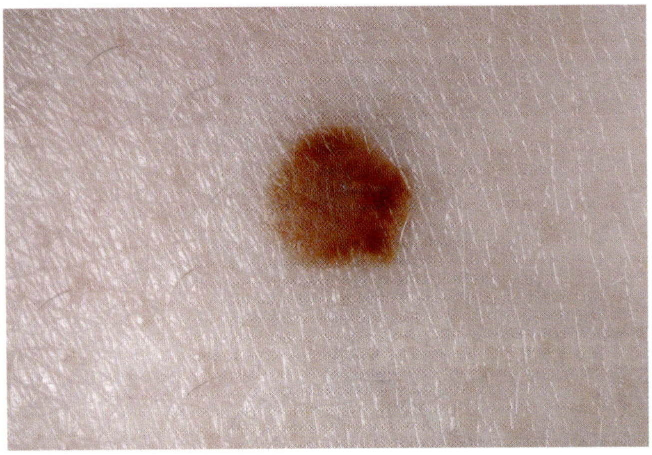

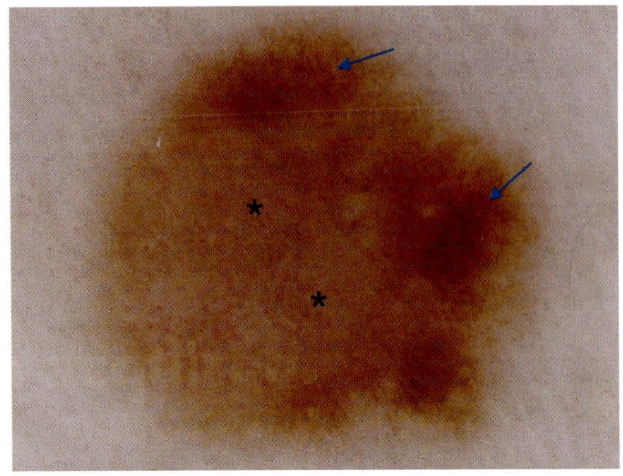

▲ **Figures 4.94, 4.95** Case 8: clinical photograph of a 5 mm brown papule on the gluteal area of a 48-year-old female patient with a history of melanoma. Dermoscopic photograph reveals a multicomponent pattern, with patchy peripheral reticulation (blue arrows) and a regression area with gray peppering, negative network, and dotted vessels (asterisks).

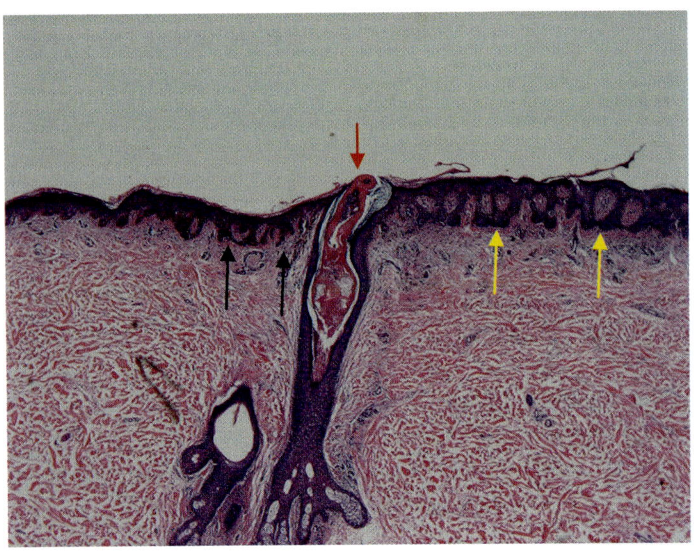

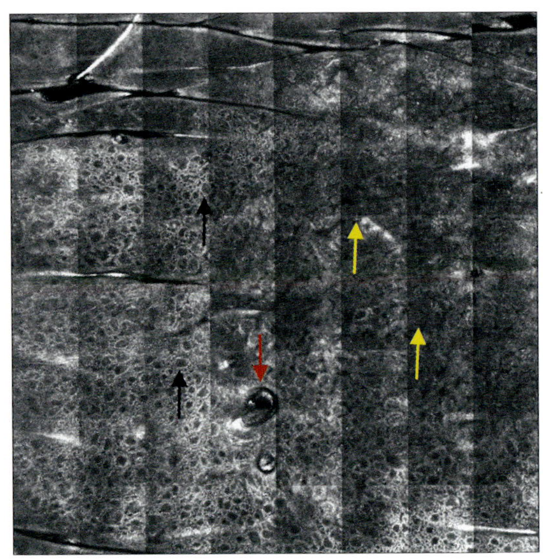

▲ **Figures 4.96, 4.97** Case 8: on histology (4×) a dilated follicle (red arrow) separates an area with thin, pigmented rete ridges with focal fusion (black arrows), from an area with an acanthotic epidermis with thick rete ridges showing frequent fusion (yellow arrows). Corresponding RCM (4 mm × 4 mm) shows a dilated follicle (red arrow) that roughly marks the border between an area with bright epidermal meshwork, edged papillae (black arrows), and a less-refractile area with non-edged papillae and thicker, closely spaced epidermal rete (yellow arrows).

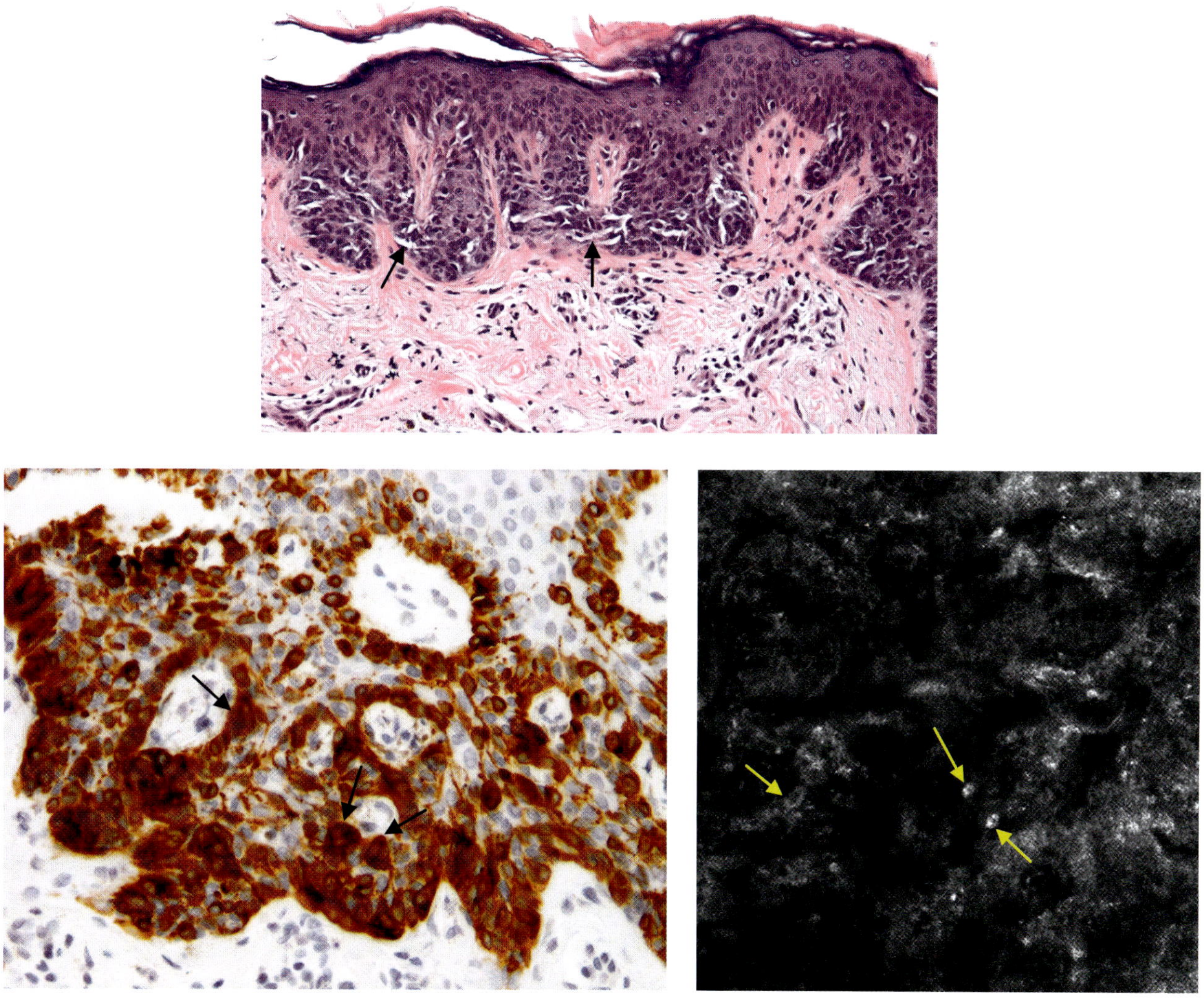

▲ **Figures 4.98–4.100** Case 8: a lentiginous melanocytic proliferation bridging adjacent rete (black arrows) is seen on histology (20×). On Melan-A immunohistochemical stain (40×), single cells (black arrows) predominate over nests. Corresponding RCM (0.5 mm × 0.5 mm) at the level of the DEJ reveals non-edged dermal papillae and prominent bright round nucleated cells (yellow arrows), compatible with enlarged atypical melanocytes within the rete.

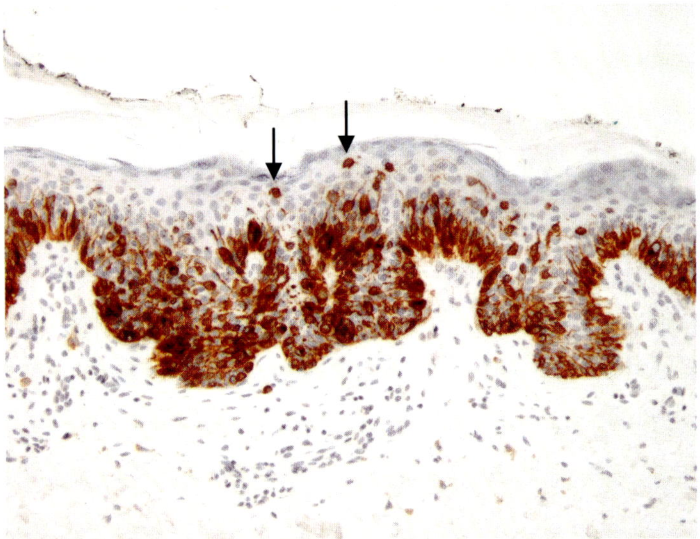

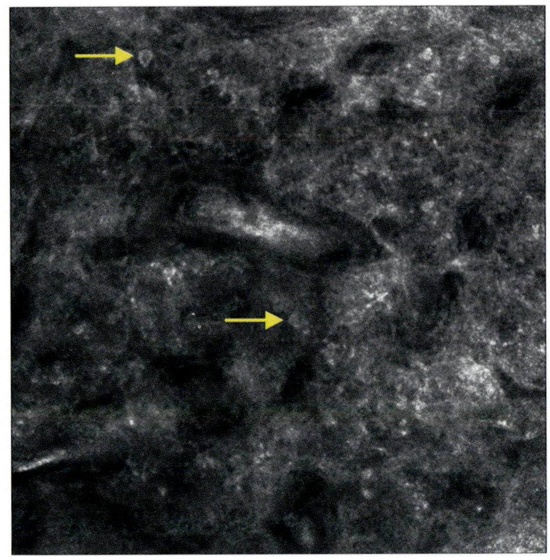

▲ **Figures 4.101, 4.102** Case 8: Melan-A immunohistochemical stain (histology, 20×) highlights the continuous and focally confluent lentiginous melanocytic proliferation with focal pagetoid spread of melanocytes (black arrows). Similarly, on RCM (0.5 mm × 0.5 mm), rare bright round cells (yellow arrows) are seen at the level of the stratum spinosum in the background of epidermal disarray, raising suspicion for evolving melanoma.

CHAPTER 4d

Malignant melanoma

Cristiane Benvenuto-Andrade, Jocelyn A Lieb, Melissa Gill, Salvador González, and Klaus J Busam

Malignant melanoma is a significant public health problem. It is estimated that 59,940 individuals will be diagnosed with melanoma in 2007, with an associated 8110 deaths.[1] Despite extensive research investigating the various clinical appearances of cutaneous melanoma, the diagnostic accuracy of dermatologists using the features of the ABCDE acronym remains suboptimal. The diagnosis of melanoma made by dermatologists when based solely on visual inspection is accurate in 65–80% of cases.[2] Dermoscopy, a non-invasive tool that permits the visualization of subsurface structures, can improve diagnostic accuracy to as high as 85% for clinicians who are trained in its use.[2] However, this accuracy level remains low for a potentially life-threatening disease.

In-vivo reflectance confocal microscopy (RCM) represents a novel technique that offers the possibility to non-invasively examine the epidermis and the superficial dermis at cellular resolution,[3] and, therefore, may improve the diagnostic accuracy for melanoma. The diagnosis of malignant melanoma by RCM relies on specific cytologic and architectural features (Table 4.1).[4–10] Furthermore, an algorithm for diagnosing melanoma has been proposed that utilizes two major criteria (non-edged dermal papillae and

Table 4.1 RCM and histopathologic features of cutaneous melanomas

Histopathologic feature	*Correlating RCM feature*
Altered epidermal background	Disarranged Pattern: disruption of the normal honeycomb and cobblestone patterns of the epidermis
Pagetoid melanocytosis	'Pagetoid' cells: bright round or dendritic cells in the spinous or granular cell layer
Atypical melanocytes	Cellular atypia: large bright cells +/- coarse dendritic processes
Increased density of solitary units	Increased number of bright cells, some of them with dendritic or roundish morphology at the dermal-epidermal junction
Disordered growth pattern of melanocytes in rete ridges	Non-edged papillae: dermal papillae without a demarcated rim of bright cells, but separated by a series of large reflecting cells
Discohesive nests, internally pleomorphic nests, or confluently aggregated melanocytes	Cell clusters with loose, dishomogenous or cerebriform morphology
Sheets of melanocytes	Sheet-like distribution of cells

Table 4.2 Pitfalls in the diagnosis of melanoma using RCM

RCM feature	*Pitfall*
'Pagetoid' cells in spinous layer	May mistake Langerhans cells for dendritic melanocytes May be benign pagetoid melanocytes of Spitz nevus, acral or traumatized/irritated nevus
Pigmented nest	May be a 'pseudonest' composed of pigmented keratinocytes (clonal seborrheic keratosis)
Non-edged papillae	May be present in nevi (dysplastic or Spitz nevi)

cytologic atypia at the dermal–epidermal junction) and four minor criteria (roundish 'pagetoid' cells, widespread 'pagetoid' infiltration in the epidermis, nucleated cells within dermal papillae, and cerebriform cell clusters in the dermis).[10,11] However potential pitfalls of this non-invasive imaging technique need to be considered (Table 4.2).

IN-SITU MELANOMA

A number of features are helpful to diagnose intraepidermal (in-situ) melanoma by RCM. Since RCM is a quasihistologic method, the morphologic criteria for the diagnosis of in-situ melanoma parallel, to a large extent, but are not limited to, the parameters used by conventional light microscopic examination. The overall symmetry or architectural gestalt (i.e. low-power view) plays an important role for the histopathologic diagnosis of a melanocytic proliferation. Therefore, on RCM, the evaluation of low-power mosaics is an important first step in the analysis of a melanocytic lesion, as it allows for the evaluation of symmetry and circumscription. However, more studies of RCM mosaics are warranted.

Key features for the diagnosis of in-situ melanoma by conventional high-power histology that can also be assessed by RCM include the predominance of solitary units of melanocytes, confluence of melanocytes along the dermal–epidermal junction (DEJ), pagetoid spread, (Figures 4.107, 4.108,4.114, 4.115, 4.119) cytologic atypia, (Figures 4.110, 4.115, 4.119) ill-defined cell borders, (Figures 4.107, 4.108, 4.114), and secondary alterations of the epidermal 'background' architecture, (Figures 4.108, 4.114, 4.115), such as effacement of rete ridges to the point of 'consumption of the epidermis'.

Features currently found to be helpful for the diagnosis of melanoma in situ by RCM are listed in Table 4.1 and illustrated in Figures 4.103–4.119. Some of the features used for the diagnosis of melanoma by RCM are more specific and sensitive than others, and many of them need to be interpreted in the context of other features for greatest diagnostic value. Based on preliminary experience by various investigators,[4,6,8,10,11] the most valuable features include epidermal disarray, non-edged papillae, 'pagetoid' cells, and cytologic atypia.

Alterations of the epidermis, which are commonly associated with melanoma, manifest under RCM as 'disarray', which refers to the disruption or loss of the normal honeycomb or cobblestone pattern of keratinocytes (Figures 4.107A, B, 4.108A, B, 4.114, 4.115). Disarray is a very helpful clue to register a lesion as abnormal and different from an ordinary nevus. However, disarray per se is a non-specific feature. It can also occur in atypical ('dysplastic') melanocytic nevi, traumatized nevi, recurrent nevi, and miscellaneous non-melanocytic tumors, such as irritated seborrheic keratoses or inflammatory dermatoses. Furthermore, it is not seen in all melanomas. Thus, the presence of disarray is neither necessary nor sufficient for melanoma. However, in the appropriate context – i.e. once a lesion is clearly identified as a melanocytic proliferation – the presence of marked epidermal disarray is one of the more valuable morphologic features to suspect melanoma.[4,8,10,11] Bright grainy particles may be present, but are non-specific, and simply reflect the presence of a pigmented lesion (Figures 4.108B, 4.114, 4.115A). However, in context with epidermal disarray, their presence favors an atypical melanocytic tumor.

Another feature useful for the diagnosis of melanoma is marked architectural disarrangement of the DEJ which has been termed non-edged papillae[11] (Figures 4.106, 4.107C, 4.108C, 4.115C). The term refers to the appearance of dermal papillae commonly seen by RCM. When a rim of bright cells forms a sharply demarcated bright ring around a dark dermal papilla, the papilla is described as 'edged'. Non-edged papillae lack a sharp demarcation rim of bright basal cells and are separated by a rete ridge containing a series of large reflecting cells.[10,11] The finding of edged vs non-edged papillae probably reflects a combination of changes in the architecture of epidermal rete ridges as well as growth pattern and density of melanocytes at the DEJ. It is possible that irregular rete ridges (focally effaced or fused) and/or abnormal growth pattern of melanocytes (variation in size and shape of nests, fusion of nests, lentiginous single cell growth alternating with nested growth) result in non-edged papillae. In contrast, the majority of ordinary nevi have edged papillae or unaltered dermal papillary rings by RCM. While non-edged papillae raise concern about melanoma, they are not specific. They may also be seen in (atypical) dysplastic nevi and Spitz nevi.

Since solitary units of melanocytes are normally confined to the DEJ, their presence in the spinous or granular cell layer is, both for conventional histology as well as RCM, an important feature to suspect (Figures 4.107B, 4.108A, 4.115A, 4.119) melanoma.[6] As with conventional histology, 'pagetoid' cells per se are not restricted to melanoma, and their presence needs to be interpreted in the appropriate clinical context. Some pagetoid melanocytosis is acceptable for nevi at acral sites, traumatized, irritated, or recurrent nevi, congenital nevi, and Spitz nevi. However, in the appropriate clinical context (e.g. changing nevus on the back in an adult with no history of trauma), the detection of pagetoid melanocytes strongly suggests in-situ melanoma, and in RCM has been reported the most relevant discriminating feature.[11]

Cytologic atypia is part of the assessment of melanomas by conventional histology. Some aspects of atypia can be assessed by RCM, but not all. Cell size, cell contour, nuclear size, and perhaps nuclear contour can be judged by RCM, but to date there is no known feature under RCM that correlates with chromatin pattern or nucleoli within melanocytes. Nonetheless, in many melanomas, cellular atypia is apparent under RCM by the presence of enlarged bright cells within the epidermis (Figures 4.107A, B, 4.108A–D, 4.110, 4.114, 4.115B, C, 4.119). While the presence of atypia adds to concerns about the lesion, atypia alone is neither sufficient nor necessary for melanoma. Lentigo malignas, for example, may contain melanocytes of normal size and shape, but have too many of them at the DEJ. On the other hand, marked atypia may be seen in dysplastic or Spitz nevi.

The parameters listed here apply in differing degrees to the intraepidermal component of both melanomas of the superficial spreading type (Figures 4.103–4.119) and the lentigo maligna melanoma (LMM) type (Figures 4.129–4.138). In superficial spreading melanoma, pagetoid melanocytosis, corresponding to bright round 'pagetoid' cells on RCM, tends to be more prominent and diagnostically useful. In LMM, pagetoid spread is less common and one has to rely more on the detection of an increased number of solitary units of melanocytes at the DEJ, with confluence of cells and extension of melanocytes into adnexal structures.

A major problem for the diagnosis of melanoma (and melanocytic nevi) by RCM is the distinction of melanocytes from bright non-melanocytic cells (Table 4.2). Although this distinction can often be made based on the morphology of the cells (nested growth pattern, fascicles of spindle cells, presence of dendrites), this is not always the case. Pigmented keratinocytes can aggregate (clonal seborrheic keratosis) and simulate a nest. Langerhans cells are dendritic and can be indistinguishable from melanocytes by RCM and can simulate pagetoid melanocytosis.[12]

Key RCM features of in-situ melanoma

- Bright round or dendritic cells in the spinous or granular cell layer (**'pagetoid' cells**)
- Increased number of bright cells, some of them with dendritic or roundish morphology, at the dermal-epidermal junction
- **Junctional thickenings** or **cell clusters** that are **loose** or **dishomogenous**
- Large bright cells with variable dendritic processes, including coarse processes (**cellular atypia**)
- Dermal papillae without a demarcated rim of bright cells, but separated by a series of large reflecting cells (**non-edged papillae**)
- Disarray of the normal architecture of the superficial layers of the epidermis; i.e., loss of the honeycomb and cobblestone pattern (**disarranged pattern**)
- Lentigo maligna type may show rare or no 'pagetoid' cells, but often shows disruption of the normal epidermal architecture at all levels including the DEJ, prominent coarse branching dendrites and atypical bright nucleated cells at the DEJ as confluent single cells and clusters with extension down adnexal structures.

INVASIVE MELANOMA

The epidermal findings of invasive melanomas are similar to those described for in-situ lesions. However, invasive tumors also contain melanocytes in the superficial dermis, as single cells or more often cell aggregates of variable size and shape (Table 4.1). Invasive melanomas are illustrated in Figures 4.120–4.128.

RCM evaluation of invasive melanomas is limited by the maximum in-vivo imaging depth, approximately 150–350 μm, which may hinder the analysis of deeper dermal areas.[13] Therefore, we may think that nodular melanomas may escape detection by RCM. However, a recent study aimed to characterize nodular melanoma by RCM reported that this imaging tool was able to detect dermal clusters in nodular melanomas and the nodular component of superficial spreading melanomas in 70% of the cases. Most cases showed dishomogeneous (Figure 4.127C) or cerebriform morphology.[14] The authors also noted that this subset of melanomas shows distinctive epidermal RCM features. While superficial spreading melanomas with a nodular component are frequently characterized by architectural disarrangement of the epidermis and 'pagetoid' infiltration (Figures 4.124A, 4.127A), purely nodular melanomas contain few 'pagetoid' cells within an unaltered epidermis. Furthermore, at the DEJ, dermal papillae were non-edged in half of the superficial spreading melanomas with a nodular component and only in 10% in the purely nodular melanomas. The lack of dermal papillae probably relates to effacement of rete ridges and possibly 'consumption' of the epidermis. The majority of the cases showed pleomorphic cells in a sheet-like distribution (Figures 4.124B, 4.128A–D). The ability of RCM to detect desmoplastic melanoma would probably be difficult, and further investigation is warranted.

Key RCM features of invasive melanoma

- RCM features of in-situ melanoma
- Individual atypical nucleated and reflective cells in the dermis
- **Dermal cell clusters** with **loose, dishomogeneous** or **cerebriform** morphology
- Cells in a **sheet-like distribution**
- Superficial spreading melanoma with a nodular component typically shows 'Pagetoid' infiltration and a disarranged pattern; about half have non-edged papillae
- Purely nodular melanoma contains few 'pagetoid' cells, little to no alteration of the epidermal architecture and non-edged papillae are infrequent
- Lentigo maligna melanoma may show few 'pagetoid' cells, but the epidermal architecture is usually disrupted; the transition from the confluent proliferation of atypical cells at the DEJ to those within the dermis may be difficult to discern due to effacement of rete ridges

AMELANOTIC MELANOMA

Amelanotic melanomas account for 2–8% of cutaneous melanomas and represent an important diagnostic pitfall for clinicians and a management problem for surgeons. Clinically amelanotic in-situ melanoma, however, can be recognized by RCM, owing to the presence of cells with melanocytic morphology in an atypical distribution and coexisting epidermal disarray. Furthermore, it is helpful if the lesional melanocytes still carry enough contrast in optical images to stand out against the background epidermal keratinocytes,[6,13] presumably because of the presence of melanosomes and/or the presence of some melanin in pre-melanosomes as well as the size of these organelles.[5,15] An example of a clinically amelanotic melanoma detectable by RCM is shown in Figures 4.139–4.141. RCM has been successfully used to map and evaluate response to treatment in these lesions.[13,16] Large studies are ongoing to determine the accuracy of RCM for the detection of amelanotic melanomas.

Key RCM features of amelanotic melanoma

- RCM features characteristic of the histological architectural subtype of melanoma, but composed of melanocytes that are only slightly reflective

METASTATIC MELANOMA

Metastatic melanoma may be detectable by RCM if it involves the superficial dermis or epidermis. Superficial dermal melanoma metastasis may appear as dense clusters of large bright cells. Epidermotropic metastases may demonstrate features similar to in-situ melanoma. Unfortunately, many melanoma metastases are too deep to detect using currently available RCM devices.

REFERENCES

1. Surveillance, Epidemiology, and End Results (SEER) Program, April 2006. June 23, 2007; http://seer.cancer.gov/csr/1975_2004/results_single/sect_01_table.01.pdf.
2. Braun RP, Saurat JH, French LE. Dermoscopy of pigmented lesions: a valuable tool in the diagnosis of melanoma. Swiss Med Wkly 2004; 134(7–8):83–90.
3. Rajadhyaksha M, Grossman M, Esterowitz D, Webb RH, Anderson RR. In vivo confocal scanning laser microscopy of human skin: melanin provides strong contrast. J Invest Dermatol 1995; 104(6):946–52.
4. Langley RG, Rajadhyaksha M, Dwyer PJ et al. Confocal scanning laser microscopy of benign and malignant melanocytic skin lesions in vivo. J Am Acad Dermatol 2001; 45(3):365–76.
5. Busam KJ, Hester K, Charles C et al. Detection of clinically amelanotic malignant melanoma and assessment of its margins by in vivo confocal scanning laser microscopy. Arch Dermatol 2001; 137(7):923–9.
6. Busam KJ, Charles C, Lohmann CM et al. Detection of intraepidermal malignant melanoma in vivo by confocal scanning laser microscopy. Melanoma Res 2002; 12(4):349–55.
7. Gerger A, Koller S, Kern T et al. Diagnostic applicability of in vivo confocal laser scanning microscopy in melanocytic skin tumors. J Invest Dermatol 2005; 124(3):493–8.
8. Gerger A, Koller S, Weger W et al. Sensitivity and specificity of confocal laser-scanning microscopy for in vivo diagnosis of malignant skin tumors. Cancer 2006; 107(1):193–200.
9. Pellacani G, Cesinaro AM, Seidenari S. In vivo assessment of melanocytic nests in nevi and melanomas by reflectance confocal microscopy. Mod Pathol 2005; 18(4):469–74.
10. Pellacani G, Cesinaro AM, Longo C, Grana C, Seidenari S. Microscopic in vivo description of cellular architecture of dermoscopic pigment network in nevi and melanomas. Arch Dermatol 2005; 141(2):147–54.
11. Pellacani G, Guitera P, Longo C et al. The impact of in vivo reflectance confocal microscopy for the diagnostic accuracy of melanoma and equivocal melanocytic lesions. J Invest Dermatol 2007; Jul 26: [epub ahead of print].
12. Busam KJ, Marghoob AA, Halpern A. Melanoma diagnosis by confocal microscopy: promise and pitfalls. J Invest Dermatol 2005; 125(3):vii.
13. Curiel-Lewandrowski C, Williams CM, Swindells KJ et al. Use of in vivo confocal microscopy in malignant melanoma: an aid in diagnosis and assessment of surgical and nonsurgical therapeutic approaches. Arch Dermatol 2004; 140(9):1127–32.
14. Segura S, Pellacani G, Puig S et al. In vivo microscopic features of nodular melanomas: dermoscopy, confocal microscopy and histologic. Arch Dermatol [epub ahead of print].
15. Rajadhyaksha M, Gonzalez S, Zavislan JM. Detectability of contrast agents for confocal reflectance imaging of skin and microcirculation. J Biomed Opt 2004; 9(2):323–31.
16. Chen CS, Elias M, Busam K, Rajadhyaksha M, Marghoob AA. Multimodal in vivo optical imaging, including confocal microscopy, facilitates presurgical margin mapping for clinically complex lentigo maligna melanoma. Br J Dermatol 2005; 153(5):1031–6.

IN-SITU MELANOMA

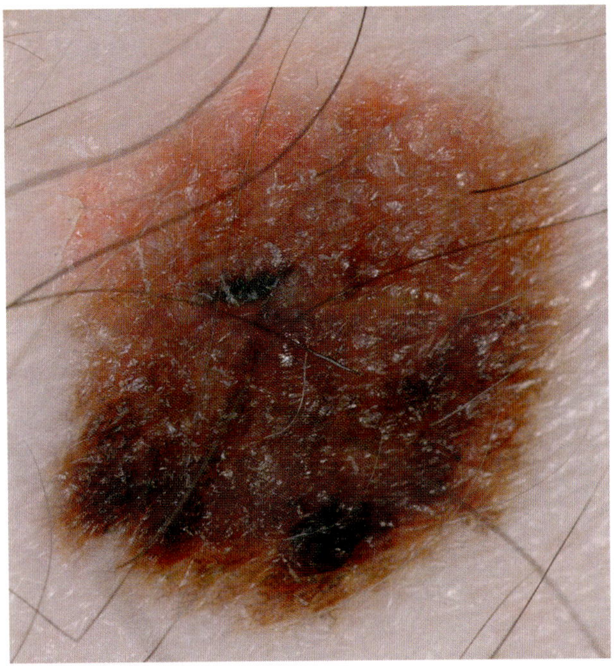

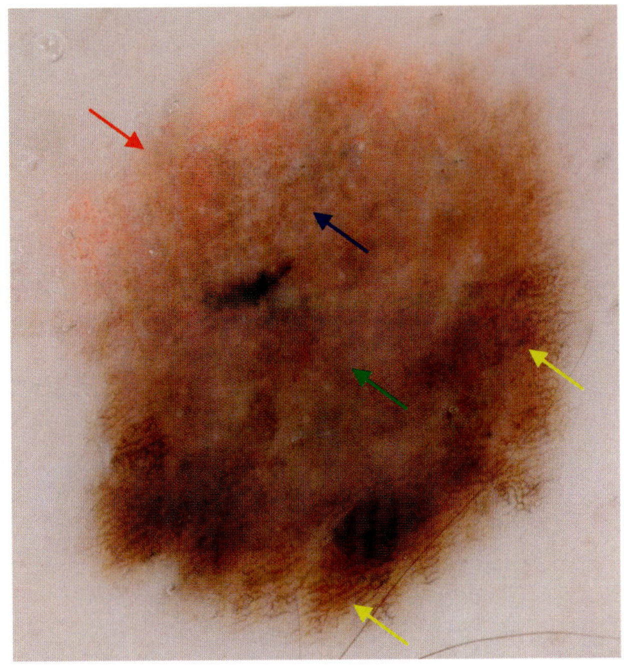

▲ **Figures 4.103, 4.104** Case 1: clinical photograph of a 12 mm brown-black macule with a reddish color on the upper pole on the left lower back. Dermoscopic image reveals multiple colors (brown, black, gray, red) and structural asymmetry with a multicomponent pattern including a peripheral patchy pigment network with branched streaks (yellow arrows), negative network (blue arrow), central regression and peppering (green arrow), and a pink veil on the superior pole with dotted and irregular vessels (red arrow).

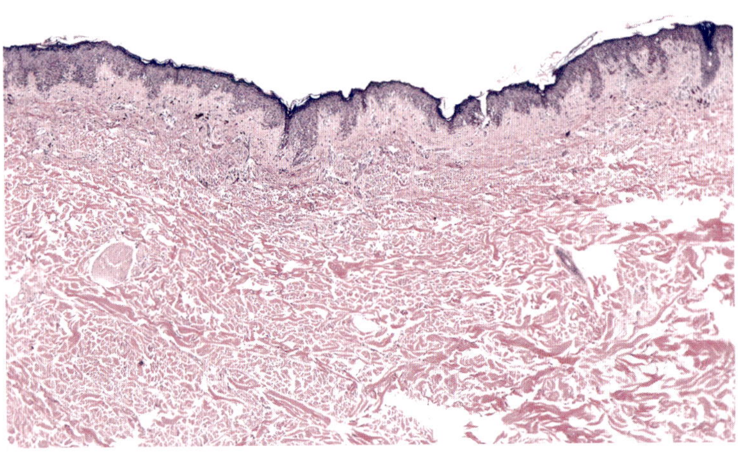

▲ **Figures 4.105, 4.106** Case 1: histology (4×) shows the silhouette of a superficial spreading melanoma. RCM mosaic (4 mm × 4 mm) at the level of the DEJ shows the distribution of scattered bright elements and disrupted DEJ architecture. Note the presence of variably non-edged papillae of irregular size distributed throughout the RCM mosaic.

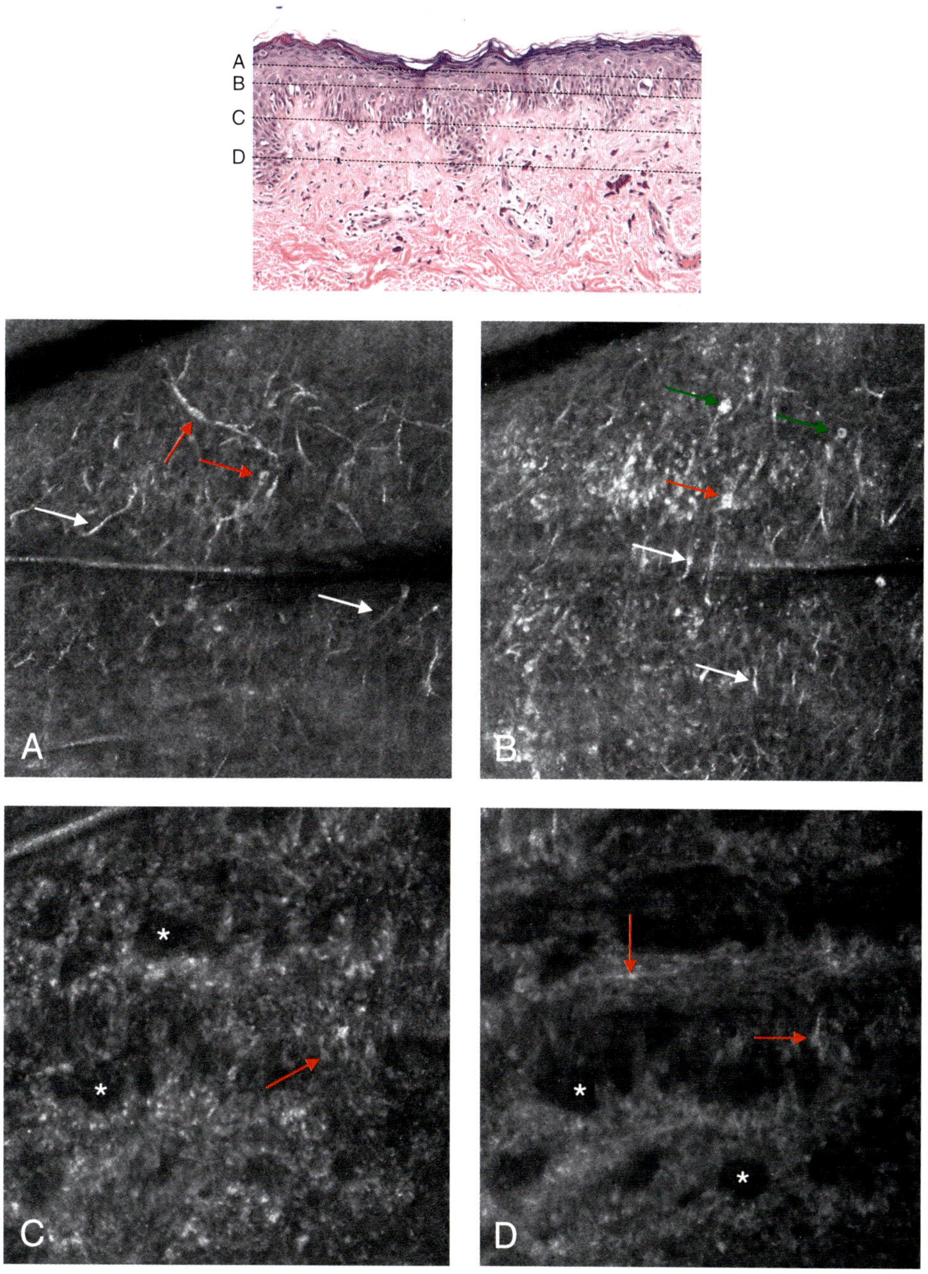

▲ **Figure 4.107** Case 1: histology (20×) shows an increased number of solitary units of melanocytes at the basal layer and within the spinous layer of the epidermis. Many of them are atypical, characterized by enlarged and hyperchromatic nuclei. Horizontal lines labeled A–D indicate from where each RCM image (0.5 mm × 0.5 mm) is captured: spinous layer (A), suprapapillary basal layer (B), superficial DEJ (C), and deep DEJ (D). Architectural disarrangement and bright dendritic structures (white arrows) are seen throughout the epidermis, including the rete ridges (A, B, C, D). Dendritic (red arrows) and round (green arrows) nucleated 'pagetoid' cells are seen in the suprabasal epidermis (A, B). An increased number of bright dendritic melanocytes (red arrows) are present within rete ridges and papillae are non-edged (asterisks) (C, D).

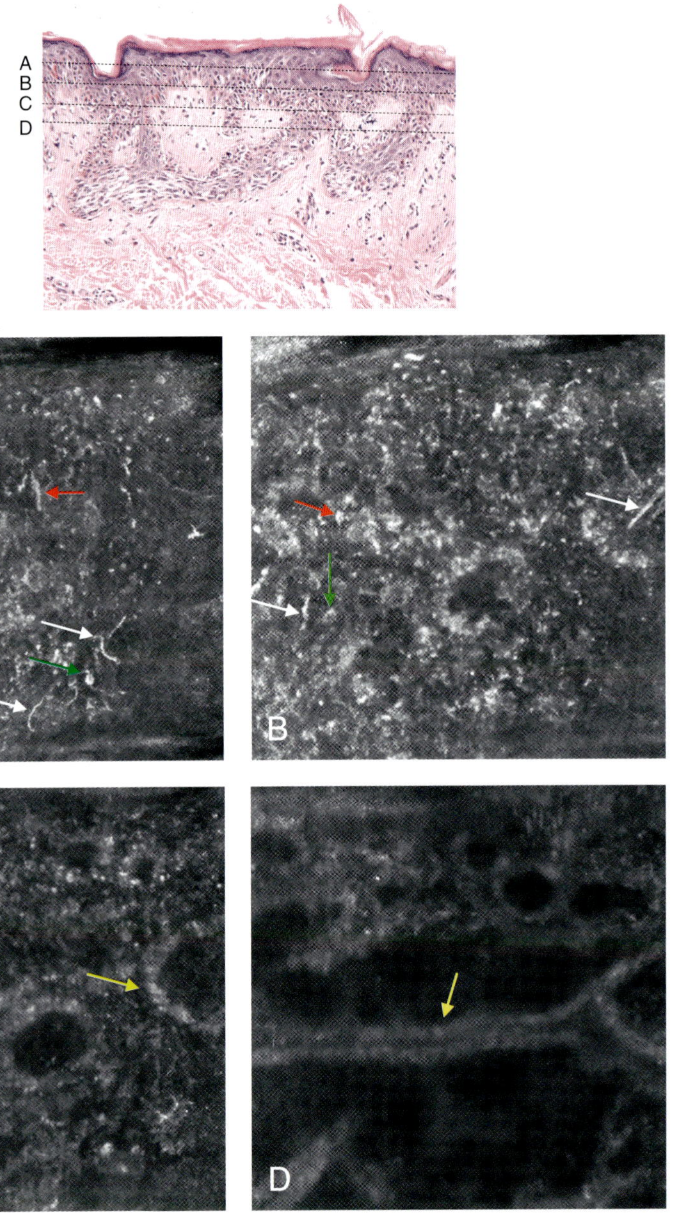

▲ **Figure 4.108** Case 1: histology (20×) shows fusion of nests of melanocytes at the DEJ associated with solitary units of melanocytes, some of which are located in the spinous cell layer (pagetoid spread). Horizontal lines labeled A–D indicate from where each RCM image (0.5 mm × 0.5 mm) is captured: granular/spinous layer (A), spinous basal layer (B), superficial DEJ (C), and deep DEJ (D). Note the bright dendritic structures (white arrows) with cell bodies (red arrows) and round nucleated 'pagetoid' cells (green arrows) within the disarranged suprabasal epidermis (A, B), and increased density of melanocytes (yellow arrows) at the DEJ and along elongated rete ridges (C, D). Non-edged papillae are noted.

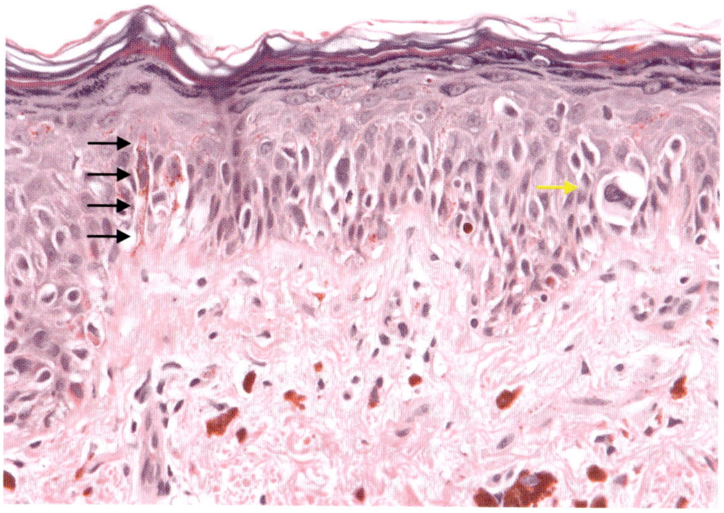

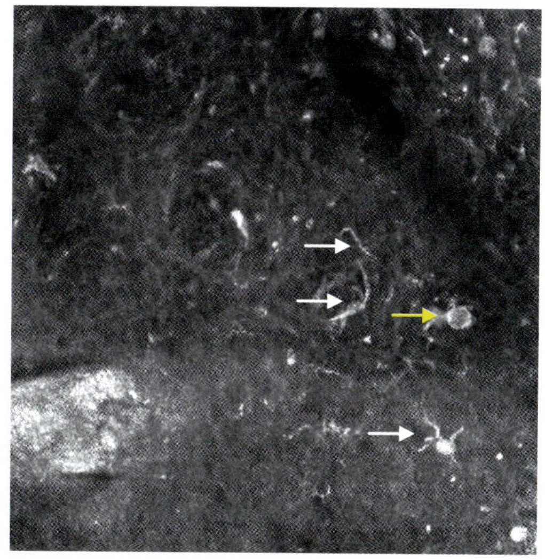

▲ **Figures 4.109, 4.110** Case 1: histology (40×) shows atypical round and dendritic melanocytes with large, hyperchromatic nuclei in the basal and spinous cell layers. Note a fusiform melanocyte with long pigmented cytoplasmic extensions (black arrows), which correspond with the dendritic processes (white arrows) and cells seen on RCM (0.5 mm × 0.5 mm). On histology, note the large round atypical melanocytes, with increased nuclear-to-cytoplasmic ratio (yellow arrow), which correspond to similar large cells seen on RCM (yellow arrow).

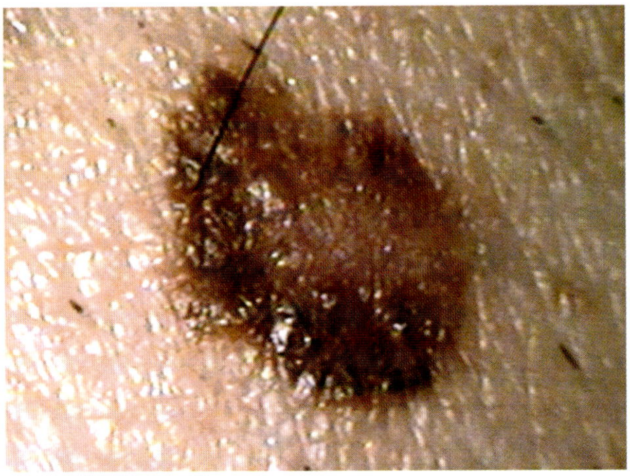

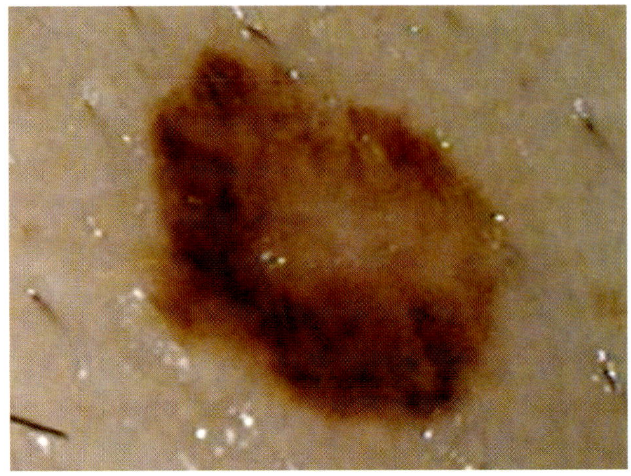

▲ **Figures 4.111, 4.112** Case 2: clinical photograph of a 7 mm brown-black macule with a pinkish center on the right upper back. Dermoscopic photograph reveals a brown, asymmetric lesion with a peripheral broken-up network and a central regression area.

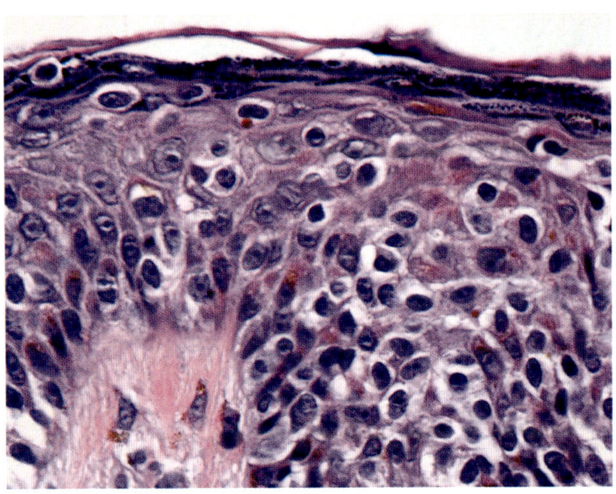

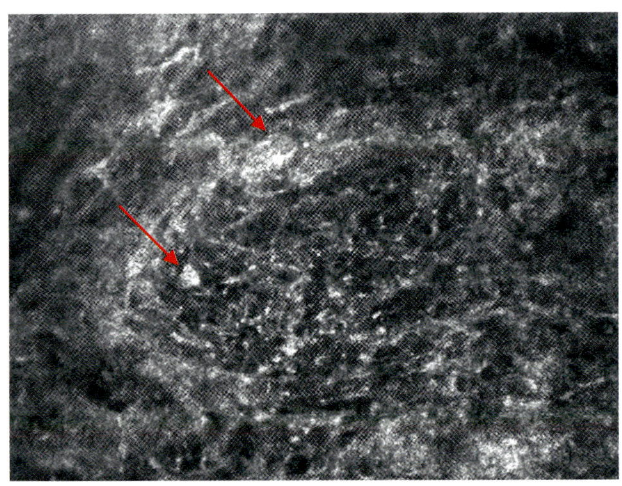

▲ **Figures 4.113, 4.114** Case 2: histology (40×) shows many solitary units of small epithelioid melanocytes in the spinous and granular layers (florid pagetoid spread). On RCM (0.27 mm × 0.2 mm), note the scattered small, bright cells and the large, bright, nucleated cells at the suprabasal level (red arrows). Clearly not all pagetoid cells are appreciated in this image, but there is marked epidermal disarrangement.

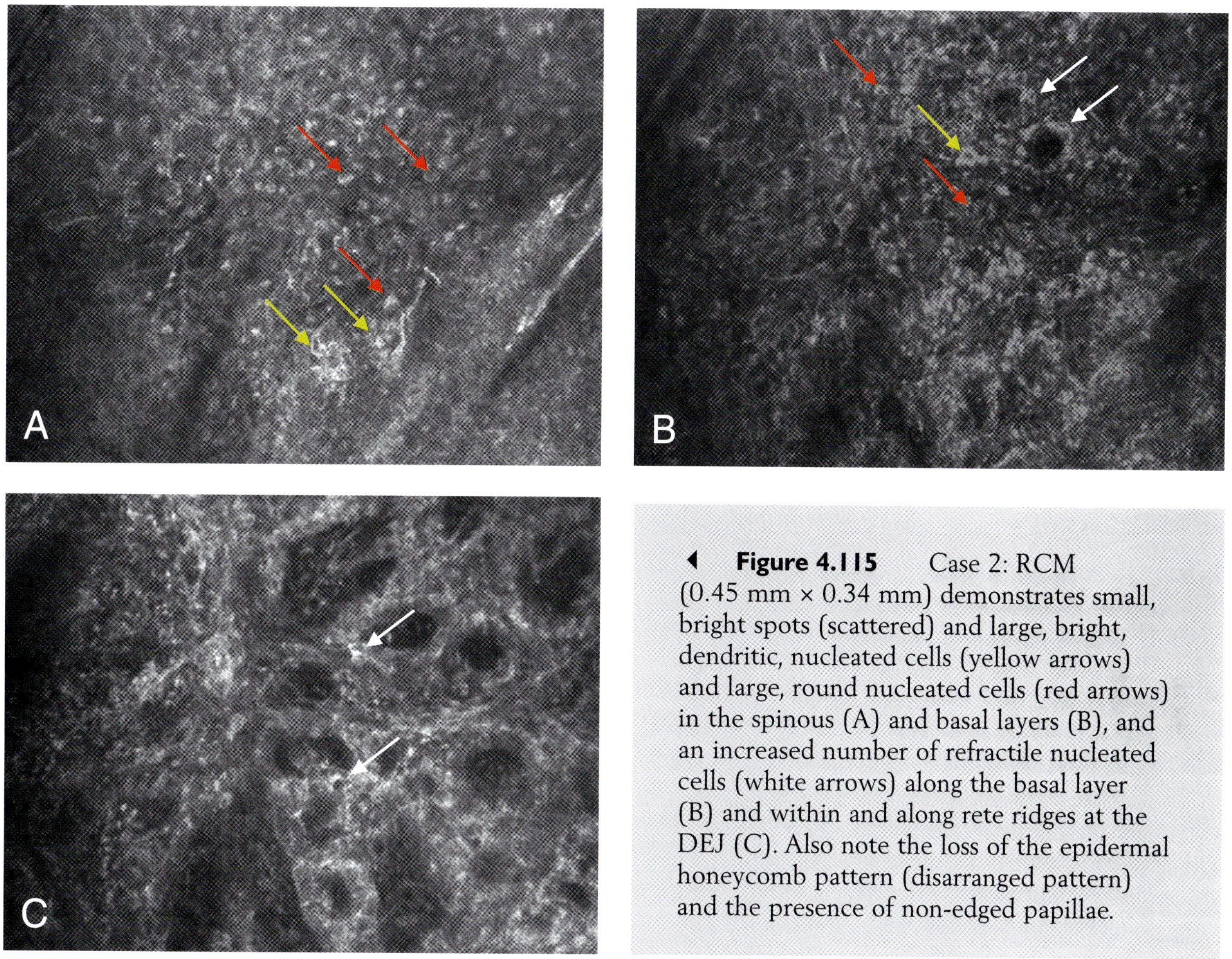

◀ **Figure 4.115** Case 2: RCM (0.45 mm × 0.34 mm) demonstrates small, bright spots (scattered) and large, bright, dendritic, nucleated cells (yellow arrows) and large, round nucleated cells (red arrows) in the spinous (A) and basal layers (B), and an increased number of refractile nucleated cells (white arrows) along the basal layer (B) and within and along rete ridges at the DEJ (C). Also note the loss of the epidermal honeycomb pattern (disarranged pattern) and the presence of non-edged papillae.

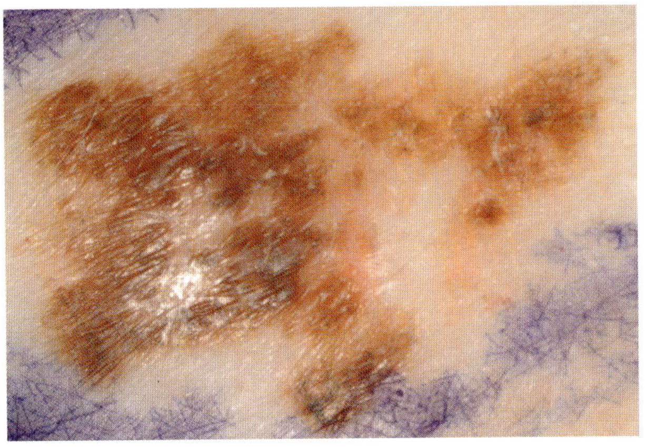

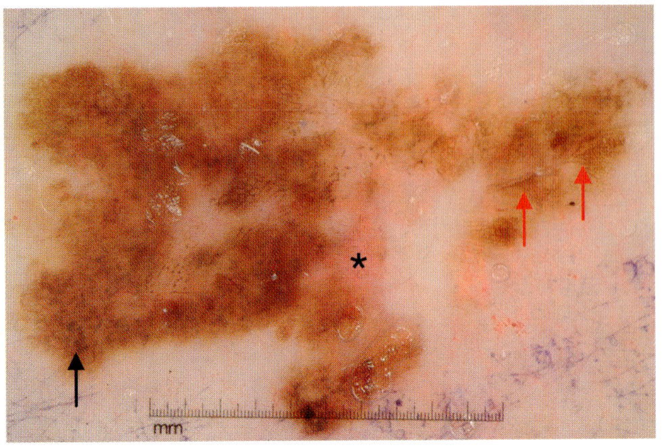

▲ **Figures 4.116, 4.117** Case 3: clinical image of an asymmetric 19 mm × 11 mm tan-brown patch with uneven pigmentation. Dermoscopic image shows an asymmetric lesion with a patchy pigment network, bluish-brown dots (black arrow), branched streaks at the periphery (red arrow), and a pink area (asterisk).

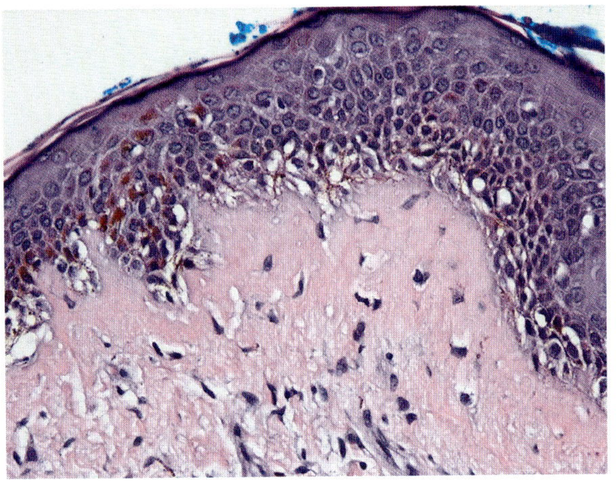

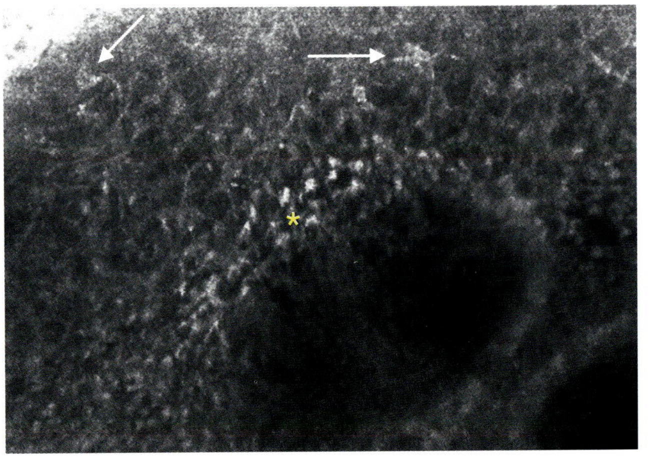

▲ **Figures 4.118, 4.119** Case 3: histology (20×) shows partial effacement of epidermal rete ridges with an increased number of solitary units of melanocytes at the DEJ and above. Note the confluence of solitary units. RCM (0.41 × 0.38 mm) demonstrates the increased density of bright stellate melanocytes at the DEJ (yellow asterisk) and large bright, irregular-shaped dendritic cells within the stratum spinosum (white arrows).

INVASIVE MELANOMA

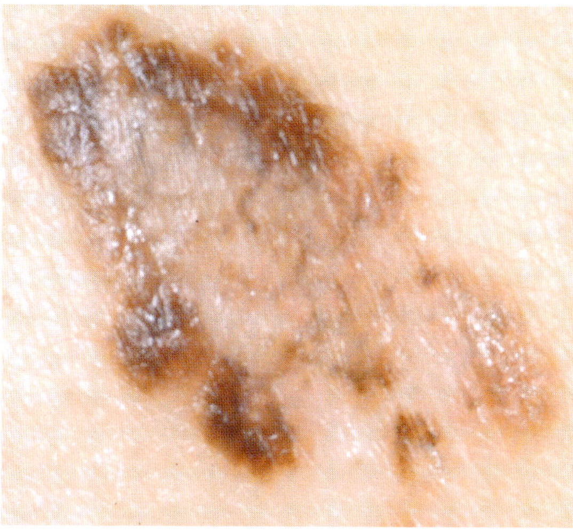

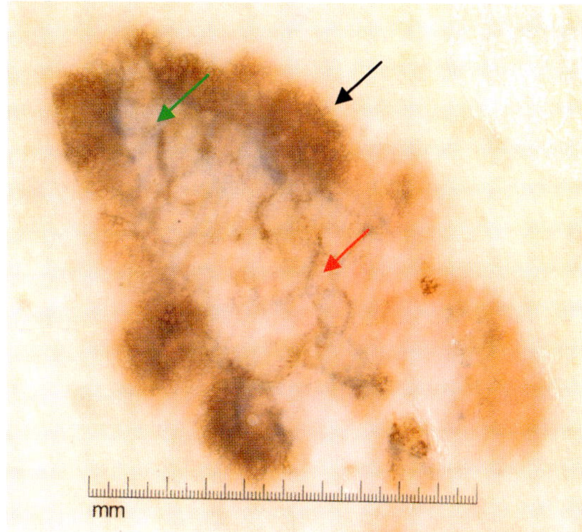

▲ **Figures 4.120, 4.121** Case 1: clinical photograph of a 15 mm × 10 mm brown macule with central pallor on the right mid back. Dermoscopic photograph reveals multiple colors (brown, gray and pink), asymmetry with a multi-component pattern including a peripheral patchy pigment network (black arrow), central regression with peppering (green arrow), and a central broken up network (red arrow).

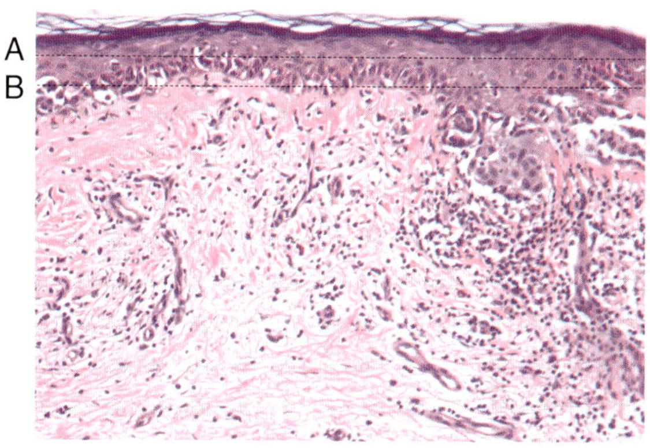

▲ **Figure 4.122** Case 1: histology (10×) shows predominance of solitary units of melanocytes at the DEJ and focally above it in the spinous layer. The superficial dermis is characterized by inflammation, small clusters of tumor cells, and features of regression. Horizontal lines labeled A and B indicate from where each RCM mosaic (2 mm × 2 mm) is captured: spinous layer (A) and DEJ (B). RCM mosaics show bright round cells with dendritic structures in the epidermis and DEJ (red asterisks) with epidermal disarray, architectural disruption of the rete ridges, and non-edged papillae (yellow asterisks).

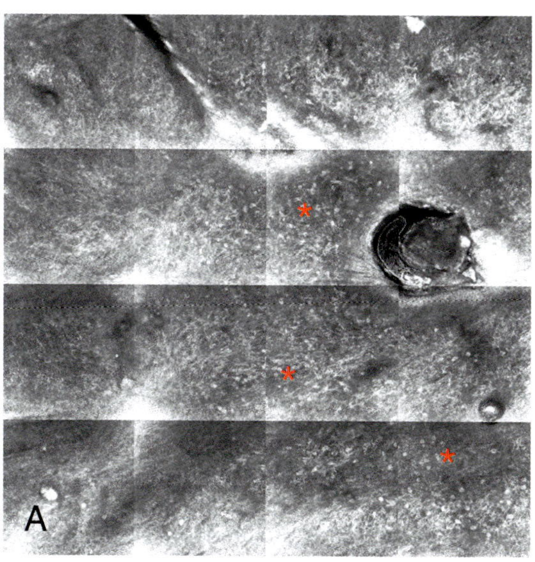

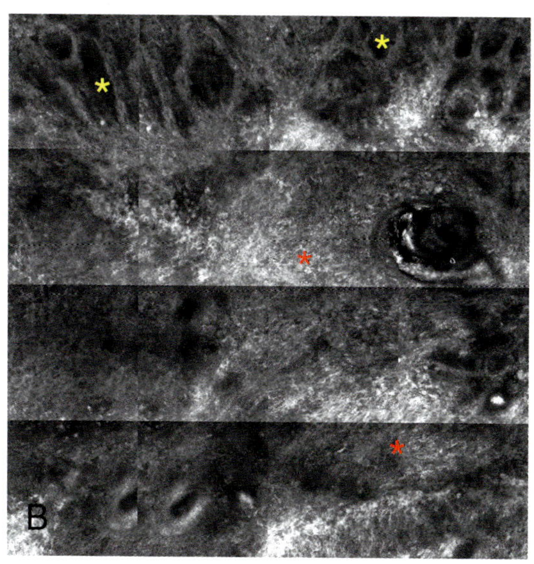

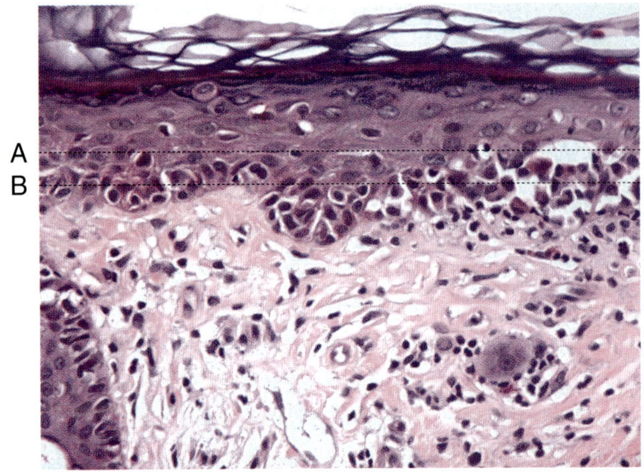

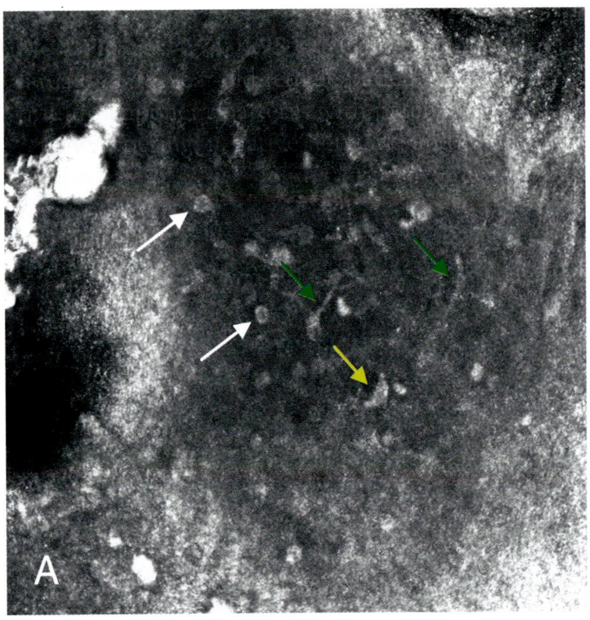

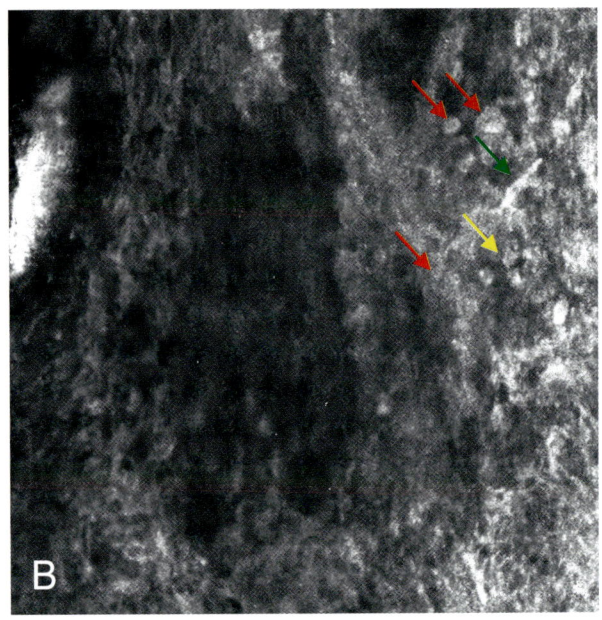

▲ **Figure 4.123** Case 1: histology (20×) shows solitary units of melanocytes at the DEJ and above. A nest with discohesive melanocytes is also seen. Horizontal lines labeled A and B indicate from where each RCM (0.5 mm × 0.5 mm) is captured: spinous layer (A) and DEJ (B). On RCM, note the severe architectural disarray with bright round nucleated 'pagetoid' cells (white arrows), dendritic structures (green arrows), stellate cells (yellow arrow), and the increased density of atypical bright nucleated cells at the DEJ (red arrows).

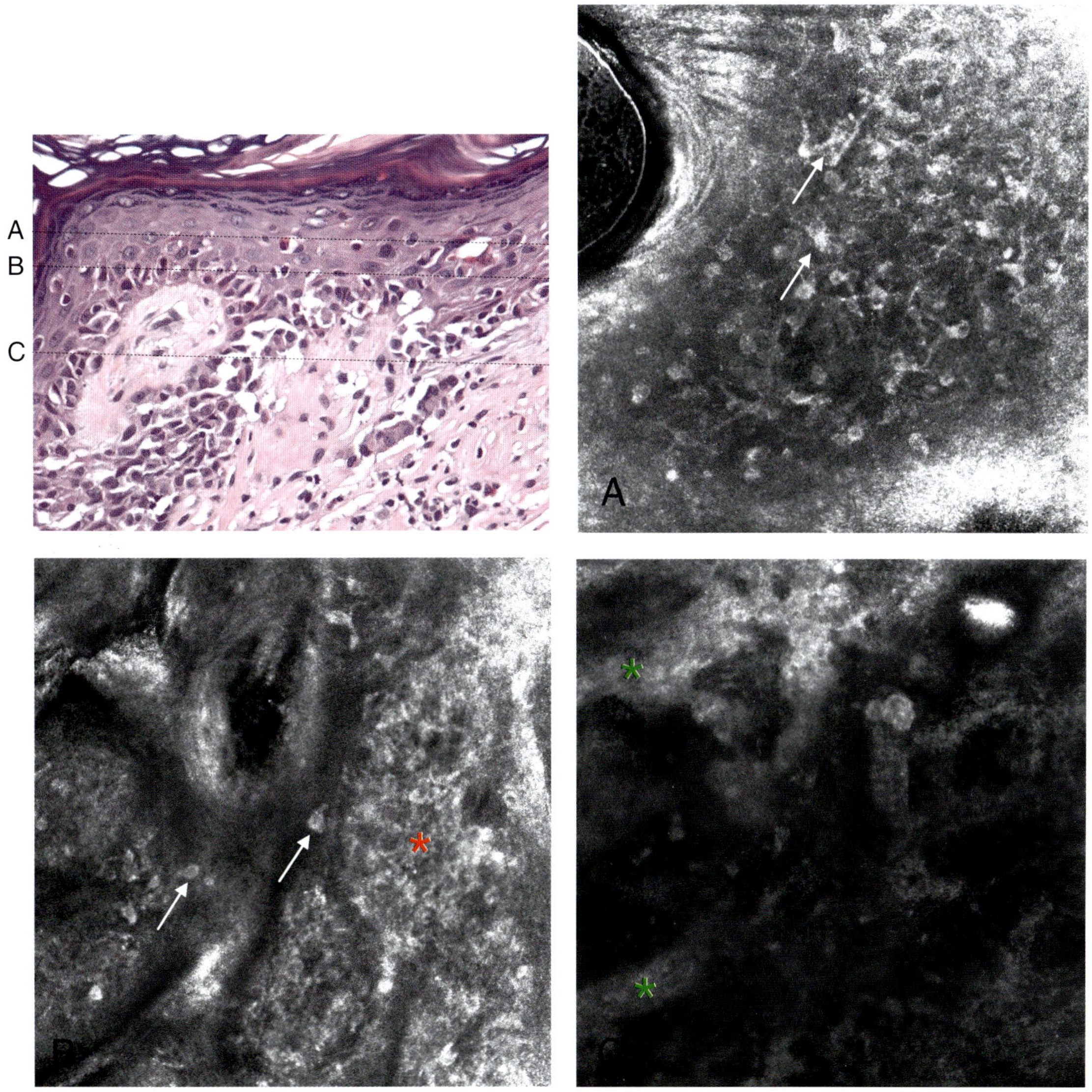

▲ **Figure 4.124** Case 1: histology (40×) shows a dense proliferation of melanocytes as solitary units and irregular nests at the DEJ. Focal pagetoid melanocytosis is seen. The melanocytes are cytologically atypical with enlarged nuclei and abundant cytoplasm. Some tumor cells are also present in the superficial dermis. There is marked cellular discohesion of melanocytes at the DEJ and in aggregates in the superficial dermis. Horizontal lines labeled A–C indicate from where each RCM (0.5 mm × 0.5 mm) is captured: spinous layer (A), basal layer (B), and DEJ (C). Note the atypical-appearing large round and stellate-shaped nucleated cells in the spinous and basal layers (white arrows), the sheet-like cell distribution of bright stellate-shaped cells in the basal layer (red asterisk), and the junctional aggregates/thickenings formed by atypical bright round nucleated cells (green asterisks) within rete ridges at the DEJ.

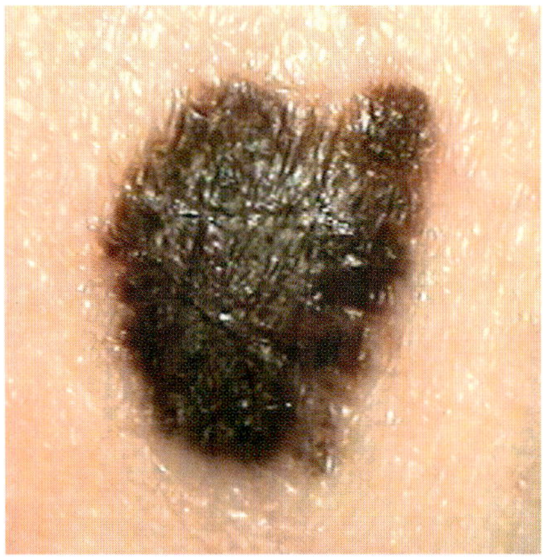

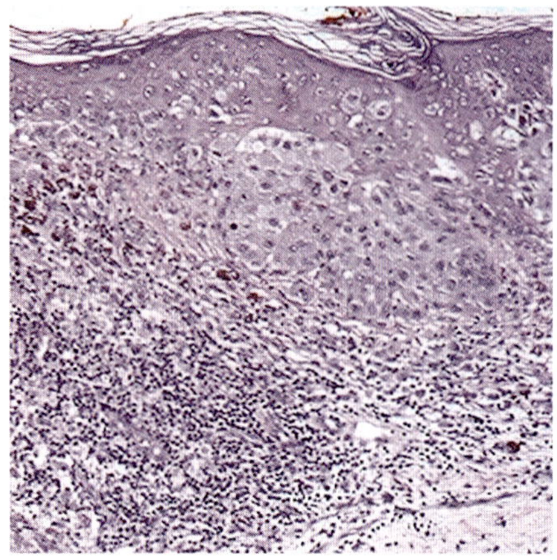

▲ **Figures 4.125, 4.126** Case 2: clinical photograph shows a large dark brown, raised lesion. Histology (10×) shows in-situ melanoma characterized by irregular nests and pagetoid spread of melanocytes as well as invasive tumor associated with a lymphocytic infiltrate.

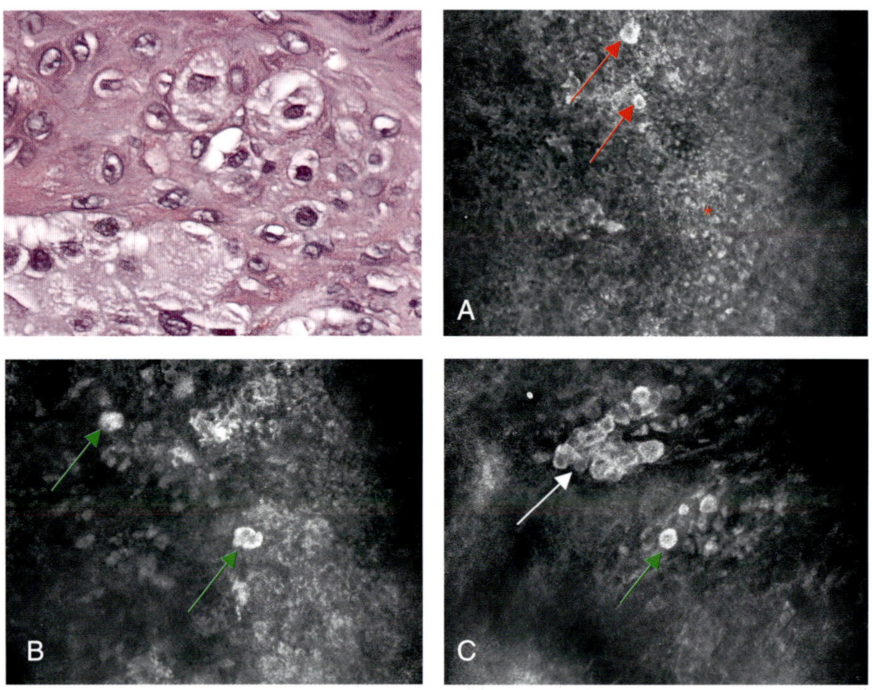

▲ **Figure 4.127** Case 2: histology (40×) shows a nest of melanoma cells and pagetoid spread of atypical epithelioid melanocytes. RCM (0.45 mm × 0.34 mm) at the level of the spinous layer (A), DEJ (B), and dermis (C) show disarrangement of the epidermal architecture with an atypical cobblestone pattern (asterisk) containing large, atypical round 'pagetoid' cells (red arrows), individual atypical large bright, round, nucleated cells (green arrows) associated with numerous smaller less refractile inflammatory cells at the DEJ and within the dermis, and a dishomogeneous dermal cell cluster (white arrow).

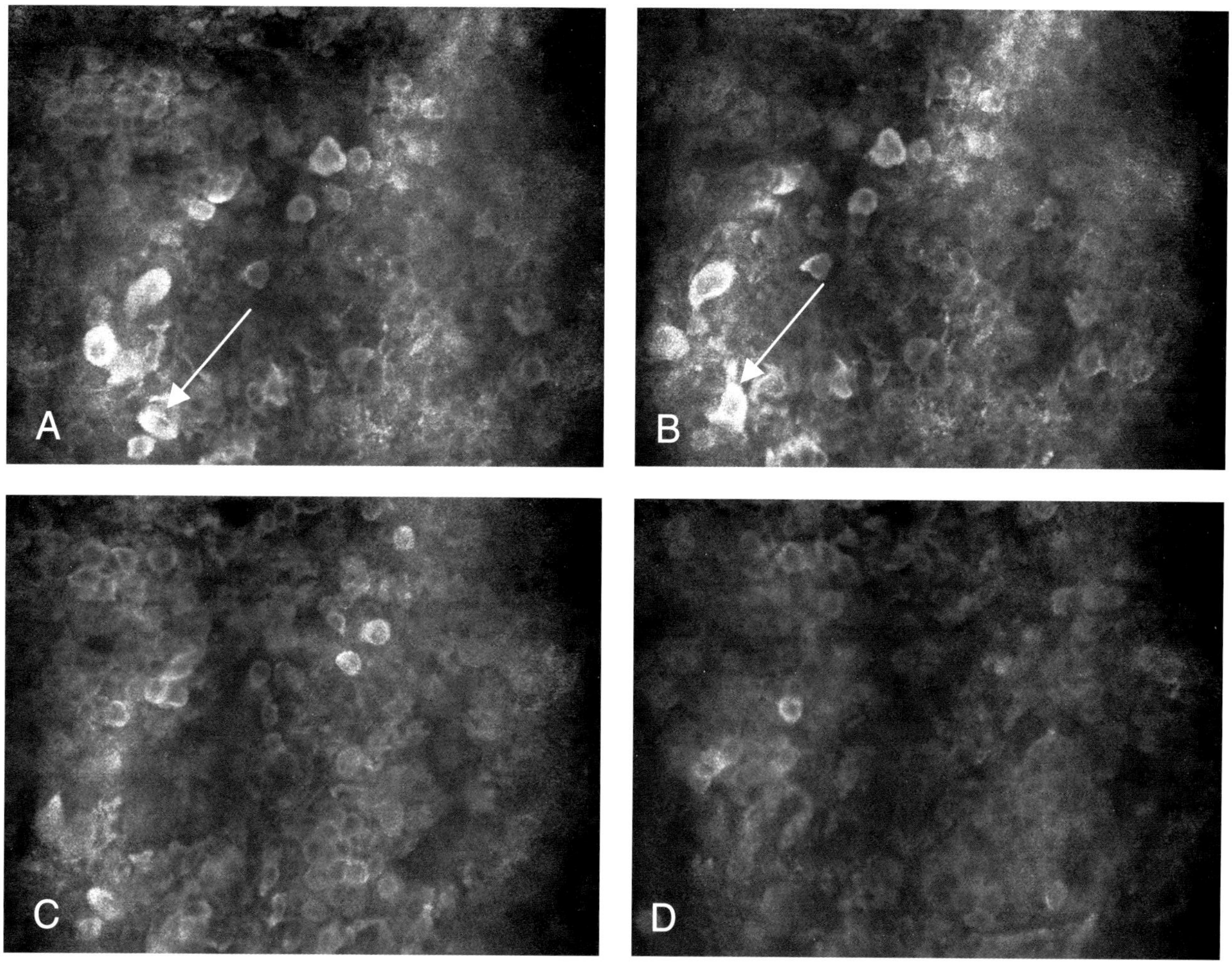

▲ **Figure 4.128** Case 2: RCM images (0.45 mm × 0.34 mm) show sheets of atypical, large, bright, round and stellate, nucleated cells (white arrows) extending from the epidermis (A, B) into the dermis (C, D). The normal skin architecture is completely obliterated such that it is impossible to determine the level of the RCM image based on RCM features alone.

LENTIGO MALIGNA

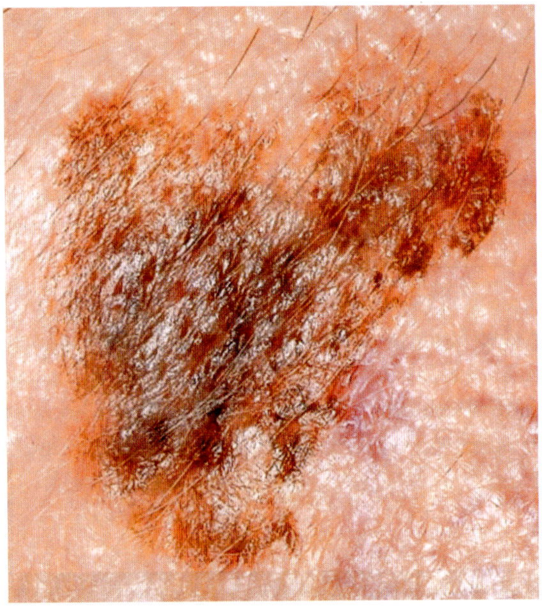

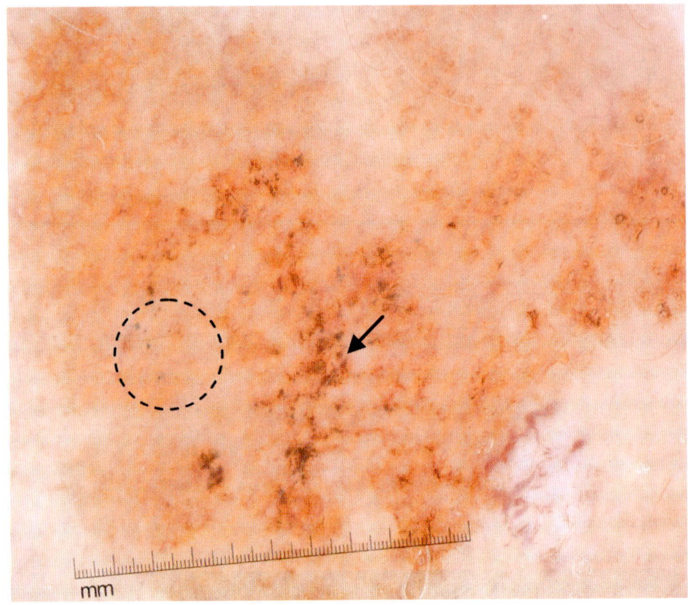

▲ **Figures 4.129, 4.130** Case 1: clinical photograph shows a 17 mm × 18 mm, asymmetric, brown to tan macule with reddish areas on the right cheek. Dermoscopic photograph reveals multiple colors (brown, red and blue-gray), asymmetry with an annular–granular pigment pattern (arrow), peppering (dashed circle), and asymmetric follicular openings.

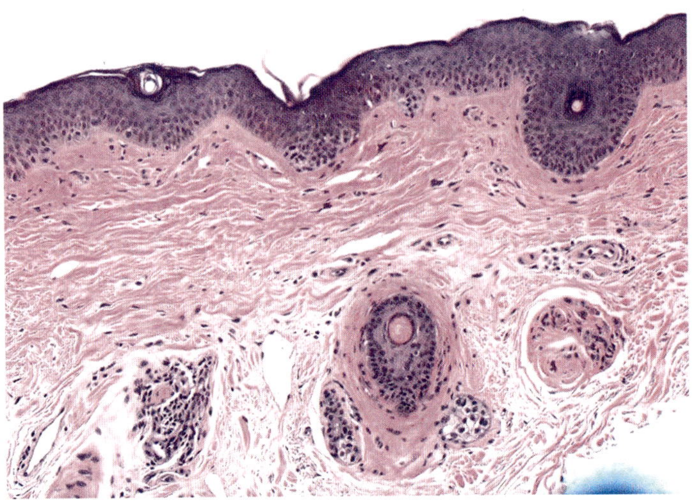

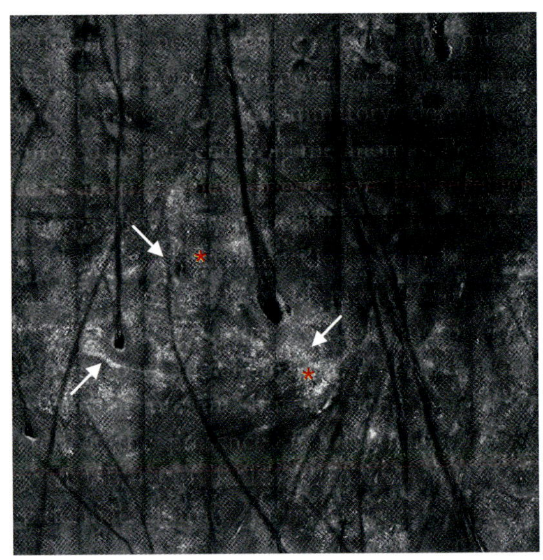

▲ **Figures 4.131, 4.132** Case 1: histology (10×) shows an increased number of melanocytes along the basal layer, tracking deep into the hair follicles. RCM mosaic (4 mm × 4 mm) at the level of the lower epidermis and DEJ (oblique image) shows scattered bright elements (asterisks), and increased brightness surrounding follicles (white arrows).

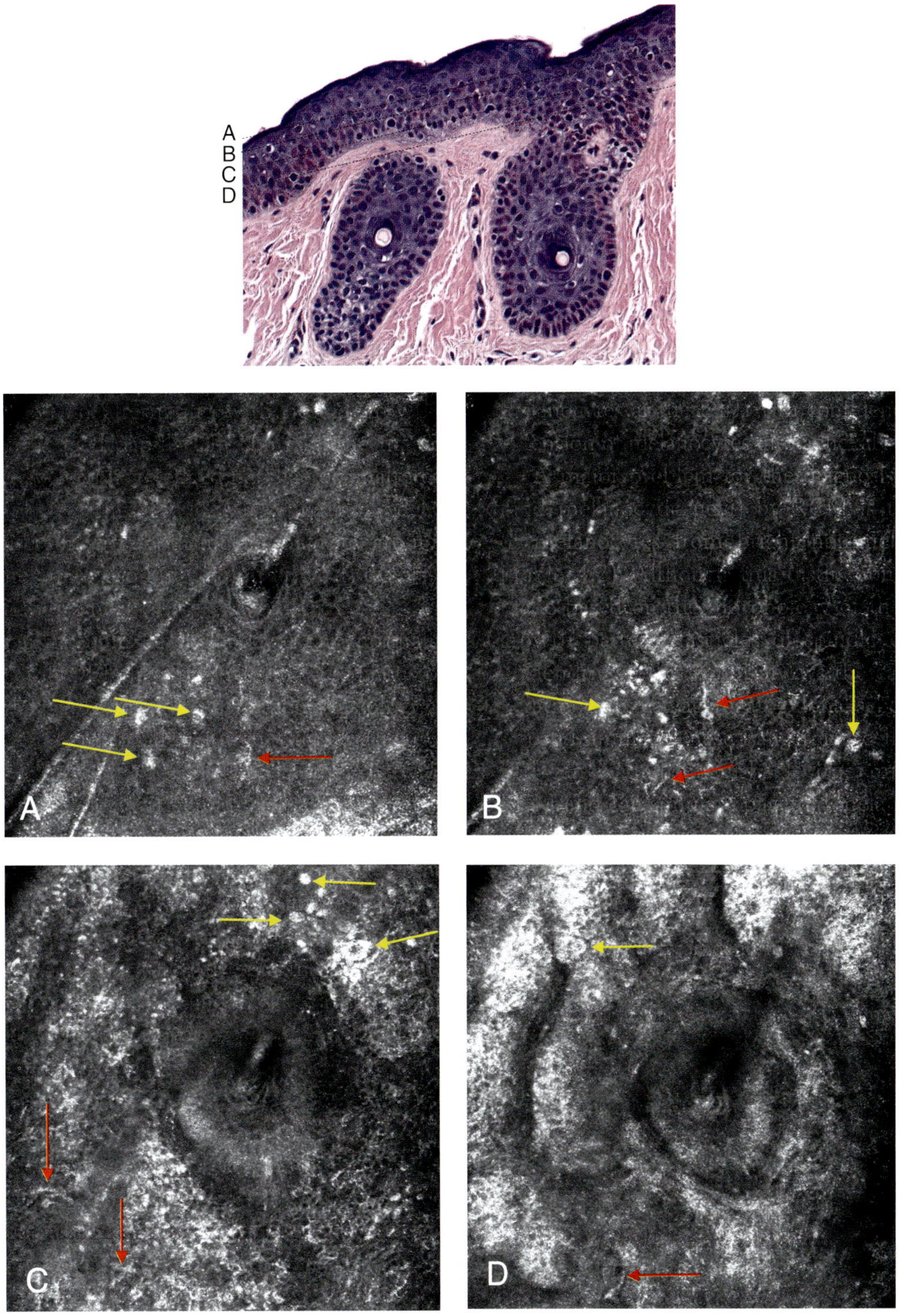

▲ **Figure 4.133** Case 1: histology (40×) shows an increased density of atypical melanocytes in the basal layer, tracking deep into the hair follicle. Horizontal lines labeled A–D indicate from where each RCM (0.5 mm × 0.5 mm) is captured: upper spinous layer (A), lower spinous layer (B), basal layer (C), and DEJ (D). Bright round (yellow arrows) and dendritic (red arrows) structures are present in the spinous layer extending into the basal layer and deep follicular epithelium. Note the preservation of the honeycomb pattern in the spinous layer.

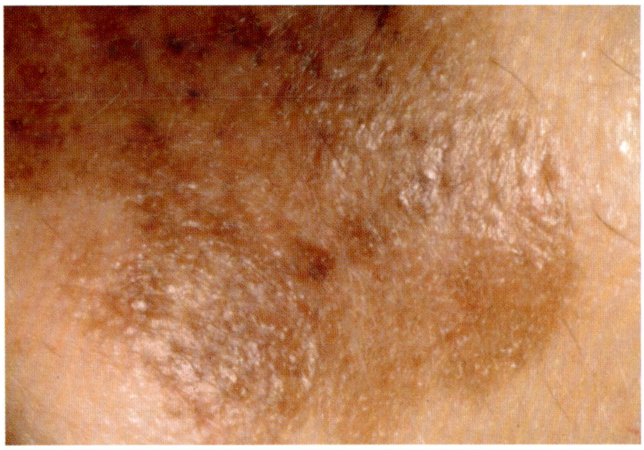
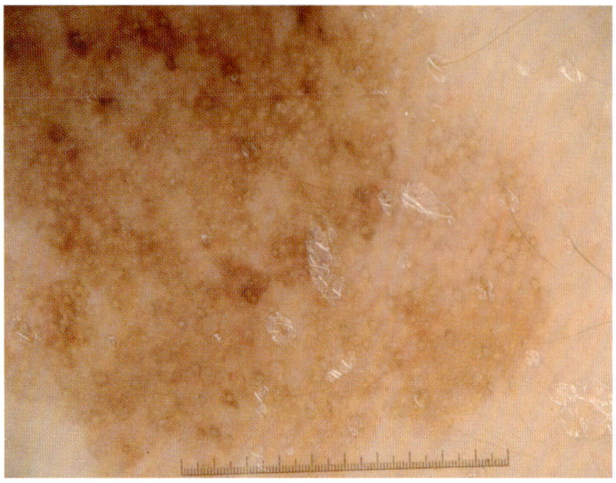

▲ **Figures 4.134, 4.135** Case 2: clinical photograph shows a poorly demarcated, asymmetric, 2 cm tan-brown patch on the left cheek. Dermoscopic photograph reveals an unevenly pigmented, poorly demarcated brown lesion with increased perifollicular pigmentation and asymmetric follicular openings.

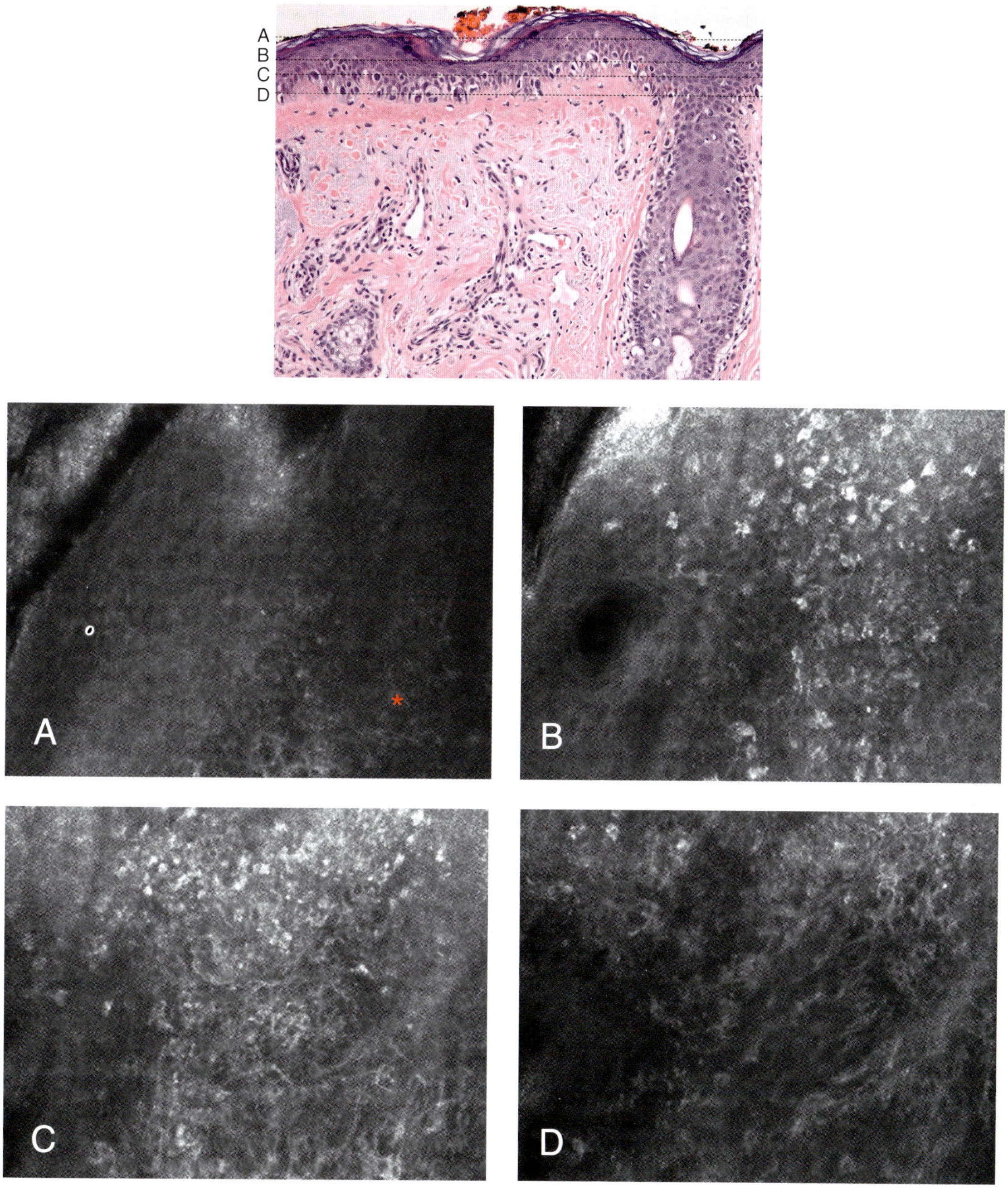

▲ **Figure 4.136** Case 2: histology (10×) shows an increased density of solitary units of melanocytes with areas of confluence. Many of the melanocytes have atypical nuclear features. The melanocytes populate the DEJ, extend along the periphery of the superficial portion of a hair follicle and a few scatter up into the suprabasal epidermis. Rete ridges are effaced and there is marked solar elastosis. Horizontal lines labeled A–D indicate from where each RCM (0.45 mm × 0.34 mm) is captured: granular/upper spinous layer (A), spinous layer (B), basal layer (C), and DEJ (D). On RCM, note the bright dendritic structures and refractile particles in the superficial epidermis (asterisk), bright stellate and round nucleated cells in the spinous and basal layers, and the destruction of the DEJ architecture.

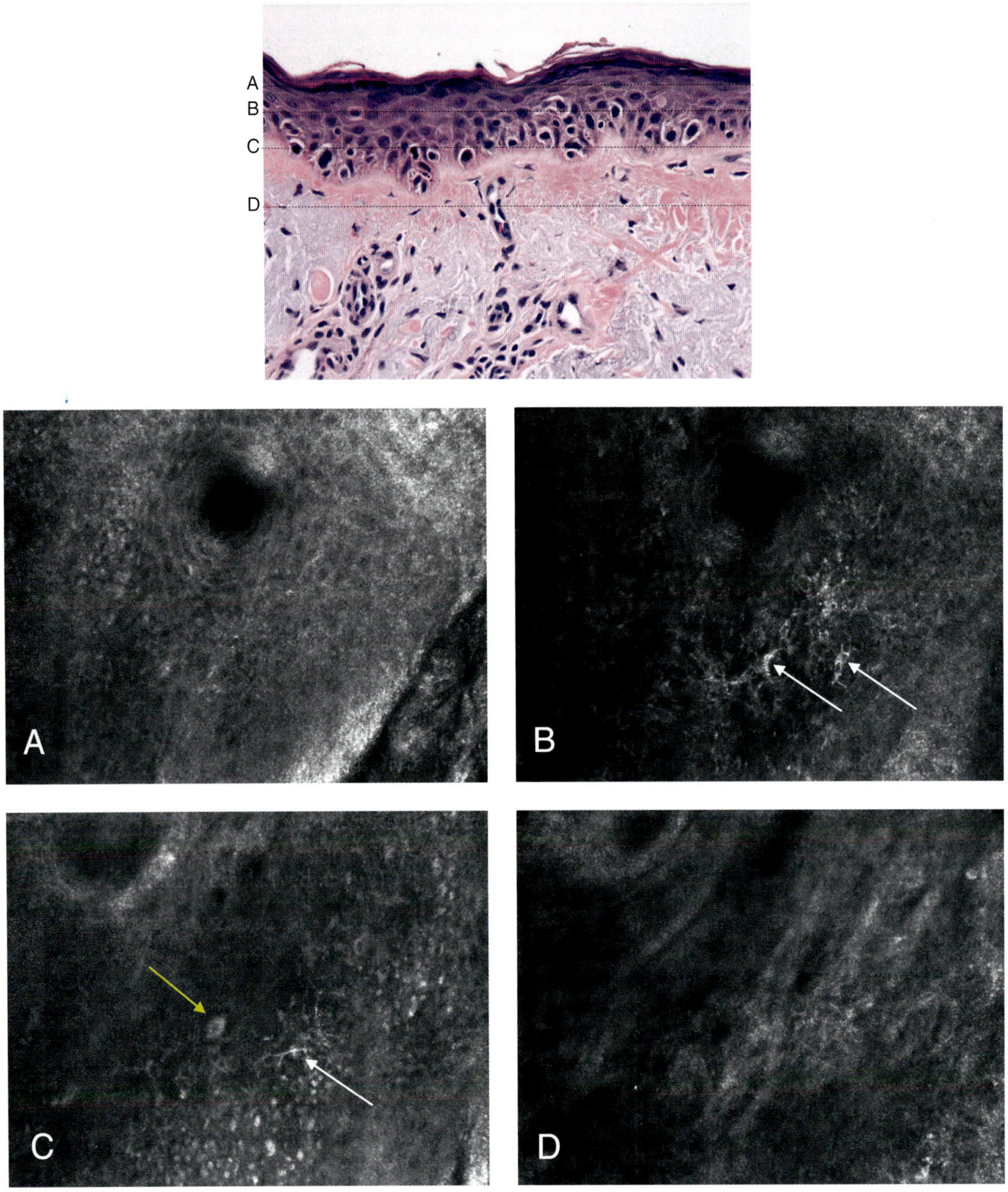

▲ **Figure 4.137** Case 2: histology (40×) shows solitary units of melanocytes at an increased density along the DEJ and slightly above it. Their nuclei are enlarged and hyperchromatic. Horizontal lines labeled A–D indicate from where each RCM (0.45 mm × 0.34 mm) is captured: granular layer (A), spinous layer (B), DEJ (C), and dermis (D). On RCM, dendritic structures and refractile particles are present at all layers of the epidermis. Bright stellate nucleated cells (white arrows) are visible in the spinous and basal layers, and bright round nucleated cells (yellow arrows) are seen in the basal layer at the DEJ level. No cells compatible with melanocytes are seen in the dermis.

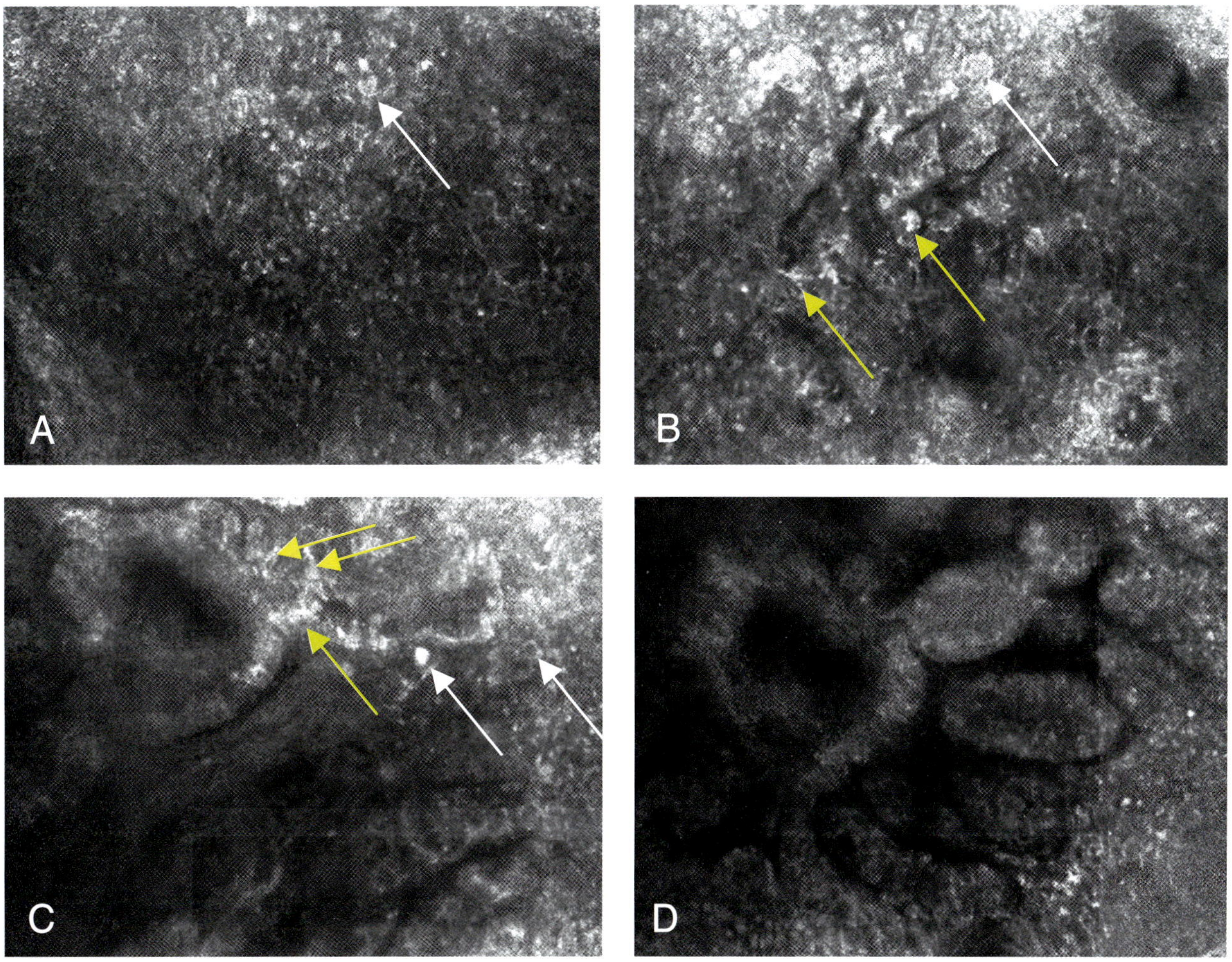

▲ **Figure 4.138** Case 2: RCM images (0.45 mm × 0.34 mm) from another area in this large lesion obtained at the upper spinous layer (A), lower spinous/basal layer (B), upper DEJ (C), and deep DEJ (D) show slightly different features. Here, bright dendritic structures and refractile particles are numerous and diffusely distort the normal epidermal architecture. An atypical, bright roundish nucleated cell (white arrow) is seen in the upper spinous layer, a few large bright stellate (yellow arrows) and round (white arrow) nucleated cells are present in the lower spinous layer, and several bright stellate (yellow arrows) and round (white arrow) cells are seen at the basal layer of the DEJ. At the level of the DEJ, the epidermal architecture is almost cerebriform, resembling a solar lentigo pattern.

AMELANOTIC MELANOMA

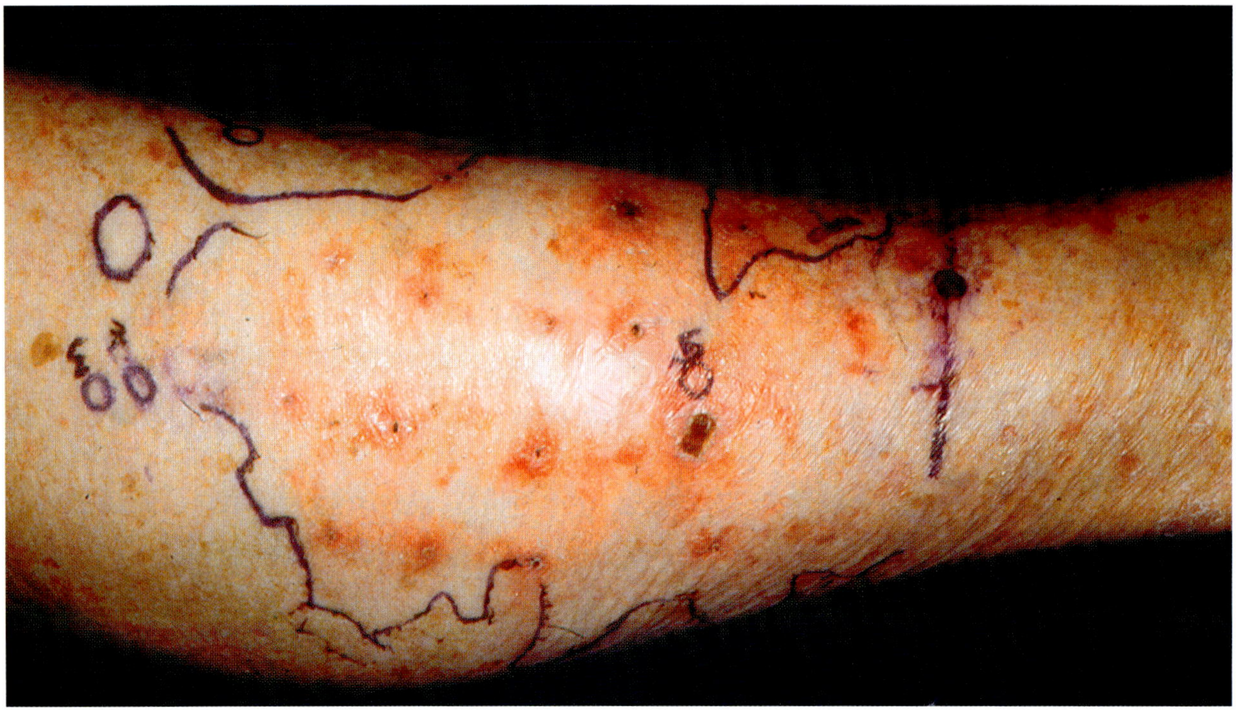

▲ **Figure 4.139** Case 1. Clinical photograph of an ill-defined, poorly demarcated patch with areas of ulceration on the lower leg.

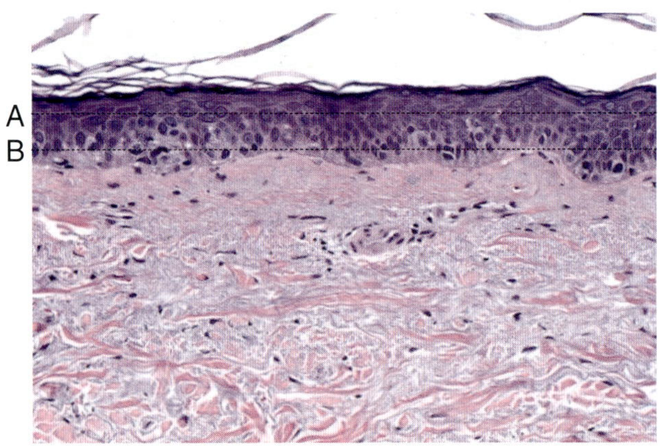

▲ **Figure 4.140** Case 1: histology (10×) shows a predominance of solitary units of melanocytes at the DEJ and above. Rete ridges are effaced. There is solar elastosis. Horizontal lines labeled A and B indicate from where each RCM mosaic (1.80 mm × 1.36 mm) is captured: spinous layer (A) and DEJ (B). RCM mosaics show scattered dendritic structures and refractile particles (white arrows) within a disarranged epidermis, a stellate cell (red arrow) in the spinous layer, and scattered large round nucleated cells (yellow arrows) at the DEJ.

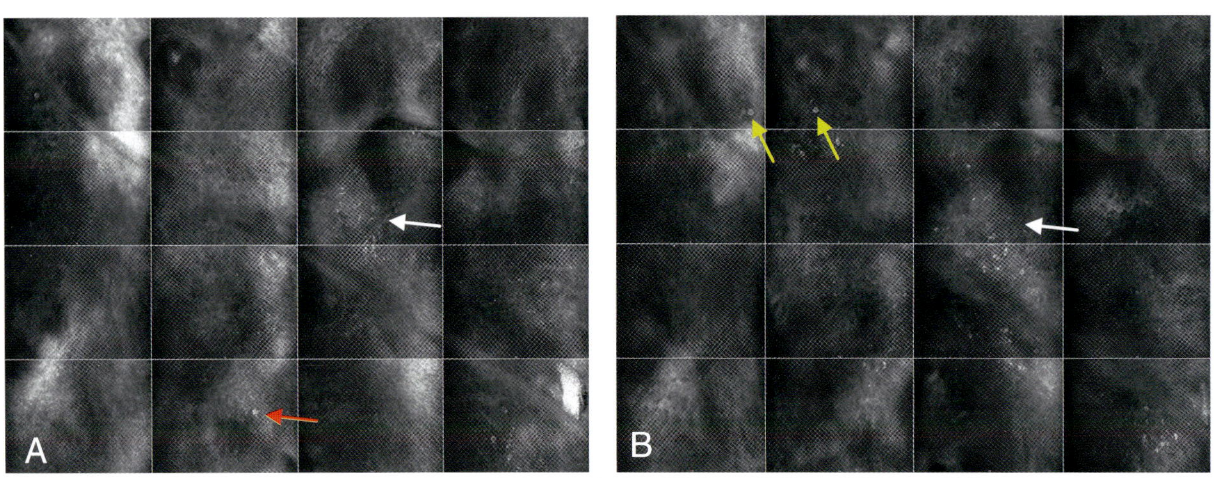

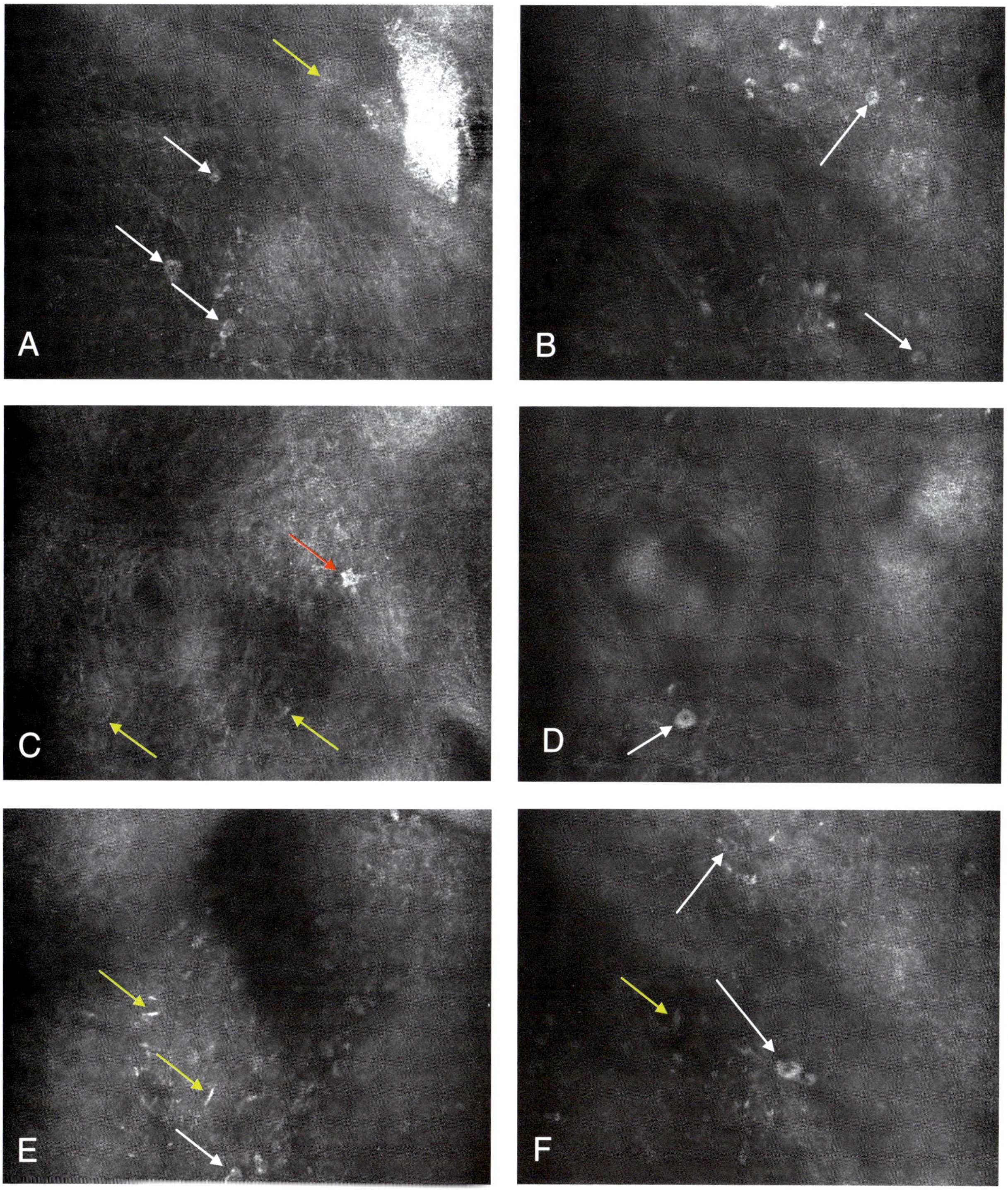

▲ **Figure 4.141** Case 1: RCM images (0.45 mm × 0.34 mm) taken at sequentially deeper levels (A–F), from the upper spinous layer to the DEJ, show large nucleated round bright cells (white arrows), dendritic structures (yellow arrows), and a bright stellate cell (red arrow). These images demonstrate that, despite the unspecific clinical appearance, atypical melanocytes can be seen on RCM.

CHAPTER 4e

Blue nevus

Marco Ardigo and Melissa Gill

Blue nevus is a dermal proliferation of pigmented dendritic melanocytes (Figures 4.144, 4.146, 4.148, 4.150, 4.154, 4.156).[1] Prevalence varies among races, suggesting a genetic predisposition; blue nevus can be identified in about 3–5% of adult Asians, 1–2% of adult Caucasians, and only rarely in blacks.[2] Blue nevus usually appears in childhood and adolescence, but it can develop at any age. Clinically, it is a small (<1 cm), well-circumscribed, blue-gray or black plaque or dome-shaped papule (Figures 4.142, 4.152). It usually occurs as a solitary lesion on the head, neck, sacral region, or dorsal aspect of the hand or foot.[3] In most cases, after a thorough history and physical examination, the diagnosis of blue nevus can be made easily. Occasionally, however, blue nevus can simulate hemangioma, basal cell carcinoma, primary melanoma, or metastatic melanoma. Dermoscopy may aid in the diagnosis of blue nevus, revealing well circumscribed, homogeneous, confluent, blue-gray to blue-black pigmentation that fades into the surrounding skin (Figures 4.143, 4.153). Moreover, identification of focal pigmented network, globules, streaks, vessels, or signs of regression on dermoscopic examination suggests the possibility of a nodular primary or metastatic melanoma.[2]

Findings on reflectance confocal microscopy (RCM) of blue nevus are subtle as the lesion occurs in the dermis. RCM shows a normal epidermal honeycomb pattern and normal dermal papillary rings or, in the case of sun-damaged skin, unaltered epidermis as compared to surrounding non-lesional skin (Figures 4.145, 4.147, 4.155). Within the dermis, brightly refractile dendritic cells are identified between moderately refractile collagen bundles, corresponding to pigmented dendritic melanocytes in a variably fibrotic stroma on histology (Figures 4.149, 4.157).[1] Melanophages, which may also be present in blue nevi, appear as scattered brightly refractile, large, plump, polygonal bright cells in the dermis on RCM (Figures 4.149, 4.151).[1] RCM examination of blue nevi is helpful when characteristic features are identified, but this imaging modality may miss deeper lesions entirely; thus, a normal RCM examination of a suspected blue nevus should always be considered non-diagnostic.

Key RCM features of blue nevus

- Normal/unaltered epidermis
- Brightly refractile, dendritic cells between collagen bundles in the dermis
- Scattered plump bright cells (melanophages) in the dermis

REFERENCES

1. Zembowicz A, Mihm MC. Dermal dendritic melanocytic proliferations: an update. Histopathology 2004; 45(5):433–51.

2. Katz B, Rao B, Marghoob A. Blue nevus/combined nevus. In: Marghoob AA, Braun RP, Kopf AW, eds. Atlas of Dermoscopy. Abingdon, UK: Taylor & Francis; 2005: 188.

3. Barnhill RL, Llewellyn K. Benign melanocytic neoplasms. Blue nevus and its variants. In: Bolognia JL, Jorizzo JL, Rapini RP, eds. Dermatology. London: Mosby; 2003: 1766.

BLUE NEVUS

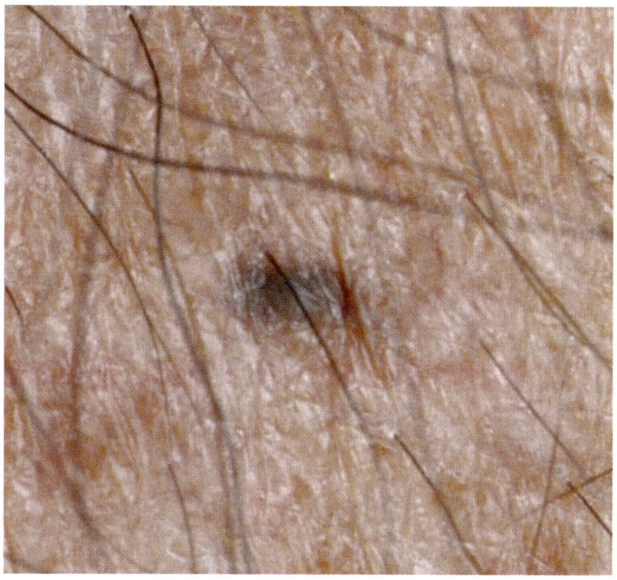

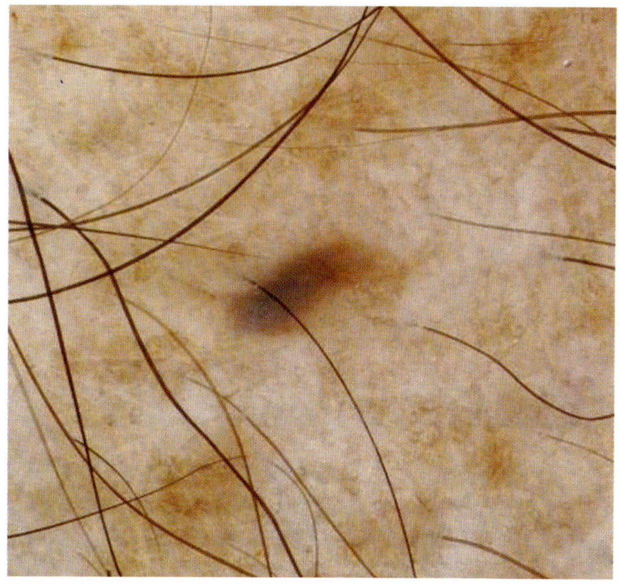

▲ **Figures 4.142, 4.143** Case 1: clinical photograph of a well-defined, blue-gray, 2 mm × 4 mm macule on the forearm of an 83-year-old man. Dermoscopy reveals homogeneous, confluent, blue-gray pigmentation that fades into the surrounding skin.

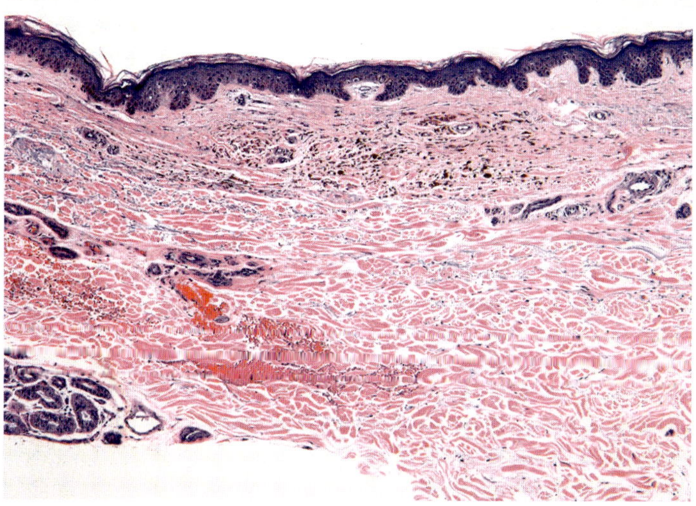

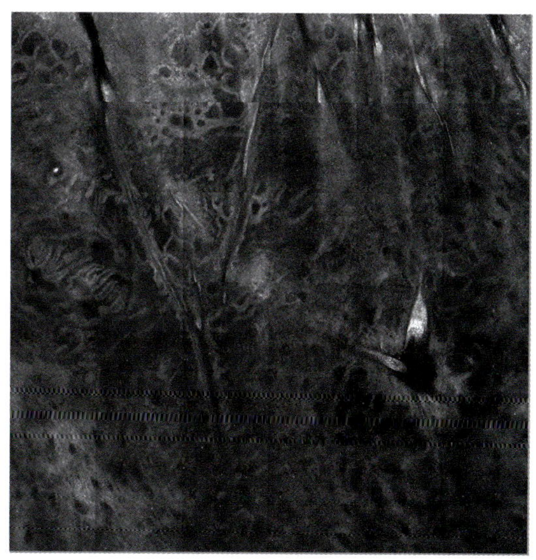

▲ **Figures 4.144, 4.145** Case 1: histology (10×) shows an entirely dermal lesion composed of pigmented cells in a fibrotic stroma. The epidermis notably lacks a melanocytic proliferation. RCM mosaic (3 mm × 3 mm) at the level of the dermal–epidermal junction/papillary dermis likewise finds no evidence of an intraepidermal melanocytic proliferation.

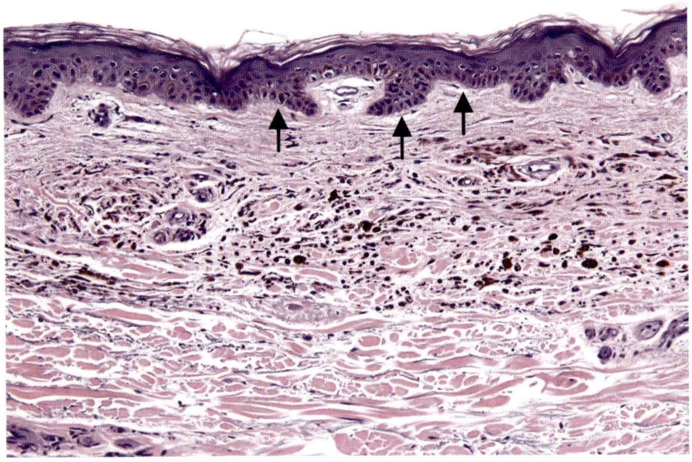

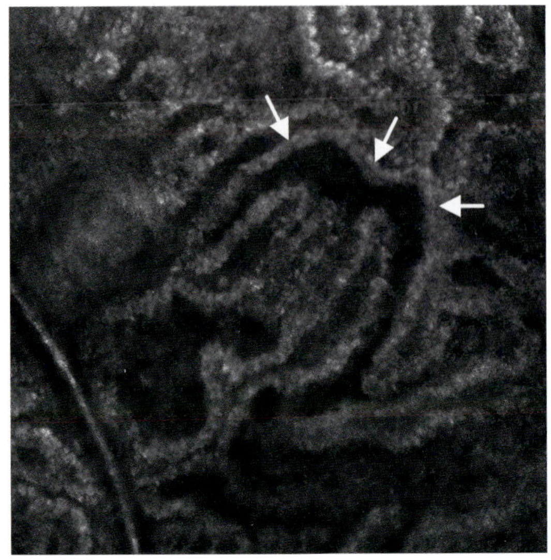

▲ **Figures 4.146, 4.147** Case 1: actinic damage, including hyperkeratosis, slight keratinocytic atypia, variable hyperpigmentation of the basal layer, and alteration of the normal rete ridge pattern (black arrows) is evident in the epidermis overlying the lesion on histology (20×). The same features are seen on RCM (0.5 mm × 0.5 mm) at the level of the dermal–epidermal junction as elongated dermal papillary rings with polymorphic, undulating contours (white arrows) and variation in refractility, size, and shape of basal keratinocytes.

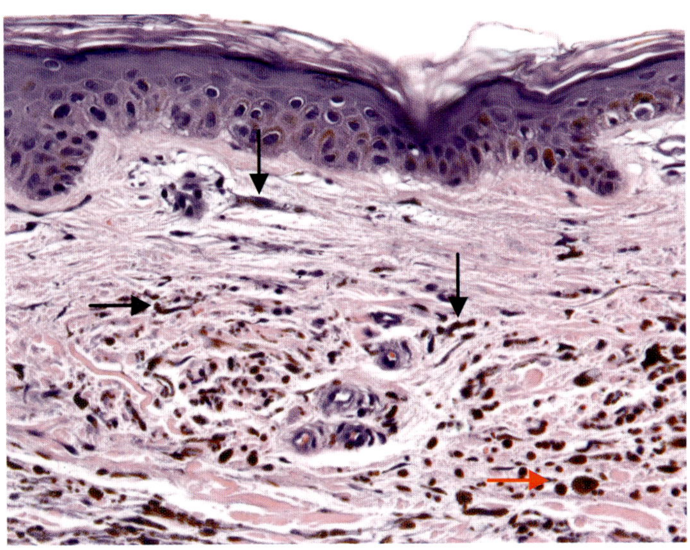

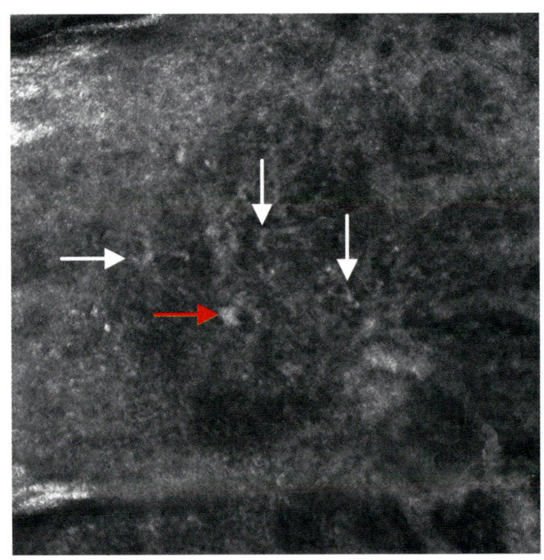

▲ **Figures 4.148, 4.149** Case 1: on histology (40×), the dermal tumor is composed of dendritic melanocytes (black arrows) in a variably fibrotic stroma, corresponding to bright dendritic cells (white arrows) between moderately refractile collagen bundles on RCM (0.5 mm × 0.5 mm). Melanophages appear as scattered large, triangular-to-polygonal bright cells (red arrows) in the dermis.

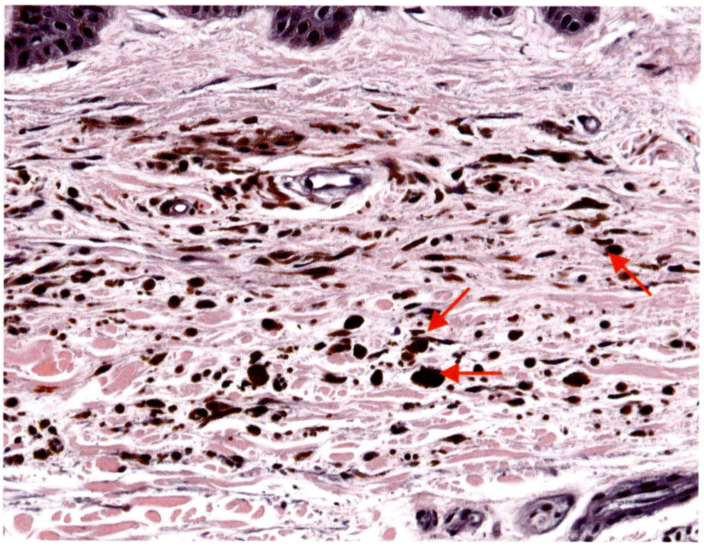

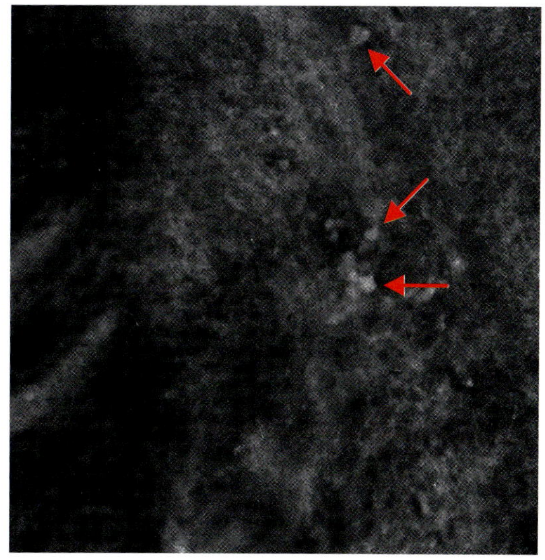

▲ **Figures 4.150, 4.151** Case 1: numerous melanophages are present singly and in clusters (red arrows), on histology (40×) and RCM (0.5 mm × 0.5 mm).

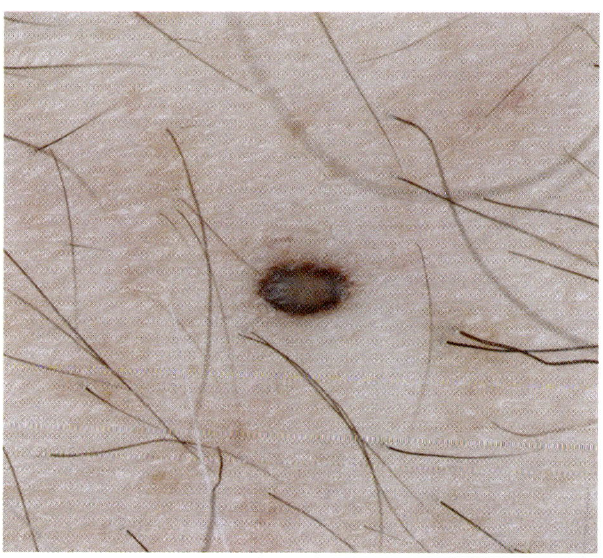

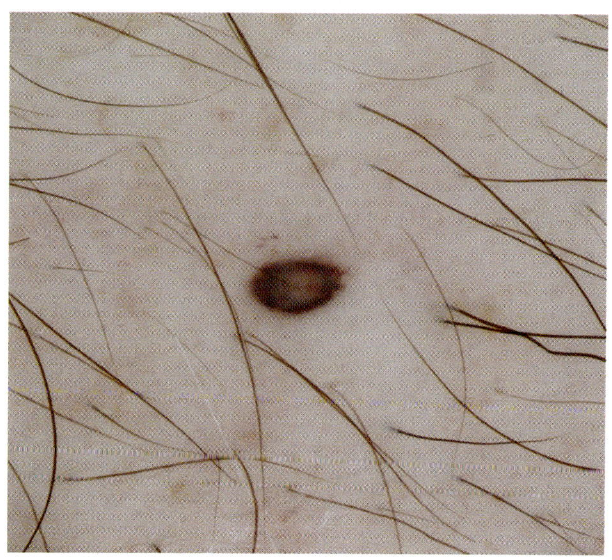

▲ **Figures 4.152, 4.153** Case 2: clinical photograph of a 4 mm blue nevus from the lower back presenting as a dome-shaped papule with a blue-gray periphery and light gray central area. Dermoscopy reveals a well-circumscribed lesion with homogeneous blue-gray peripheral pigmentation and confluent central pallor.

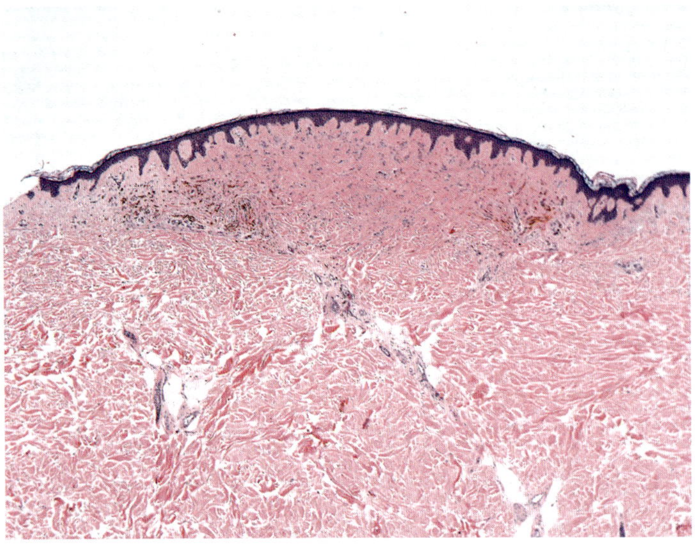
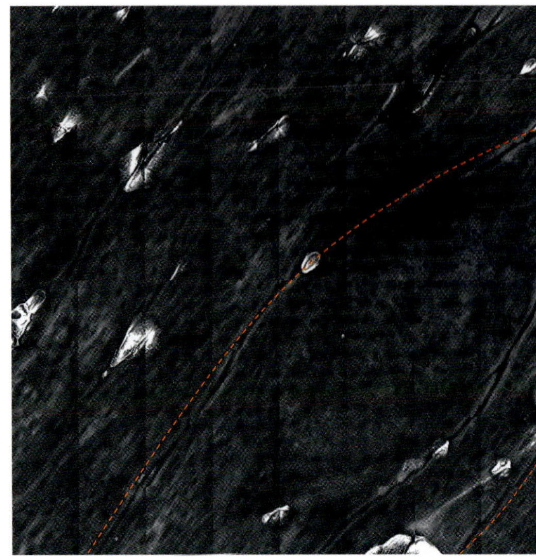

▲ **Figures 4.154, 4.155** Case 2: on histology (4×), the dome-shaped surface contour is evident. The tumor appears as a wedge-shaped, pigmented lesion with central fibrosis in the upper dermis. As the lesion is elevated and fibrotic, thus not compressible, one can identify the contour of the nevus (red dashed line) on RCM mosaic (4 mm × 4 mm): the lesion is seen at the level of the dermal–epidermal junction, allowing for visualization of dermal papillary rings, while the surrounding normal skin is seen at the level of the lower stratum spinosum, allowing for only occasional visualization of superficial tips of dermal papillae. Notably, no melanocytic proliferation is identified in the epidermis on RCM.

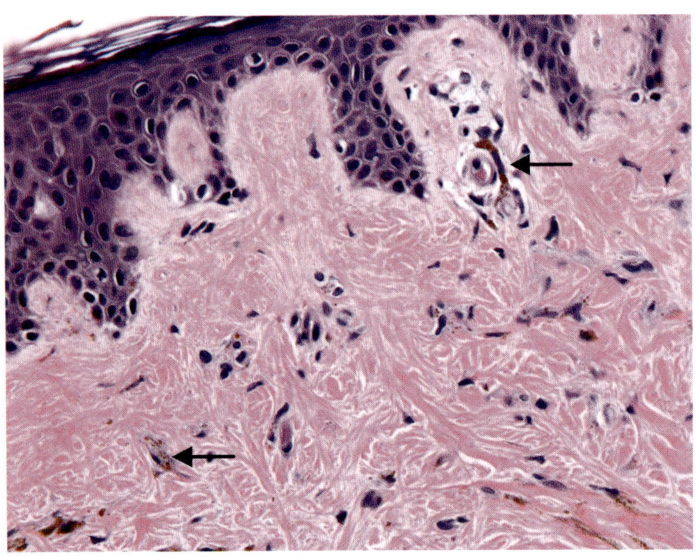
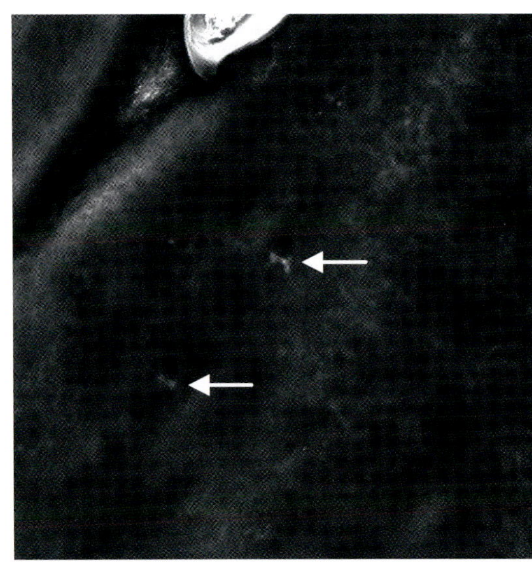

▲ **Figures 4.156, 4.157** Case 2: on histology (40×), the superficial portion of the nevus shows sparse, variably pigmented, dendritic melanocytes (black arrows) embedded in a stroma with haphazard fibrosis. Corresponding RCM (0.5 mm × 0.5 mm) of the upper dermis shows scattered brightly refractile dendritic cells (white arrows) in a stroma composed of moderately refractile, haphazardly arranged bundles.

CHAPTER 4f

Spitz nevus

Giovanni Pellacani, Caterina Longo, Sara Bassoli, and Stefania Seidenari

First described by Sophie Spitz,[1] epithelioid and/or spindled cell nevi share some clinical and histologic features with melanomas. Subsequently, a deeply pigmented melanocytic lesion, predominantly in young adults on the lower extremities, was described.[2] Since the clinicopathologic distinction between pigmented Spitz nevus and Reed nevus is highly controversial,[3] the term spindle and/or epithelioid cell nevus[4] and the term Spitz nevus have been employed as unifying definitions for this diagnostic category. Usually, Spitz nevi appear clinically as solitary, firm, dome-shaped, round-to-oval papules or nodules, in a wide spectrum of colors, including red, tan, or dark brown, located on the lower extremities and the face (Figures 4.158, 4.164).[5] The lesion is frequently observed in children, although more than half of the cases occur in patients >14 years old.[6] Dermoscopy, which enables the in-vivo observation of subsurface structures, increases the diagnostic accuracy for Spitz nevi, identifying characteristic features which correlate with specific histologic findings (Figures 4.159, 4.165).[7,8] However, some cases are still impossible to distinguish from dysplastic nevi or melanomas.[9,10] Histologically, these lesions are defined by a set of characteristic features, including several features which overlap with melanoma. In spite of their bizarre histology, Spitz nevi can usually be differentiated from melanomas by well-demarcated lateral margins, the presence of a distinctive, symmetrical pattern of growth, maturation of cells with increasing depth, uniform nuclei, and by the absence of atypical mitoses and deep dermal invasion.[11]

Findings on reflectance confocal microscopy (RCM) of Spitz nevi[12,13] include the presence of 'pagetoid' cells within the superficial layers of the epidermis in approximately half of the cases. In comparison to melanoma, pagetoid melanocytosis is usually less abundant, predominantly located in the center of the lesion, and constituted by small, elongated cells with short dendritic-like branches.[14] Moreover, thin elongated cells with peripheral dendritic processes at the extremities are frequently observed in the basal and suprabasal layers, corresponding to spindle cells on histology (Figures 4.162, 4.163). A rim of dense nests regularly distributed at the lesion's perimeter is observed in many cases and directly correlates with the peripheral globules seen on dermoscopy and the peripheral melanocytic nests sharply demarcating the lesion's border on histology (Figures 4.160, 4.161, 4.165–4.169). Numerous large melanocytic dense clusters are found throughout the whole lesion in Spitz nevi, showing a globular appearance on dermoscopy (Figures 4.165–4.171).[15] Spitz nevi presenting a homogeneous diffuse pigmentation and/or pigment network on dermoscopy are predominantly characterized by non-edged papillae at the dermal–epidermal junction (DEJ), sometimes with the presence of atypical cells within the epidermal basal layer.[16] In a small proportion of cases, the lesions show roundish rings of refractive cells surrounding dermal papillae, called edged papillae, corresponding to regular rete ridges with elongated cristae on histology.[16] Numerous plump bright cells, corresponding to melanophages, may be seen in the dermis and blood vessels and are frequently observable in the upper dermis.[17] The asymmetric silhouette, which usually makes distinction from melanoma impossible on dermoscopy, corresponds in some cases to melanophages aggregated at one pole of the lesion. In nodular lesions, large confluent irregular clusters of cells, non-homogeneous in shape and reflectivity, are observed in the upper dermis and correspond to ovoid nests composed of densely clustered large epithelioid cells on histology. In conclusion, RCM enables the in-vivo evaluation of cytologic and architectural features of Spitz nevi, which correlate with histology. Nevertheless, the limited imaging depth prevents complete examination of the dermal component for features such as deep mitoses and cellular maturation, and does not permit a definite differentiation from melanoma in most cases.

Key RCM features of Spitz nevus

- 'Pagetoid' melanocytosis, predominantly constituted by small dendritic cells
- Rim of dense cell clusters at the periphery
- Dense cell clusters distributed throughout the lesion
- Non-edged papillae and atypical cells in the basal layer and dermal–epidermal junction
- Regular roundish edged papillae
- Increased vascularity
- Large confluent irregular dermal clusters of reflective polygonal cells

REFERENCES

1. Spitz S. Melanomas of childhood. Am J Pathol 1948; 24: 591–609.
2. Reed RJ, Ichinose H, Clark WH Jr et al. Common and uncommon melanocytic nevi and borderline melanomas. Semin Oncol 1975; 2:119–47.
3. Barnhill RL, Barnhill MA, Berwick M et al. The histologic spectrum of pigmented spindle cell nevus: a review of 120 cases with emphasis on atypical variants. Hum Pathol 1991; 22:52–8.
4. Kernen JA, Ackerman LV. Spindle cell nevi and epithelioid cell nevi (so-called juvenile melanomas) in children and adults: a clinicopathological study of 27 cases. Cancer 1960; 13:612–25.
5. Dal Pozzo V, Benelli C, Restano L et al. Clinical review of 247 case records of Spitz nevus (epithelioid cell and/or spindle cell nevus). Dermatology 1997; 194:20–5.
6. Weedon D, Little JH. Spindle and epithelioid cell nevi in children and adults. A review of 211 cases of the Spitz nevus. Cancer 1977; 40:217–25.
7. Ferrara G, Argenziano G, Soyer HP et al. The spectrum of Spitz nevi: a clinicopathologic study of 83 cases. Arch Dermatol 2005; 141:1381–7.
8. Steiner A, Pehamberger H, Binder M et al. Pigmented Spitz nevi: improvement of the diagnostic accuracy by epiluminescence microscopy. J Am Acad Dermatol 1992; 27:697–701.
9. Argenziano G, Scalvenzi M, Staibano S et al. Dermatoscopic pitfalls in differentiating pigmented Spitz naevi from cutaneous melanomas. Br J Dermatol 1999; 141:788–93.
10. Pellacani G, Cesinaro AM, Seidenari S. Morphological features of Spitz naevus as observed by digital videomicroscopy. Acta Derm Venereol 2000; 80:117–21.
11. Ackerman AB, Magana-Garcia M. Naming acquired melanocytic nevi. Unna's, Miescher's, Spitz's, Clark's. Am J Dermatopathol 1990; 12:193–209.
12. Pellacani G, Cesinaro AM, Grana C et al. In vivo confocal scanning laser microscopy of pigmented Spitz nevi: comparison of in vivo confocal images with dermoscopy and routine histopathology. J Am Acad Dermatol 2004; 51:371–6.
13. Pellacani G, Cesinaro AM, Seidenari S. Reflectance-mode confocal microscopy of pigmented skin lesions – improvement in melanoma diagnostic specificity. J Am Acad Dermatol 2005; 53:979–85.
14. Pellacani G, Cesinaro AM, Seidenari S. Reflectance-mode confocal microscopy for the in vivo characterization of pagetoid melanocytosis in melanomas and nevi. J Invest Dermatol 2005; 125:532–7.
15. Pellacani G, Cesinaro AM, Seidenari S. In vivo assessment of melanocytic nests in nevi and melanomas by reflectance confocal microscopy. Mod Pathol 2005; 18:469–74.
16. Pellacani G, Cesinaro AM, Longo C et al. Microscopic in vivo description of cellular architecture of dermoscopic pigment network in nevi and melanomas. Arch Dermatol 2005; 141:147–54.
17. Busam KJ, Charles C, Lee G et al. Morphologic features of melanocytes, pigmented keratinocytes, and melanophages by in vivo confocal scanning laser microscopy. Mod Pathol 2001; 14:862–8.

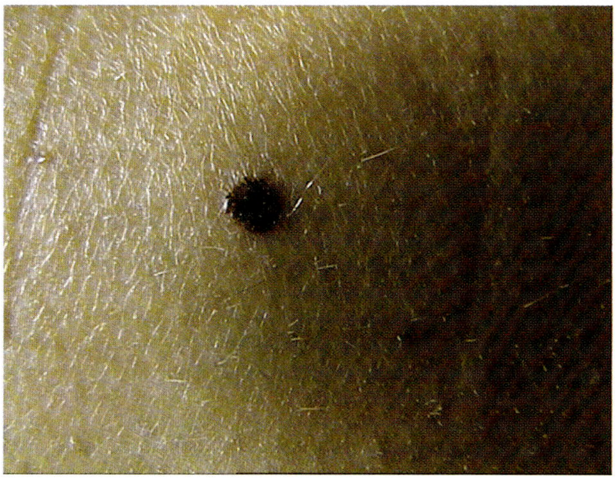

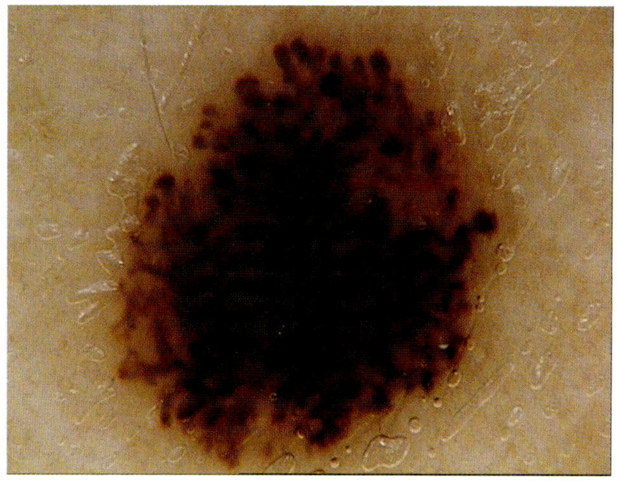

▲ **Figures 4.158, 4.159** Case 1: clinical photograph of a 5 mm Spitz nevus on the lower limb of a 25-year-old woman shows well-defined borders, dome shape, and brown color. The corresponding dermoscopic photograph shows the typical starburst pattern.

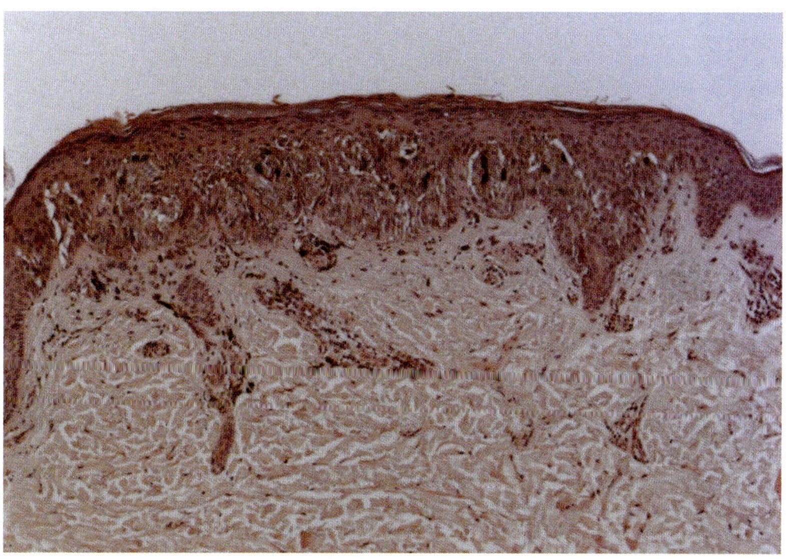

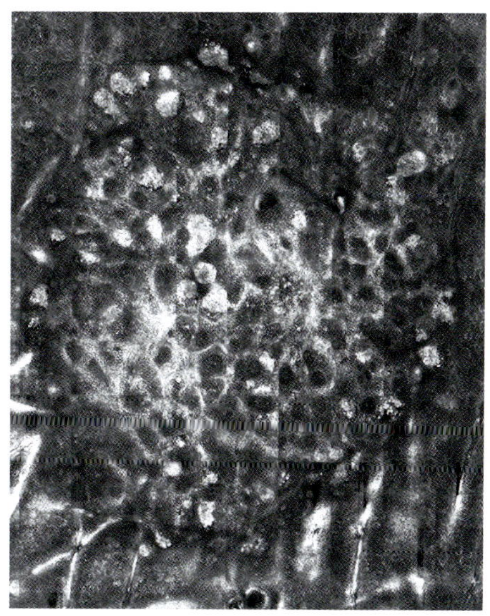

▲ **Figures 4.160, 4.161** Case 1: histology (5×) shows a compound Spitz nevus. RCM mosaic (4.5 mm × 5.5 mm) at the level of the DEJ reveals dense cell clusters, particularly evident at the periphery.

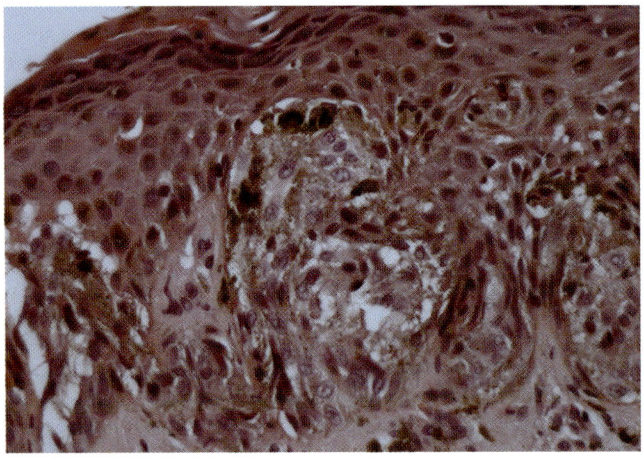

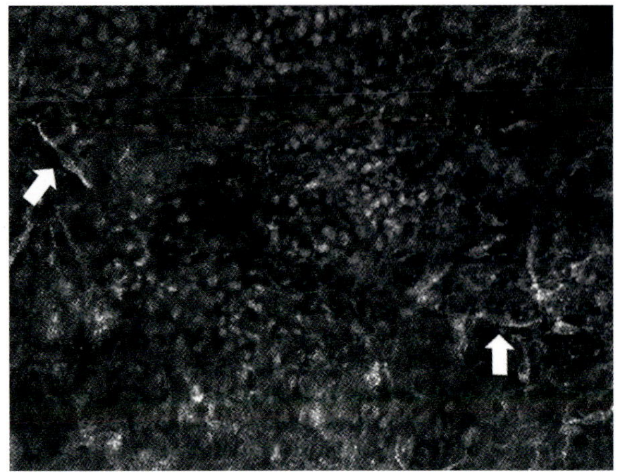

▲ **Figures 4.162, 4.163** Case 1: histology (20×) shows spindle cells located at the DEJ, often clustered into nests. RCM image (0.45 mm × 0.34 mm) at superficial levels reveals thin, elongated cells with dendritic processes at the extremities (white arrows).

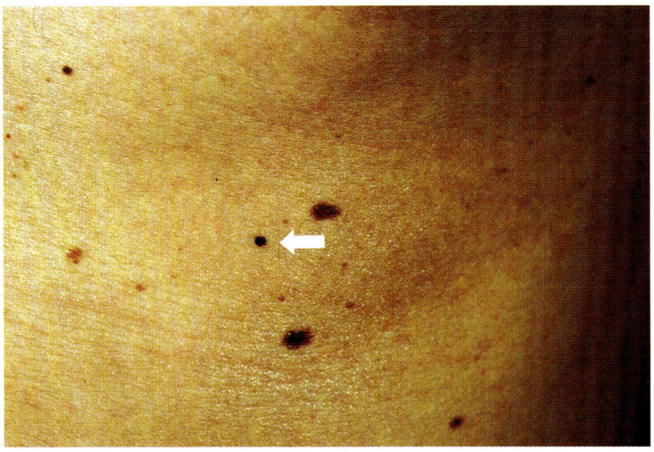

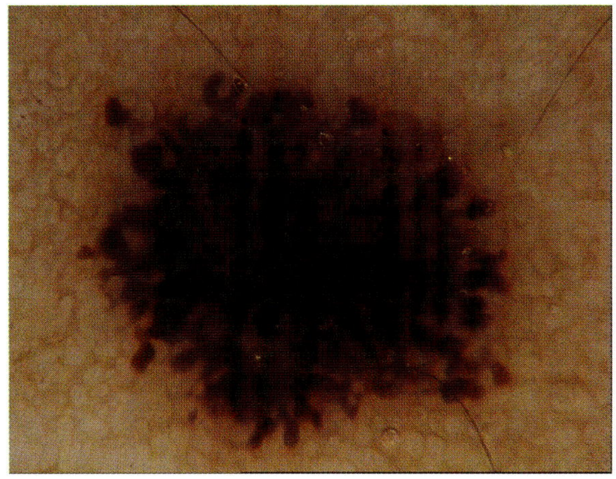

▲ **Figures 4.164, 4.165** Case 2: clinical photograph of a 4.5 mm darkly pigmented Spitz nevus (arrow) on the trunk of a 32-year-old man. Dermoscopic photograph shows this Spitz nevus is characterized by pigmented peripheral globules.

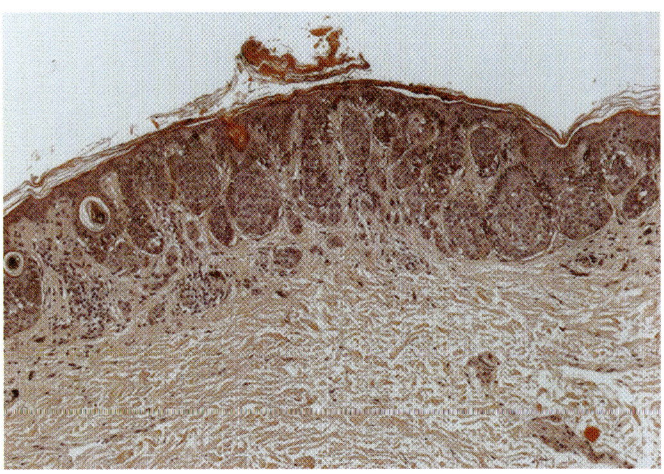

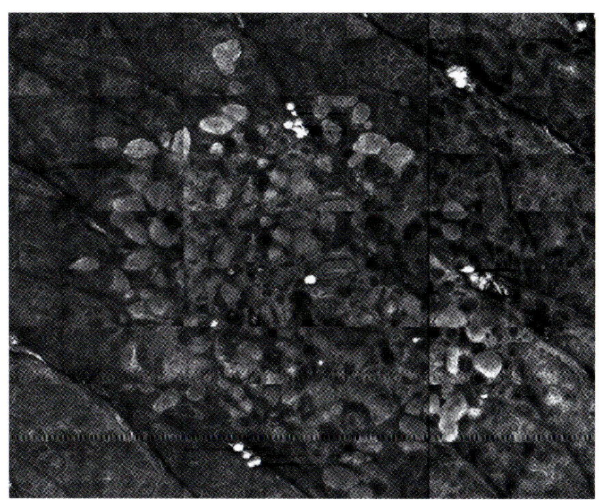

▲ **Figures 4.166, 4.167** Case 2: histology (5×) shows a compound Spitz nevus composed of regular nests of melanocytes mainly at the tips of rete ridges and within the dermis. The surrounding epidermis is highly pigmented and there is overlying pigmented parakeratosis. RCM mosaic (3.5 mm × 2.8 mm) at the level of the DEJ captures the entire lesion, which is predominantly constituted by dense cell clusters.

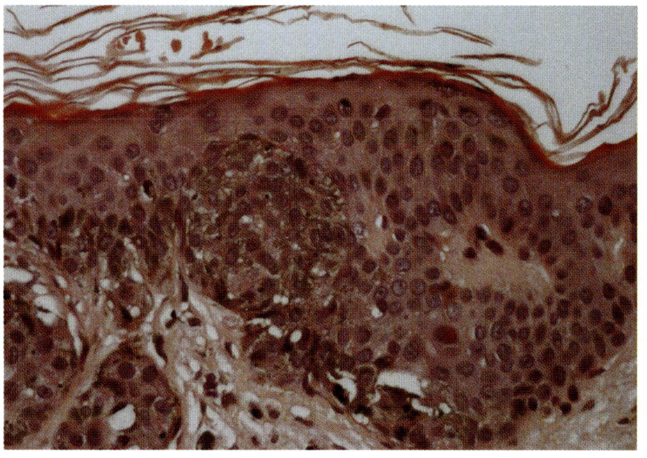
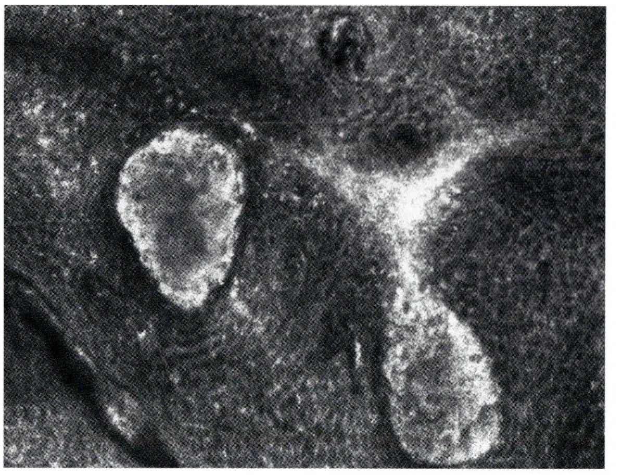

▲ **Figures 4.168, 4.169** Case 2: histology (20×) from the periphery of the lesion shows melanocytic nests sharply demarcating the border. Corresponding RCM (0.45 mm × 0.34 mm) reveals peripheral regular dense cell clusters immediately below the epidermal basal layer corresponding to the peripheral nests on histology. Of note, surrounding these nests a preserved honeycomb pattern of the spinous layer is seen.

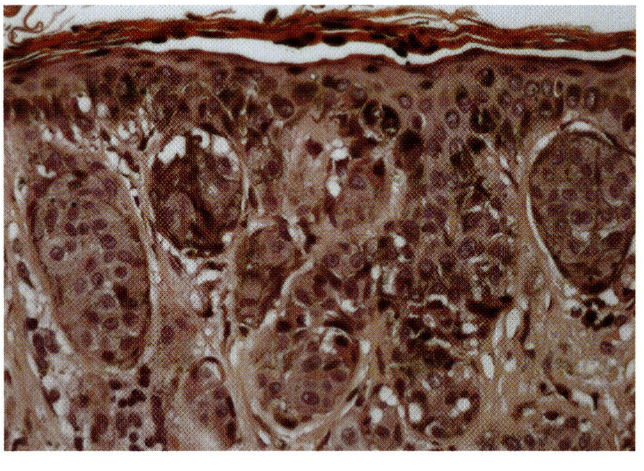
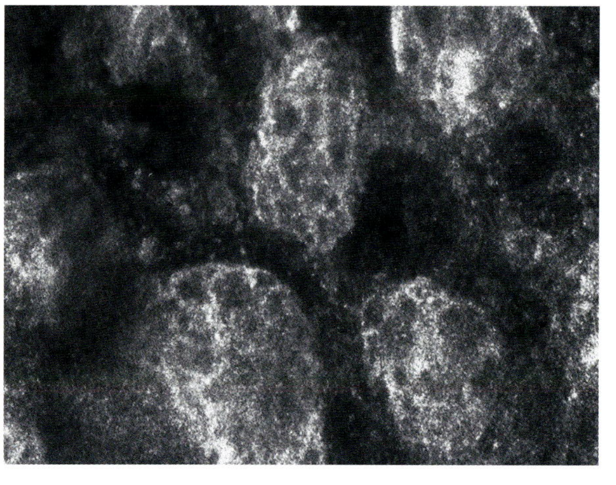

▲ **Figures 4.170, 4.171** Case 2: histology (20×) from the center shows well-defined nests located both at the DEJ and in the upper dermis. RCM (0.45 mm × 0.34 mm) at the superficial dermis shows numerous medium-to-large melanocytic dense nests throughout the whole lesion.

CHAPTER 5a

Trichoepithelioma

Marco Ardigo and Melissa Gill

Trichoepithelioma (TE) is a benign adnexal tumor of follicular germinative derivation.[1] Although trichoepitheliomas can occur singly and sporadically, most are multiple and seen in patients with multiple familial trichoepithelioma (MFT) or Brooke–Spiegler syndrome (BSS).[1,2] Both syndromes are inherited in an autosomal dominant fashion and are caused by mutations in the CYLD tumor suppressor gene on chromosome 16q12-q13.[3] BSS is characterized by a combination of trichoepitheliomas, cylindromas, and spiradenomas, whereas MFT is characterized by the development of trichoepitheliomas alone.[2] Trichoepitheliomas develop in early adulthood and gradually increase in size and number over time. Clinically, they appear as firm, skin-colored papules on the central face (Figure 5.1).[2] On dermoscopy, TE appears as a well-circumscribed homogeneous whitish papule. Trichoepitheliomas may bear superficial telangiectasias, more clearly seen on dermoscopy, leading to misdiagnosis as basal cell carcinoma (Figure 5.2).[4]

Desmoplastic trichoepithelioma (DTE), originally called sclerosing epithelial hamartoma, is a non-familial variant of TE with extensive stromal sclerosis.[5] DTE is more common in women and usually presents in early adulthood. The tumor most commonly occurs on the cheek as a solitary, non-ulcerated, annular, firm, skin-colored or whitish plaque with a central depression (Figure 5.13).[6] On dermoscopy, DTE is very similar in appearance to morpheaform basal cell carcinoma, showing an ivory white, scar-like plaque with surface telangiectasias (Figure 5.14).[4]

Reflectance confocal microscopy (RCM) of TE and DTE identifies many of the features seen on histology. Mosaic images at the level of the dermis show a lesion composed of islands of tumor ramified by brightly refractile coarse collagen arranged in parallel bundles (Figures 5.4, 5.16). On RCM, TE shows tumor islands with knobby extensions composed of small, round, nucleated cells (Figures 5.6, 5.8). Variable peripheral palisading of brighter basaloid cells with oval nuclei, reminiscent of basal cell carcinoma, is identified (Figure 5.10). Tumor islands are wrapped in a brightly refractile stroma (Figure 5.8). Corresponding histology shows basaloid tumor cells arranged in islands (Figure 5.5) with branching nests and abortive hair follicle formation within a fibrotic stroma (Figure 5.3). This characteristic fibrotic stroma concentrically encases tumor islands in parallel bands, creating an 'onion skin' appearance (Figure 5.7). Occasionally, peripheral palisading of basaloid cells, mimicking basal cell carcinoma, is identified (Figure 5.9).[5,7] DTE shows similar features to TE, but has much smaller tumor cell nests and cords scattered within more abundant, brightly refractile stroma, corresponding to the histologic findings of small basaloid nests and cords tightly embedded in a sclerotic stroma (Figures 5.15–5.20).[5] Both TE and DTE show some tumor islands containing round black spaces filled with brightly refractile material, corresponding to tricholemmal horn cysts on histology (Figures 5.11, 5.12, 5.15–5.20).[4,5]

Key RCM features of trichoepithelioma

- Dermal basaloid tumor cell islands tightly wrapped in stroma
- Brightly refractile stroma arranged in parallel bundles
- Horn cysts within tumor islands

REFERENCES

1. McCalmont T. Adnexal neoplasms. In: Bolognia JL, Jorizzo JL, Rapini RP, eds. Dermatology. London: Mosby; 2003: 1738–9.
2. Lee DA, Grossman ME, Schneiderman P, Celebi JT. Genetics of skin appendage neoplasms and related syndromes. J Med Genet 2005; 42(11):811–9.
3. Bowen S, Gill M, Lee DA et al. Mutations in the CYLD gene in Brooke–Spiegler syndrome, familial cylindromatosis, and multiple familial trichoepithelioma: lack of genotype–phenotype correlation. J Invest Dermatol 2005; 124(5):919–20.
4. Ardigo M, Zieff J, Scope A et al. Dermoscopic and reflectance confocal microscope findings of trichoepithelioma. Dermatology 2007; 215:354–8.
5. Klein W, Chan E, Seykora J. Tumors of the epidermal appendages. In: Elder DE, Elenitzas R, Johnson BL Jr, Murphy GF, eds. Lever's Histopathology of the Skin. Philadelphia: Lippincott, Williams & Wilkins; 2005: 873–6.
6. Brownstein MH, Shapiro L. Desmoplastic trichoepithelioma. Cancer 1977; 40(6):2979–86.
7. Bettencourt MS, Prieto VG, Shea CR. Trichoepithelioma: a 19-year clinicopathologic re-evaluation. J Cutan Pathol 1999; 26(8):398–404.

TRICHOEPITHELIOMA

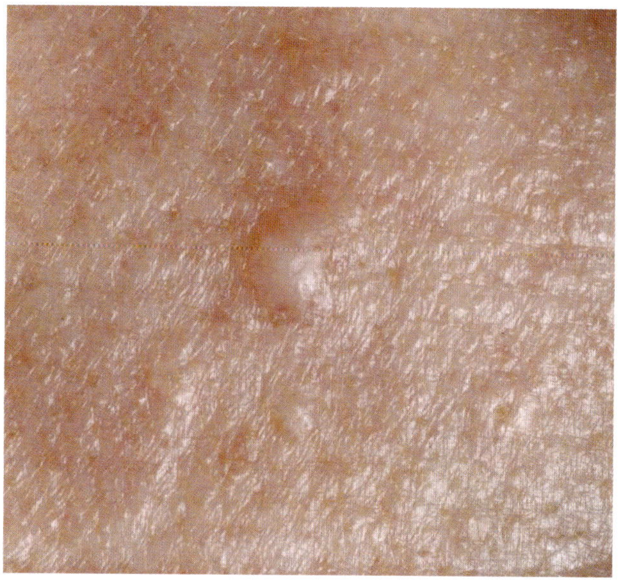

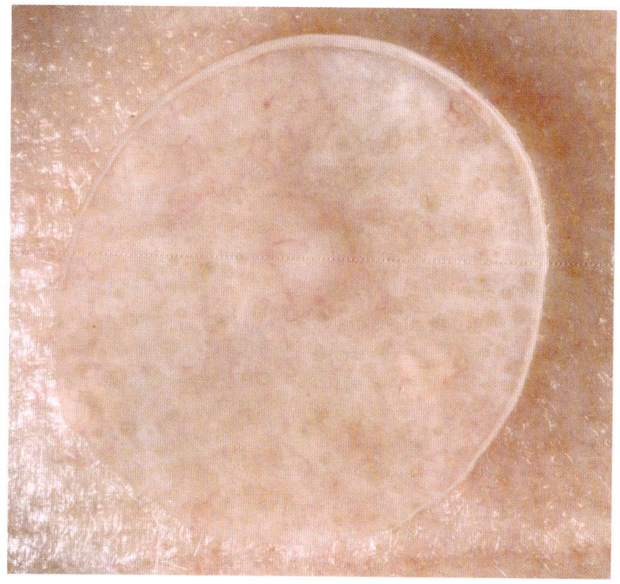

▲ **Figures 5.1, 5.2** Clinical photograph of a 3 mm, skin-colored, firm, papule on the central forehead of a 60-year-old woman with multiple familial trichoepithelioma. Dermoscopic photograph shows a lesion with a milk-white hue and a few telangiectatic surface vessels. Reproduced with permission of S. Karger AG, based from Ardigo M, Zieff J, Scope A et al. Dermoscopic and reflectance confocal microscope findings of trichoepithelioma. Dermatology 2007; 215:354–8.

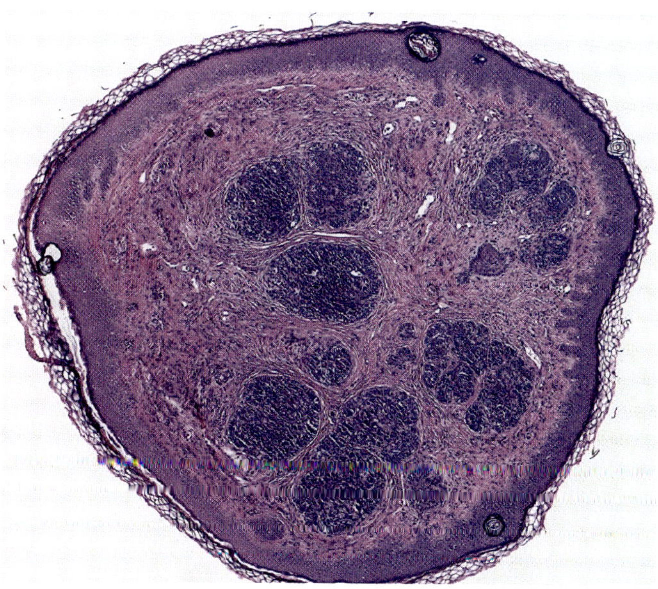

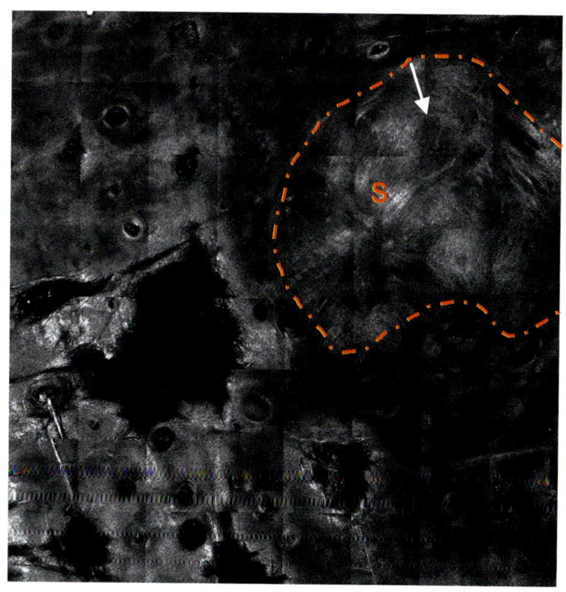

▲ **Figures 5.3, 5.4** Histology (2×, horizontal section) shows islands of basaloid tumor cells embedded in a fibrotic stroma. RCM mosaic (4 mm × 4 mm) at the level of the dermis, reveals a circumscribed lesion composed of tumor islands (white arrow within red dashed circle) in a brightly refractile stroma (S). Reproduced with permission of S. Karger AG, based from Ardigo M, Zieff J, Scope A et al. Dermoscopic and reflectance confocal microscope findings of trichoepithelioma. Dermatology 2007; 215:354–8.

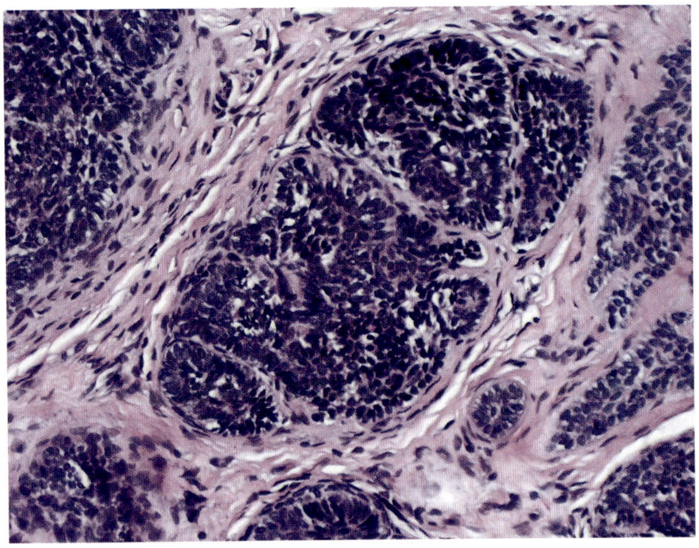

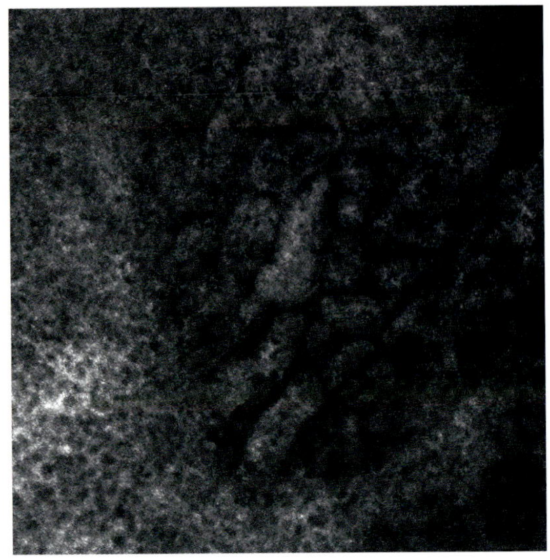

▲ **Figures 5.5, 5.6** Histology (20×) shows basaloid tumor islands composed of branching and budding nests, recapitulating follicular germs, corresponding to small round tumor cells arranged in islands with knobby extensions on RCM (0.5 mm × 0.5 mm).

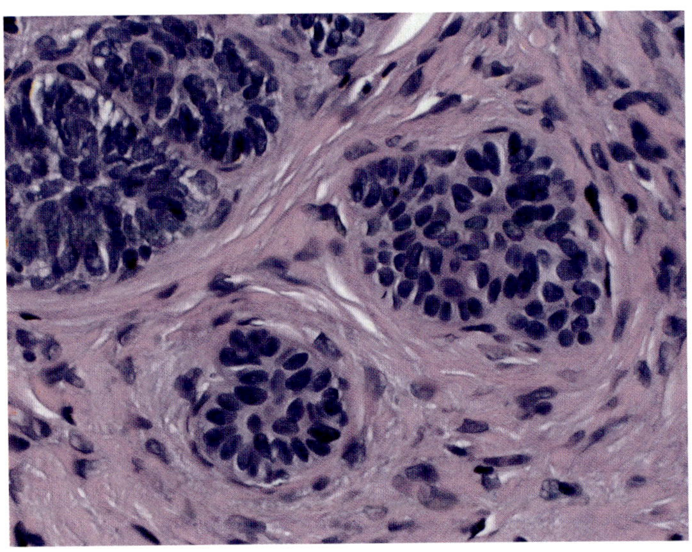

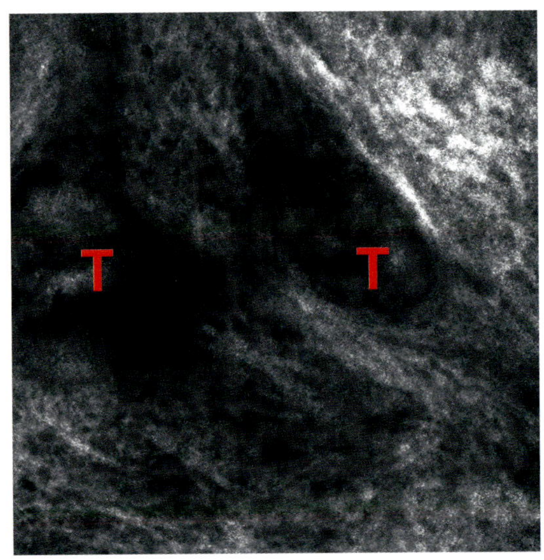

▲ **Figures 5.7, 5.8** On histology (40×), fibrotic stroma concentrically ramifies tumor islands. Corresponding RCM (0.5 mm × 0.5 mm) reveals brightly refractile collagen arranged in parallel bundles, which encases tumor islands (T). Reproduced with permission of S. Karger AG, based from Ardigo M, Zieff J, Scope A et al. Dermoscopic and reflectance confocal microscope findings of trichoepithelioma. Dermatology 2007; 215:354–8.

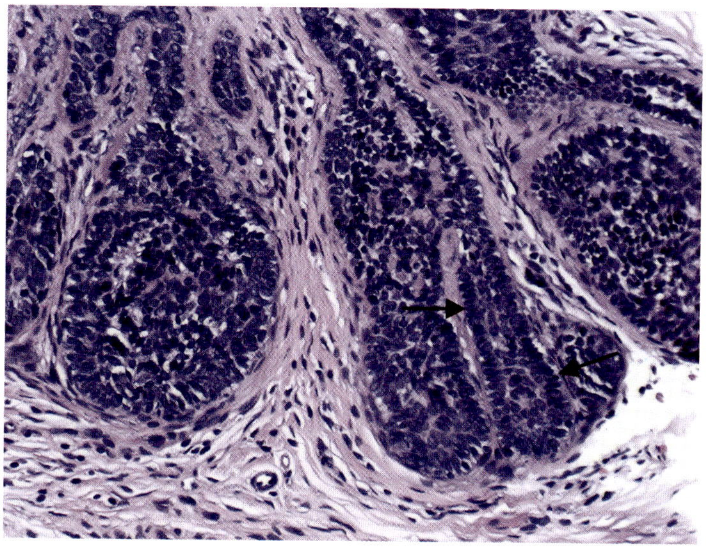

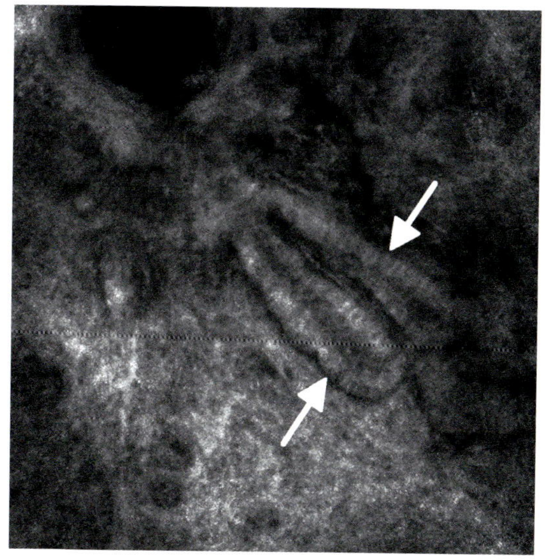

▲ **Figures 5.9, 5.10** Histology (20×) finds peripheral palisading of basaloid tumor cells in some islands (arrows), which can also be seen on RCM (0.5 mm × 0.5 mm).

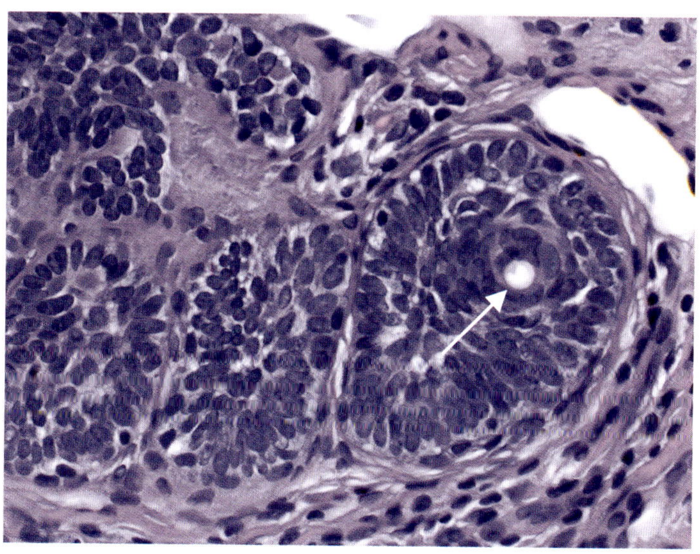

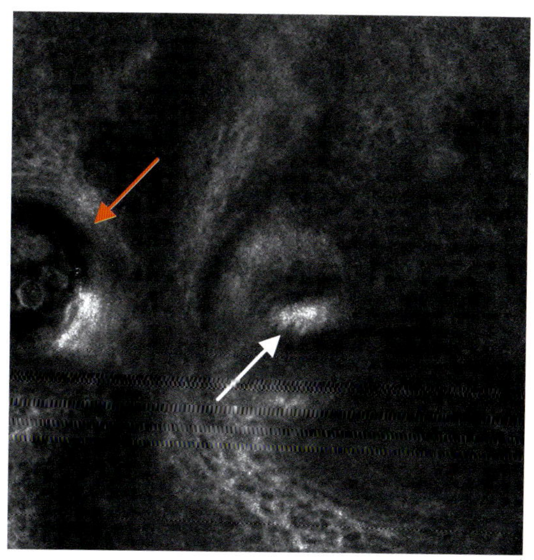

▲ **Figures 5.11, 5.12** On histology (40×), the center of a tumor nest shows an early horn cyst (white arrow), which is identified on RCM (0.5 mm × 0.5 mm) as a round black space filled with brightly refractile material in the center of a tumor island (white arrow). By contrast, a true follicle can be seen to the left of the tumor island (red arrow).

DESMOPLASTIC TRICHOEPITHELIOMA

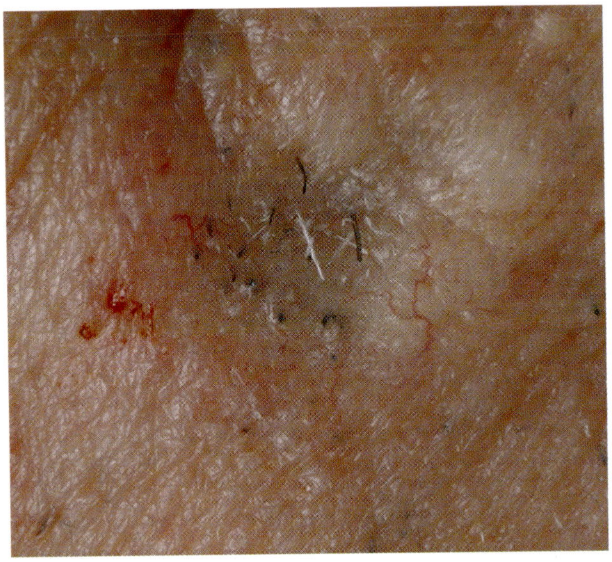

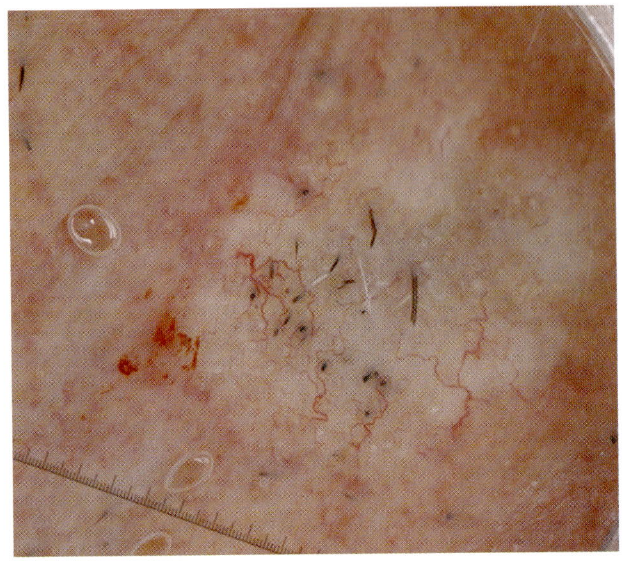

▲ **Figures 5.13, 5.14** Clinical photograph of a 14 mm, hard, annular, telangiectatic, scar-like plaque on the right chin of an 83-year-old man. The center of the lesion is depressed, but not ulcerated. Dermoscopy shows an ivory white, scar-like lesion with arborizing, telangiectatic surface vessels. Reproduced with permission of S. Karger AG, based from Ardigo M, Zieff J, Scope A et al. Dermoscopic and reflectance confocal microscope findings of trichoepithelioma. Dermatology 2007; 215:354–8.

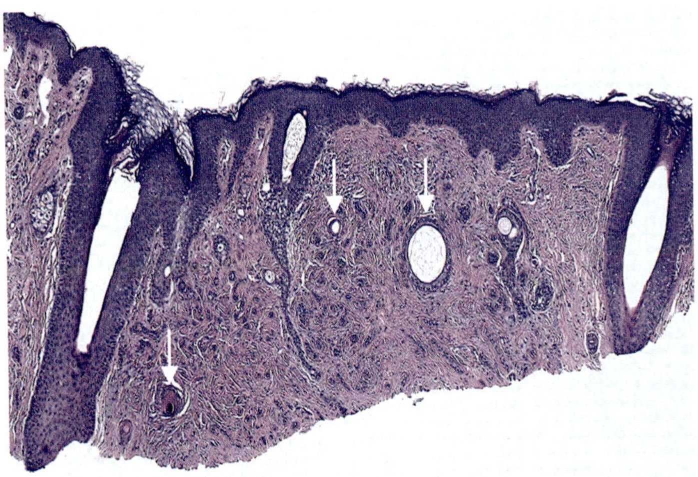

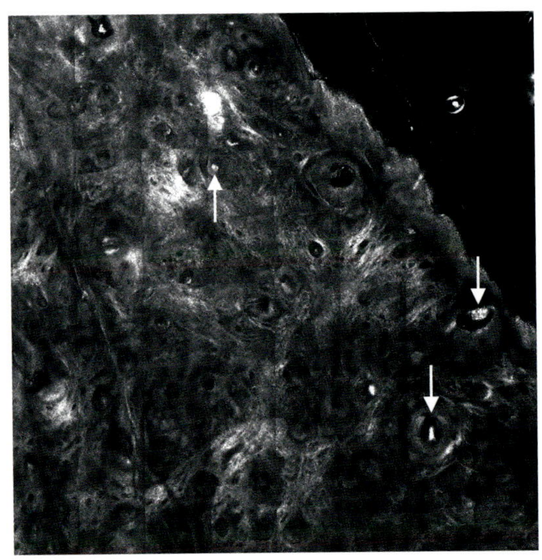

▲ **Figures 5.15, 5.16** On histology (4×), the tumor is composed of small nests and cords of tumor cells embedded in a sclerotic stroma. Corresponding RCM mosaic (4 mm × 4 mm) shows dark small round and elongated tumor nests in a brightly refractile stroma arranged in parallel bundles. Horn cysts are readily visible by both modalities (white arrows). Reproduced with permission of S. Karger AG, based from Ardigo M, Zieff J, Scope A et al. Dermoscopic and reflectance confocal microscope findings of trichoepithelioma. Dermatology 2007; 215:354–8.

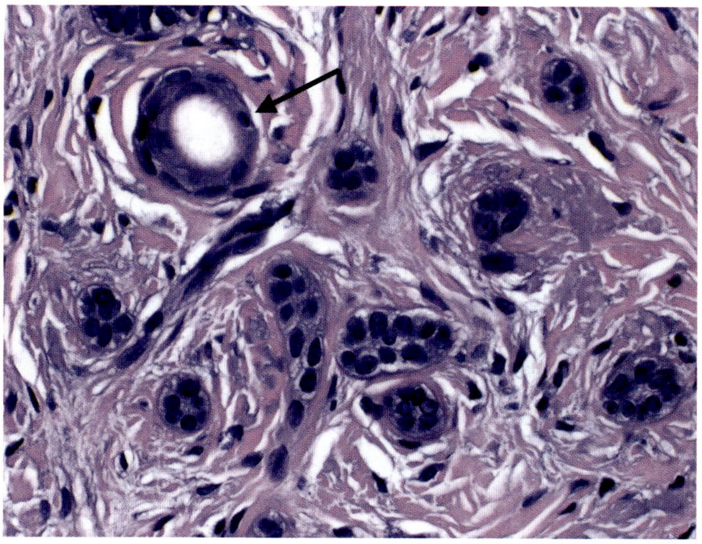

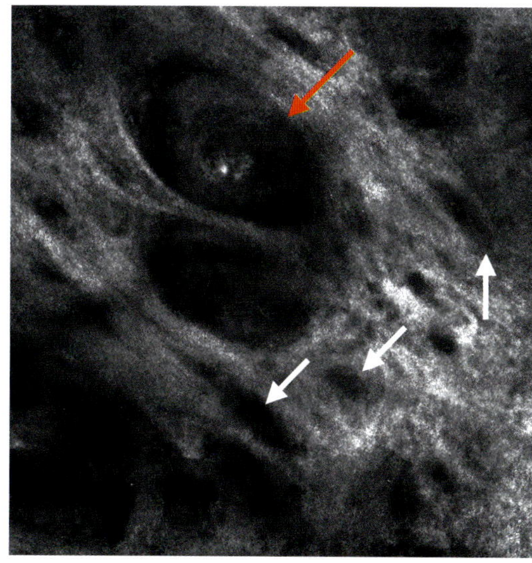

▲ **Figures 5.17, 5.18** Histology (40×) shows small nests and cords of basaloid tumor cells encased in a sclerotic stroma. A horn cyst is just starting to form inside one nest (black arrow). On RCM (0.5 mm × 0.5 mm), tumor nests appear as small round, oval and elongated, dark gray islands. Small round, weakly refractile tumor cells are visible within these nests (white arrows). The stroma is composed of brightly refractile parallel bundles which tightly wrap around the tumor islands. A larger tumor nest (red arrow) contains a small, central, round black space containing brightly refractile material, corresponding to an early horn cyst. Reproduced with permission of S. Karger AG, based from Ardigo M, Zieff J, Scope A et al. Dermoscopic and reflectance confocal microscope findings of trichoepithelioma. Dermatology 2007; 215:354–8.

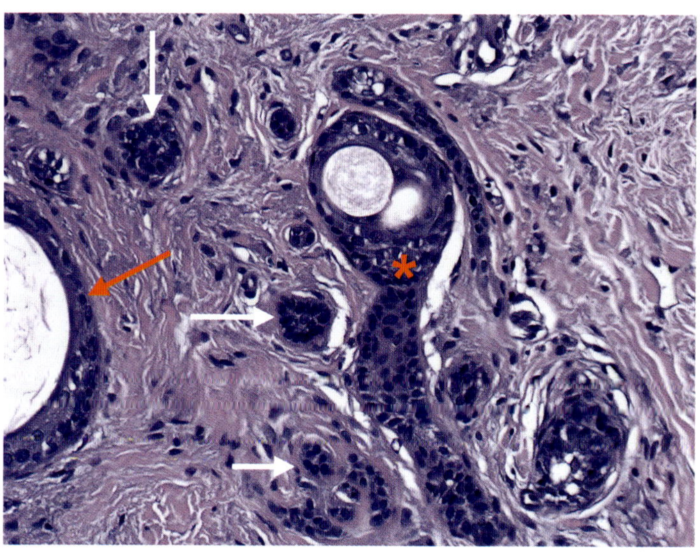

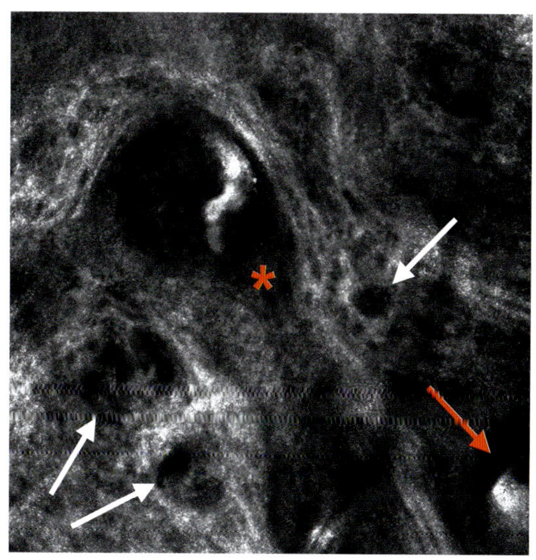

▲ **Figures 5.19, 5.20** Histology (20×) shows an entrapped eccrine duct (asterisk) in the center and a tumoral horn cyst (red arrow) on the left. Nest and cords of tumor cells (white arrows) are also present. Corresponding RCM (0.5 mm × 0.5 mm) has similar findings, but the horn cyst, a round black space filled with brightly refractile material, is seen on the right (red arrow).

CHAPTER 5b

Sebaceous hyperplasia

Josep Malvehy and Susana Puig

Sebaceous hyperplasia (SH) is a common benign tumor that typically occurs on the face, chiefly the forehead and cheeks, in middle age and the elderly. Either one or more, frequently multiple, elevated, small, soft, yellowish, slightly umbilicated papules are present. They exhibit telangiectatic vessels that may cause some lesions to clinically resemble basal cell carcinoma. On dermoscopic examination, SH shows a typical pattern with yellow-white central globular structures, corresponding to the hyperplastic sebaceous lobules. Distributed around these structures are prominent vessels called 'crown vessels' because of their morphology and distribution[1–3] (Figure 5.21). These tumors appear early and in great number in the setting of immunosuppression, in familial cases, and in some genodermatoses such as Muir–Torre syndrome and pachydermoperiostosis. Histologic examination of SH finds a tumor composed of enlarged, lobulated sebaceous glands connecting to widened sebaceous ducts which empty into a central dilated follicular infundibulum commonly plugged with sebum and keratin, forming the umbilicated portion of the tumor (Figures 5.22, 5.23, 5.26).[4]

Reflectance confocal microscopy (RCM) of sebaceous hyperplasia exhibits characteristic features that correlate well with findings on dermoscopy and histology. Imaging at the level of the epidermis reveals a dilated follicular infundibulum containing a keratotic plug with sebum (Figure 5.26A–C). In the dermis, crown vessels surrounding the duct are seen as dilated dark tubular structures containing weakly refractile round cells (erythrocytes) and brightly refractile round cells (granulocytes) (Figure 5.24). Occasionally, the surface of enlarged sebaceous glands can be seen at the level of the superficial dermis as morula-like clusters of round cells with glistening brightly refractile speckled cytoplasms (Figures 5.25, 5.26C).[5–7] RCM has been used for the monitoring of laser treatment in sebaceous hyperplasia.[5,7]

Key RCM features of sebaceous hyperplasia

- Dilated central follicular infundibulum
- Enlarged morula-like clusters of round cells with bright speckled cytoplasms (sebaceous lobules)
- Crown vessels

REFERENCES

1. Zaballos P, Ara M, Puig S et al. Dermoscopy of sebaceous hyperplasia. Arch Dermatol 2005; 141:808.
2. Argenziano G, Zalaudek I, Corona R et al. Vascular structures in skin tumors: a dermoscopy study. Arch Dermatol 2004; 140:1485–9.
3. Bryden AM, Dawe RS, Fleming C. Dermatoscopic features of benign sebaceous proliferation. Clin Exp Dermatol 2004; 29:676–7.
4. Luderschmidt C, Plewig G. Circumscribed sebaceous gland hyperplasia: autoradiographic and histoplanimetric studies. J Invest Dermatol 1978; 70:207–9.
5. Aghassi D, Gonzalez E, Anderson RR et al. Elucidating the pulsed-dye laser treatment of sebaceous hyperplasia

in vivo with real-time confocal scanning laser microscopy. J Am Acad Dermatol 2000; 43:49–53.

6. Propperova I, Langley RG. Reflectance-mode confocal microscopy for the diagnosis of sebaceous hyperplasia in vivo. Arch Dermatol 2007; 143(1):134.

7. Gonzalez S, White WM, Rajadhyaksha M et al. Confocal imaging of sebaceous gland hyperplasia in vivo to assess efficacy and mechanism of pulsed dye laser treatment. Lasers Surg Med 1999; 25:8–12.

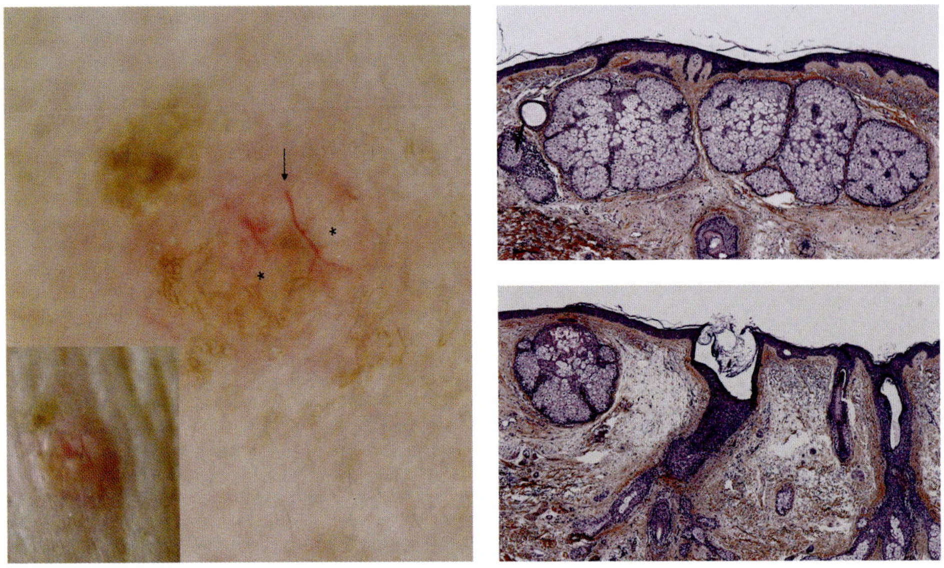

▲ **Figures 5.21–5.23** Clinical photograph (inset) of sebaceous hyperplasia on the forehead of a 71-year-old patient. Dermoscopy shows pale yellow central structures (asterisks) corresponding to the sebaceous lobules and typical crown vessels (arrow). Histology (4×) shows an increased number of enlarged sebaceous glands in the superficial dermis (above) and, at a different level, the associated, plugged follicular infundibula, from which the hyperplastic sebaceous glands emanate.

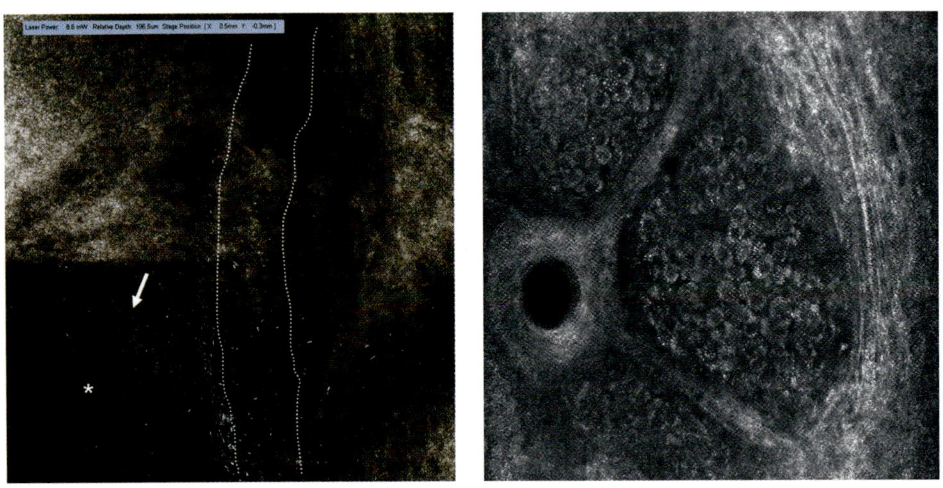

▲ **Figures 5.24, 5.25** RCM (left, 0.5 mm × 0.5 mm) at the level of the upper dermis shows a crown vessel (demarcated by interrupted white lines) adjacent to a dilated sebaceous duct (asterisk). The edge of a few refractile sebocytes (white arrow) are seen at the edge of the duct. RCM (right, 0.5 mm × 0.5 mm) from another lesion at the level of the upper dermis shows morula-like lobules of round cells with glistening brightly refractile speckled cytoplasms and central round, dark nuclei, corresponding to hyperplastic sebaceous lobules. The lobules are separated by bands of collagen and arranged around a central sebaceous duct.

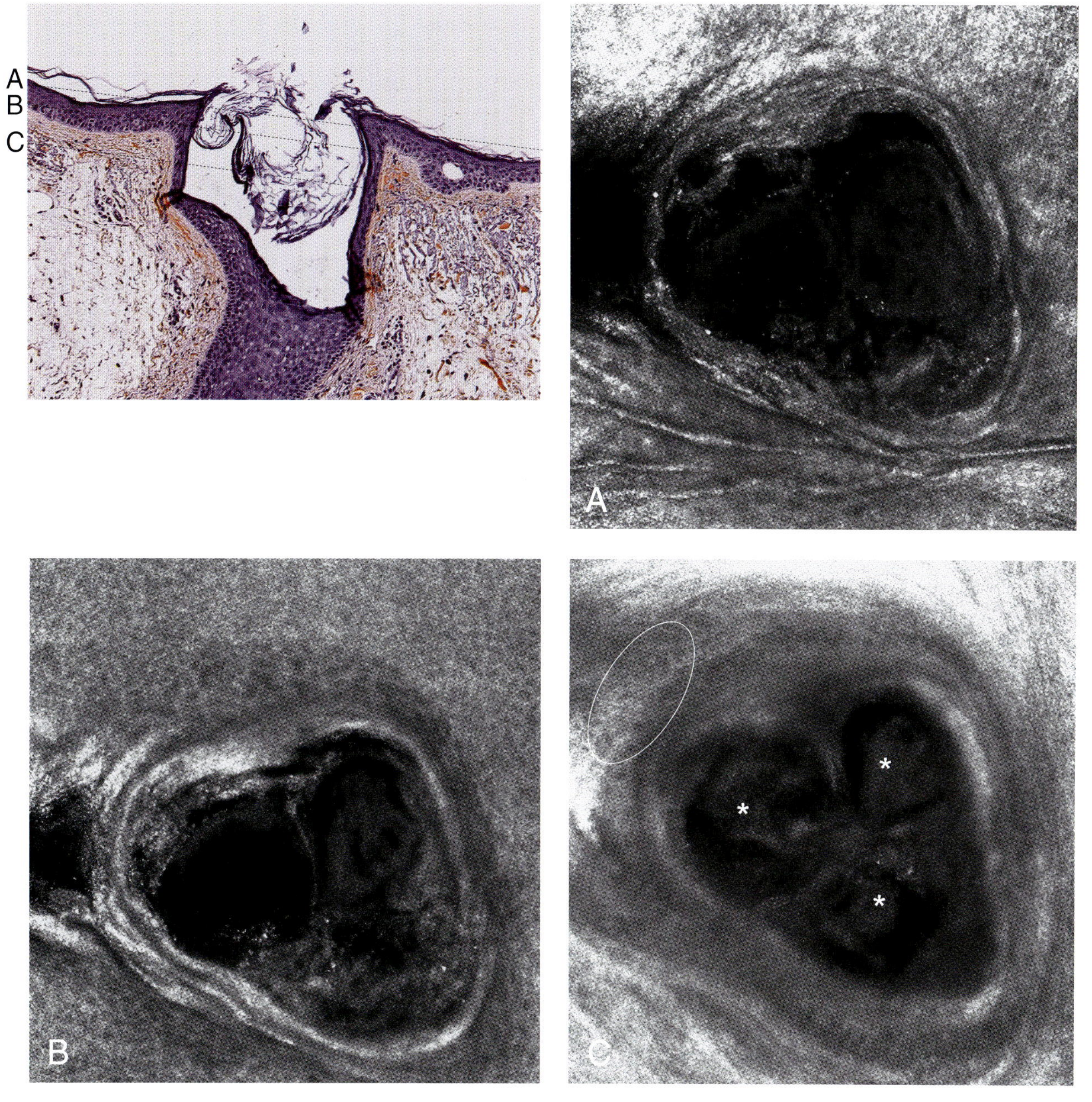

▲ **Figure 5.26** Histology (20×) shows a dilated follicular infundibulum containing a keratin plug. Horizontal lines labeled A, B, and C indicate from where each RCM image (0.5 mm × 0.5 mm) is captured. RCM at the level of the stratum corneum (A) reveals a dilated follicular orifice. At the level of the stratum spinosum (B), one begins to see the sebaceous ducts as they connect into the dilated follicular infundibulum. At the level of the dermis (C), sebaceous ducts (asterisks) are clearly visible and the edge of a sebaceous lobule (circled), with glistening round cells corresponding to sebocytes, is just emerging.

CHAPTER 5c

Dermatofibroma

Juan Luis Santiago Sánchez-Mateos, Lorea Bagazgoitia, Pedro Jaen, Marco Ardigo, and Salvador González

Dermatofibroma (DF) is a common benign dermal fibrohistiocytic tumor that can arise at any age and in any gender, but is more typically seen in young adult women. The origin is unknown; both reactive and neoplastic theories have been proposed.[1–3] Recent investigations have demonstrated clonality, supporting the neoplastic theory.[4] Clinically, DF presents as a solitary (less frequently multiple), slowly growing, firm, dome-shaped nodule, ranging from 0.5 to 1 cm in diameter, located on an extremity, generally the leg. The lesion can range in color from skin tone to gray, yellow, pink, red, blue, brown, or black, or as any combinations of these colors (Figures 5.27, 5.35, 5.43, 5.53). The majority of the lesions are asymptomatic, but pruritus is not unusual. DF almost always persists indefinitely and remains unchanged during life. Darkly pigmented lesions can simulate dysplastic nevi or melanoma. On dermoscopy, dermatofibroma generally shows a central white, scar-like area with a surrounding peripheral network with brown pigmentation (Figures 5.28, 5.36, 5.44, 5.54).[5] On histology, DF usually shows a hyperplastic epidermis with hyperpigmentation of the basal layer and elongated rete ridges (Figures 5.31, 5.33, 5.47, 5.49). In the subjacent dermis, a proliferation of spindled fibroblast-like cells and histiocytes with peripheral entrapping of thick collagen bundles is seen (Figures 5.29, 5.37, 5.39, 5.41, 5.45, 5.51). Numerous small blood vessels may also be present (Figure 5.41).[6]

Reflectance confocal microscopy (RCM) of DF reveals a normal epidermal honeycomb or cobblestone pattern and an increased density of homogeneously bright dermal papillary rings (Figures 5.30, 5.32, 5.34, 5.38, 5.42, 5.46, 5.48, 5.50, 5.55, 5.56). Within the dermis, collagen bundles are brighter and thicker than those seen in normal skin (Figures 5.40, 5.42, 5.52, 5.56). In some cases, collagen bundles appear tethered to the dermal papillary rings (Figure 5.56). An increased number of variably ectatic vessels are generally seen on confocal examination of the superficial dermis (Figures 5.42, 5.50). The fibrohistiocytic proliferation is generally too deep to visualize in vivo using currently available reflectance confocal microscopes, but future iterations of the device may allow for imaging of deeper dermal tissues. At present, the RCM features of DF are non-specific, but combined with clinical and dermoscopic features can suggest the diagnosis. Moreover, confocal allows for distinction from superficial melanocytic lesions, which occasionally enter the clinical differential diagnosis.

Key RCM features of dermatofibroma

- Normal honeycomb or cobblestone pattern of the epidermis
- Increased density of bright dermal papillary rings
- Thickened, refractile collagen bundles
- Variable tethering of dermal papillary rings by sclerotic collagen bundles

REFERENCES

1. Chen TC, Kuo T, Chan HL. Dermatofibroma is a clonal proliferative disease. J Cutan Pathol 2000; 27(1): 36–9.

2. Evans J, Clarke T, Mattacks CA, Pond CM. Dermatofibromas and arthropod bites: is there any evidence to link the two? Lancet 1989; 2(8653): 36–7.

3. Vanni R, Marras S, Faa G et al. Cellular fibrous histiocytoma of the skin: evidence of a clonal process with different karyotype from dermatofibrosarcoma. Genes Chromosomes Cancer 1997; 18(4):314–17.

4. Hui P, Glusac EJ, Sinard JH, Perkins AS. Clonal analysis of cutaneous fibrous histiocytoma (dermatofibroma). J Cutan Pathol 2002; 29(7):385–9.

5. Katz B, Rao B, Marghoob A. Cellular fibrous histiocytoma of the skin: evidence of a clonal process with different karyotype from dermatofibrosarcoma. In: Marghoob AA, Braun RP, Kopf AW, eds. Atlas of Dermoscopy Abingdon, UK: Taylor & Francis; 2005:81–5.

6. Heenan P. Tumors of fibrous tissue involving the skin. In: Elder DE, Elenitsas R, Johnson BL Jr, Murphy GF, eds. Lever's Histopathology of the Skin, 9th edn. Philadelphia: Lippincott, Williams & Wilkins; 2005: 979.

DERMATOFIBROMA

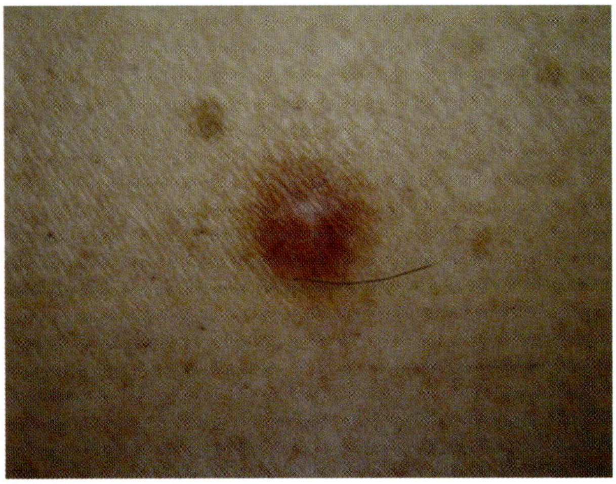
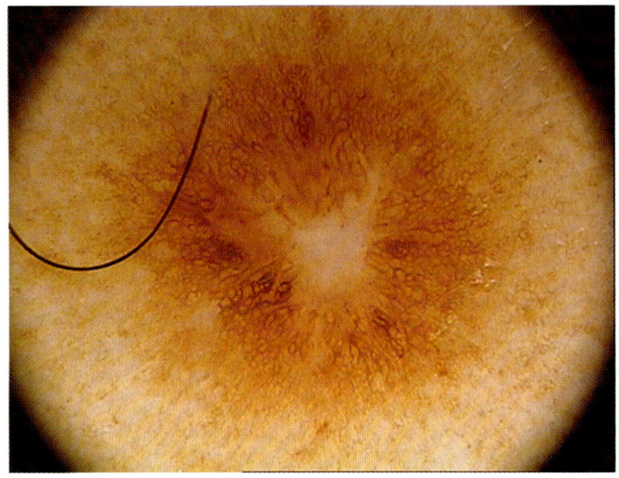

▲ **Figures 5.27, 5.28** Case 1: erythematous, pigmented papular lesion on the right leg of a 56-year-old female. Dermoscopy shows a brown pigmented network surrounding a central scar-like area, suggestive of dermatofibroma.

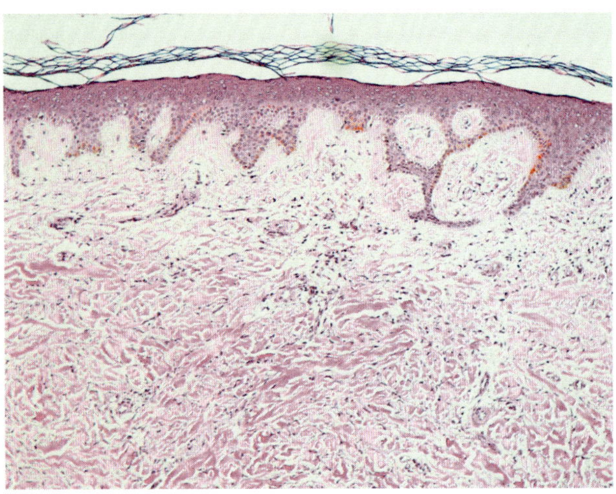
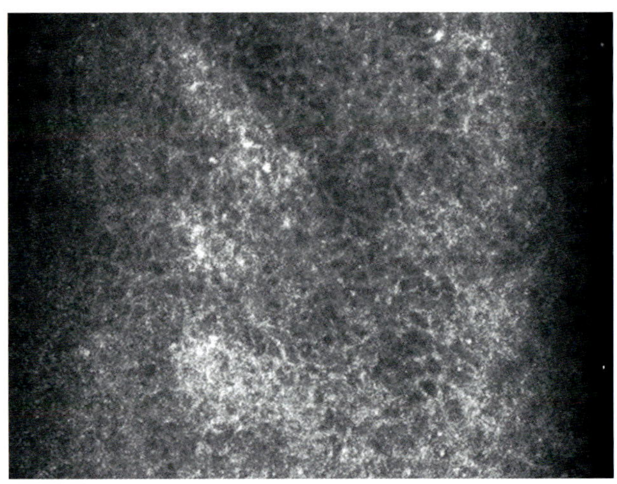

▲ **Figures 5.29, 5.30** Case 1: on histology (10×), hyperplastic epidermis without atypia and with hyperpigmentation of the basal layer is evident over a dermal proliferation of fibroblasts around thickened collagen bundles. RCM (0.45 mm × 0.34 mm) shows a normal honeycomb pattern of the epidermis.

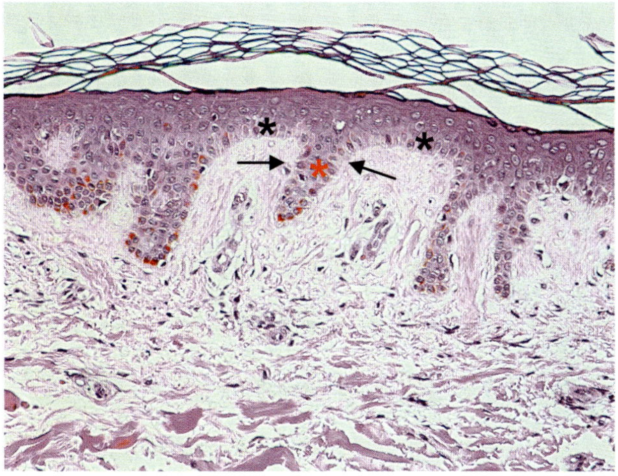

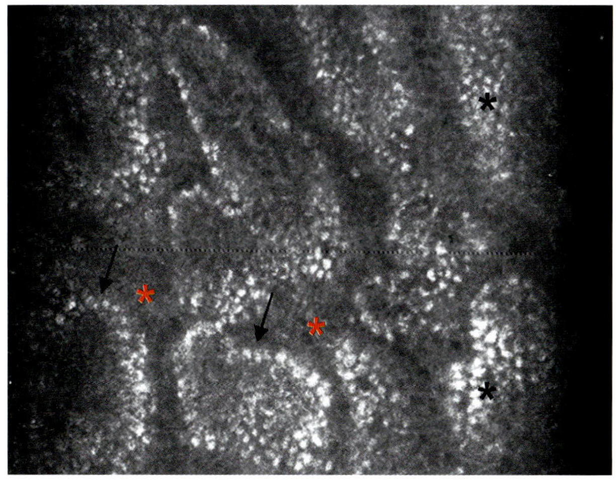

▲ **Figures 5.31, 5.32** Case 1: on higher-power histology (20×), hyperpigmentation of basal keratinocytes in the absence of a melanocytic proliferation is confirmed. Note how thin and long the rete ridges are. RCM (0.45 mm × 0.34 mm) at the level of the lower stratum spinosum/surface of the basal layer demonstrates a cobblestone pattern created by the highly refractile supranuclear melanin caps within basal keratinocytes in suprapapillary plates (black asterisks) and surrounding the narrow rete ridges (red asterisks) (arrows).

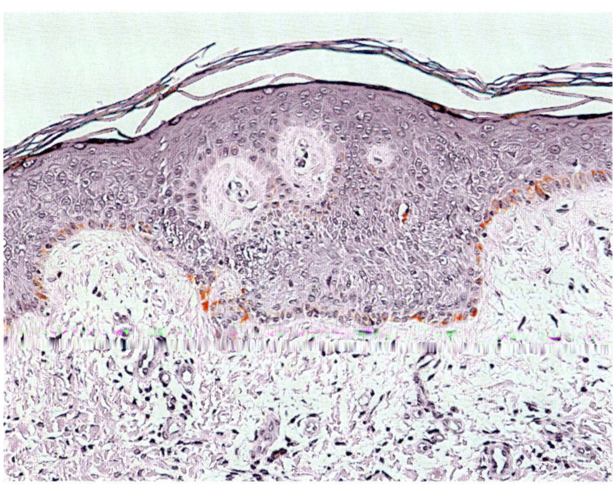

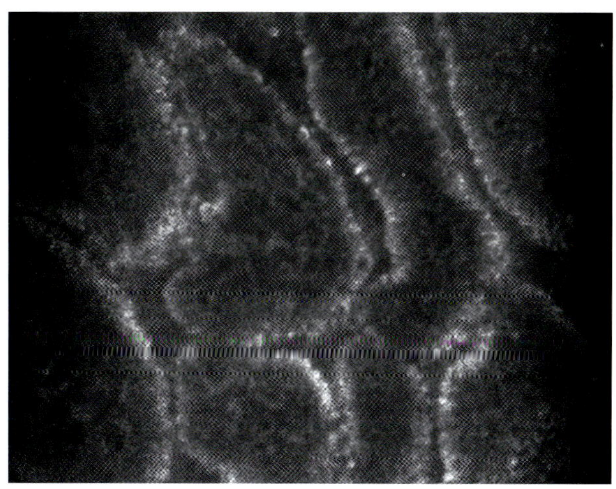

▲ **Figures 5.33, 5.34** Case 1: histology (20×) shows irregular acanthosis of the epidermis and hyperpigmentation of the basal layer. RCM (0.45 mm × 0.34 mm) at the level of the DEJ demonstrates bright dermal papillary rings with irregular elongated contours, which are closely opposed to one another.

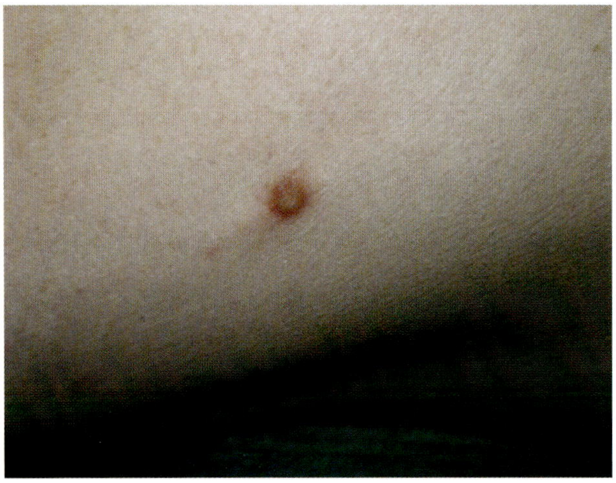

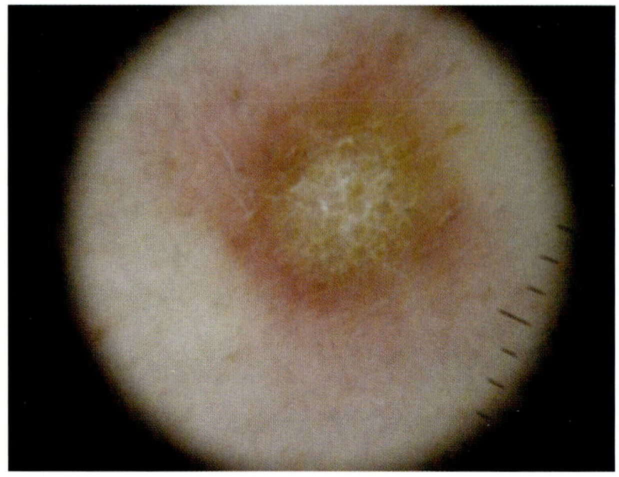

▲ **Figures 5.35, 5.36** Case 2: erythematous, pigmented papule on the right leg of a 65-year-old male. Dermoscopy shows a brown pigmented network surrounding a scar-like area.

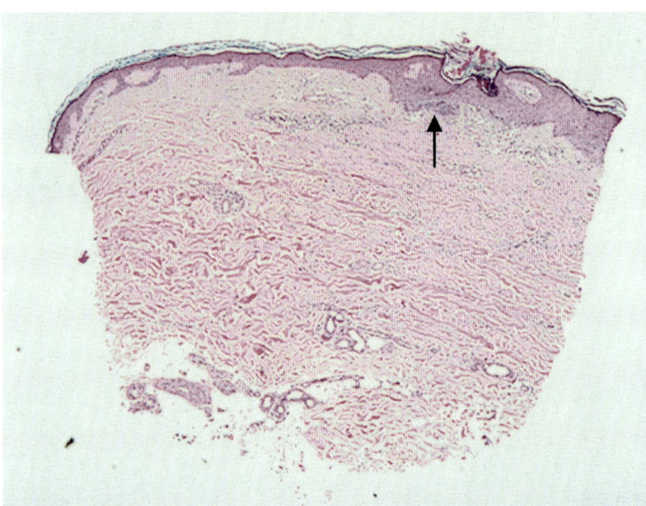

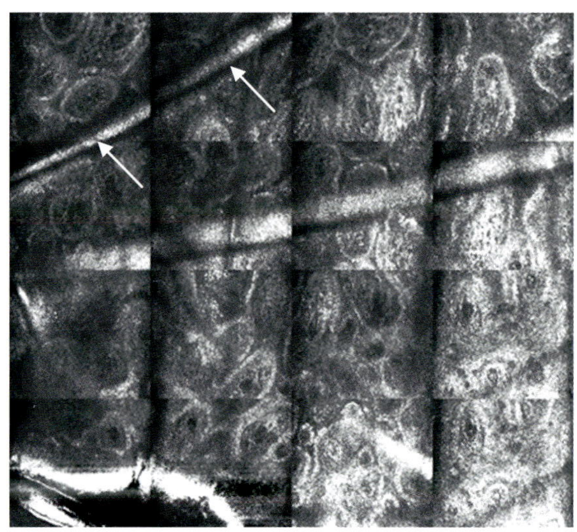

▲ **Figures 5.37, 5.38** Case 2: histology (4×) shows hyperplastic epidermis with hyperpigmentation of the basal layer, and focal elongation and thinning of rete ridges. Focally, follicular induction is seen (arrow). The subjacent dermis shows hypercellularity and sclerotic collagen bundles. RCM mosaic (2 mm × 2 mm) at the level of the DEJ demonstrates homogeneously bright dermal papillary rings and a hair shaft (arrows).

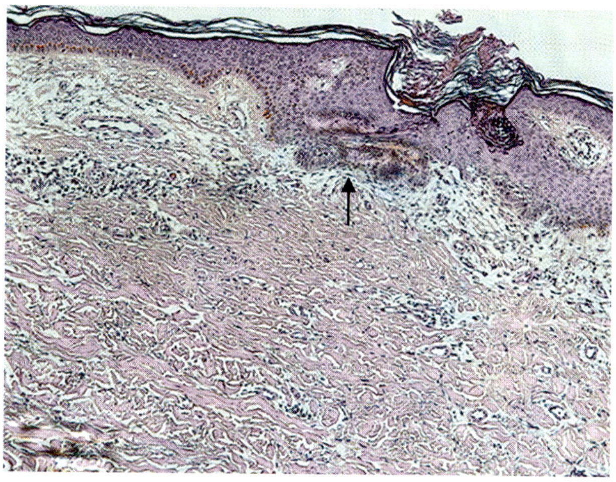

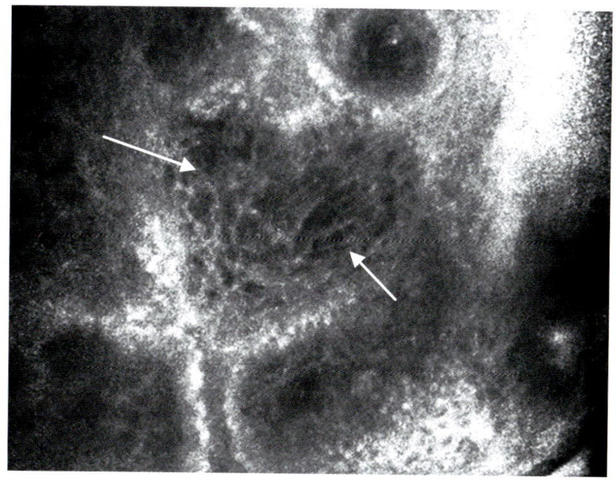

▲ **Figures 5.39, 5.40** Case 2: higher-power histology (10×) of the area with follicular induction shows characteristic buds of basaloid cells with peripheral palisading of nuclei and subjacent mesenchymal condensations (arrow). Hyperpigmentation of the basal layer and a dermal proliferation of spindled cells surrounding thickened collagen bundles are also seen. RCM image (0.45 mm × 0.34 mm) demonstrates hyperpigmentation of the basal keratinocytes forming dermal papillary rings and thickened, hyperrefractile collagen bundles in the papillary dermis (arrows).

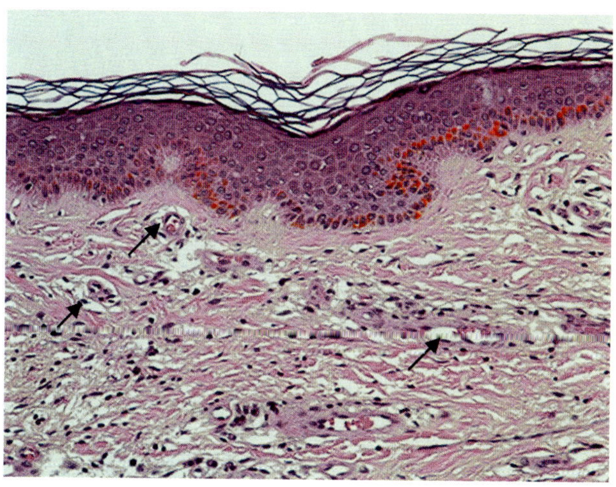

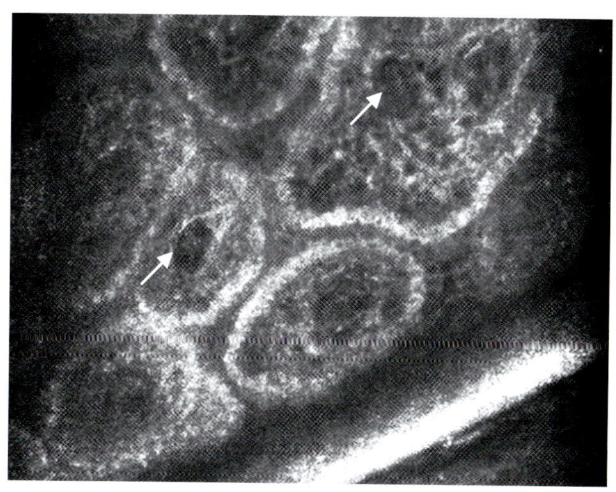

▲ **Figures 5.41, 5.42** Case 2: histology (20×) shows hyperpigmentation of basal keratinocytes in the epidermis and prominent, somewhat ectatic small blood vessels (arrows) and sclerotic collagen bundles in the dermis. RCM (0.45 mm × 0.34 mm) at the level of the DEJ shows homogeneously bright dermal papillary rings and prominent blood vessels (arrows) surrounded by focally thickened, bright collagen bundles in the dermal papillae.

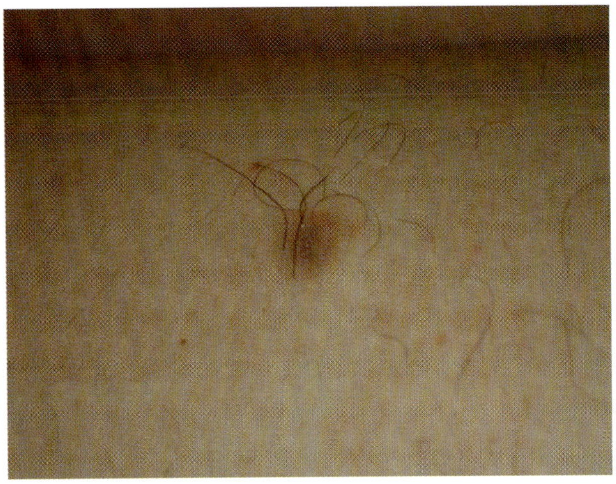

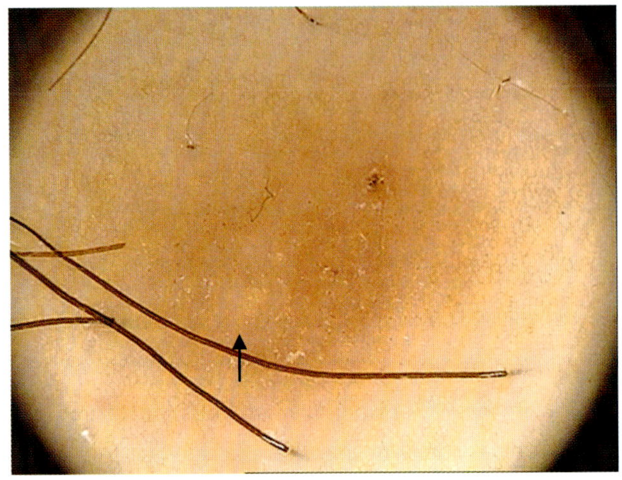

▲ **Figures 5.43, 5.44** Case 3: erythematous mildly pigmented nodule on the left leg of a 45-year-old female. Dermoscopy shows subtle features suggestive of dermatofibroma, including brown pigment surrounding a scar-like area (arrow).

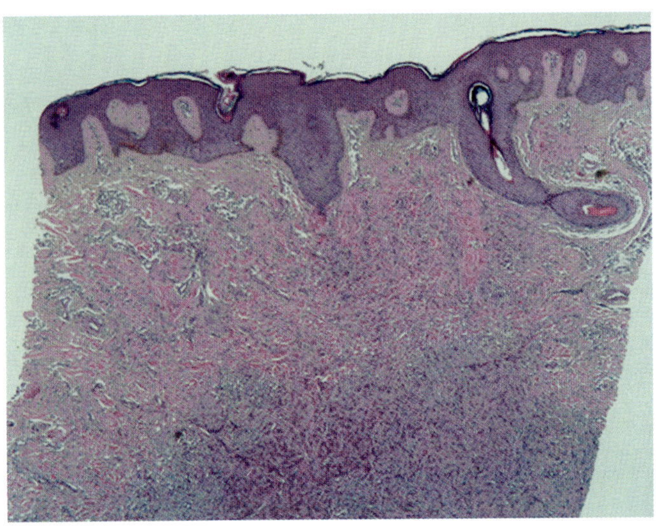

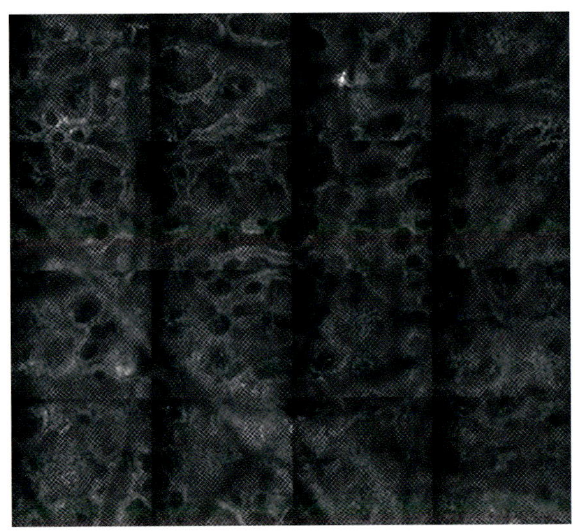

▲ **Figures 5.45, 5.46** Case 3: histology (4×) shows hyperplastic epidermis with interanastomosing, elongated rete ridges and mild pigmentation of the basal layer. In the dermis, increased cellularity and thickened collagen bundles can be seen. RCM mosaic (2 mm × 2 mm) at the level of the DEJ demonstrates an increased number of irregularly shaped, mildly refractile dermal papillary rings. Note that the rete ridges appear broader than those seen in Cases 1 and 2, where the rete ridges were also thinner on histology.

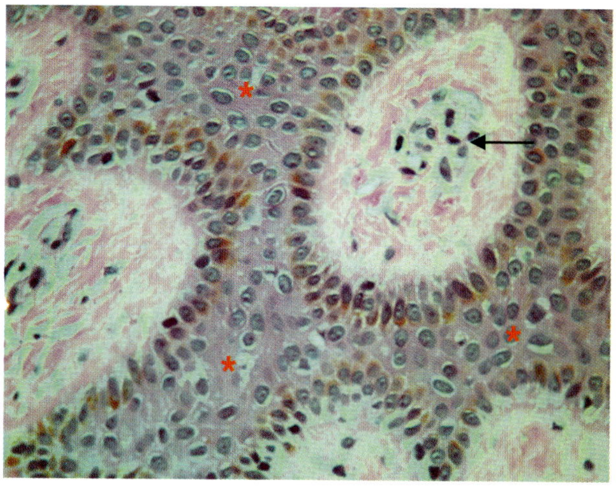

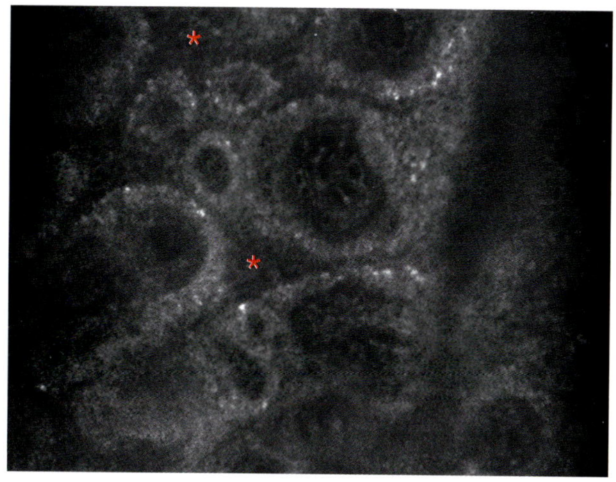

▲ **Figures 5.47, 5.48** Case 3: high-power histology (40×) confirms the presence of pigmented basal keratinocytes in the absence of a melanocytic proliferation. RCM (0.45 mm × 0.34 mm) at the level of the upper DEJ shows variably sized, mildly refractile dermal papillary rings and a normal honeycomb pattern in the rete ridges (asterisks).

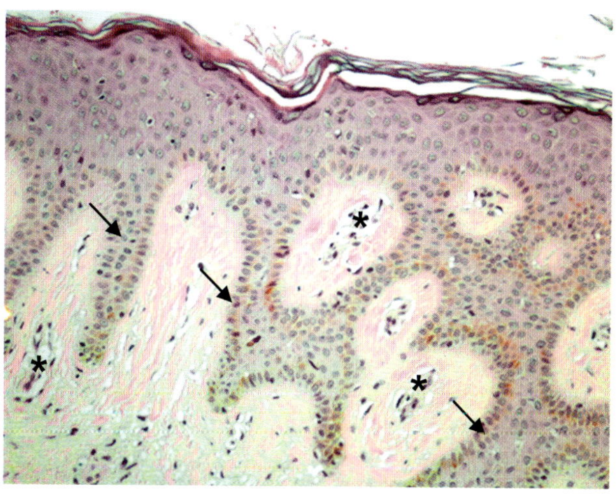

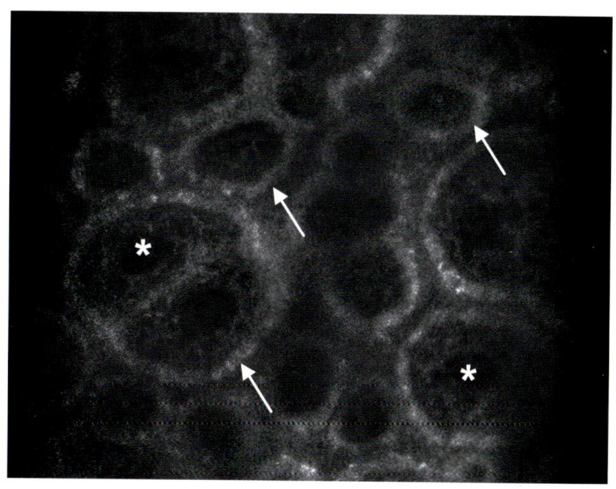

▲ **Figures 5.49, 5.50** Case 3: histology (20×) shows irregular acanthosis of the epidermis (arrows) and mild hyperpigmentation of the basal layer with dilated vessels in the upper dermis (asterisks). RCM image (0.45 mm × 0.34 mm) at the level of the lower DEJ shows crowding and variation in size and shapes of the dermal papillary rings and variability in the thickness of the rete ridges, corresponding to irregular acanthosis. Dermal papillary rings are mildly hyperrefractile (arrows). Within the dermal papillae, dilated blood vessels (asterisks) surrounded by focally thickened collagen bundles are seen.

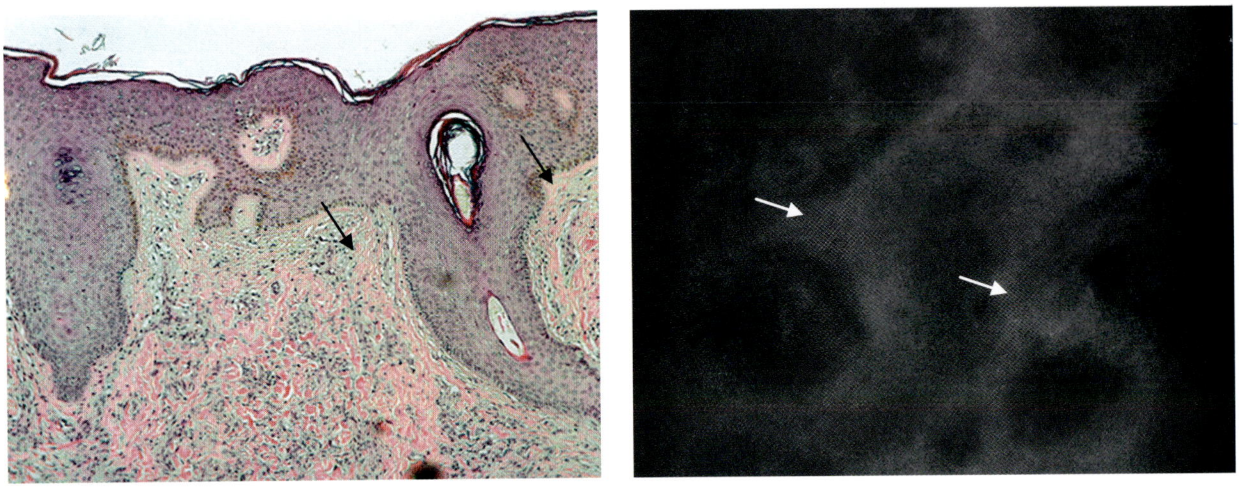

▲ **Figures 5.51, 5.52** Case 3: sclerotic collagen bundles (arrows) seen on histology (10×) appear as smudged, moderately refractile, thick bands (arrows) on RCM (0.45 mm × 0.34 mm) at the level of the superficial dermis.

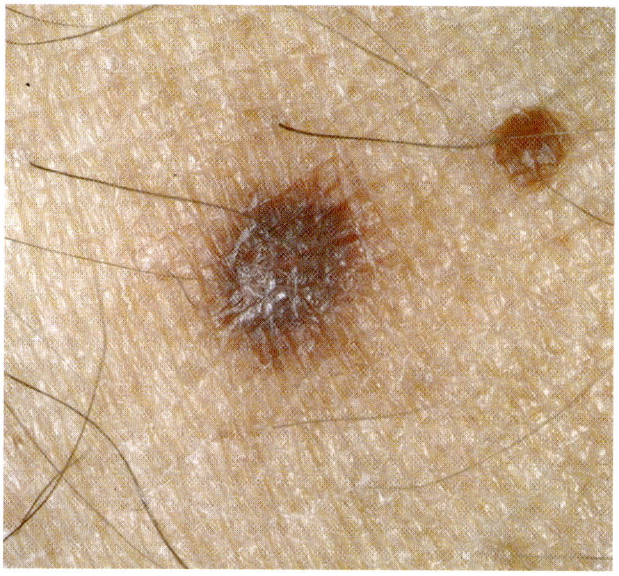

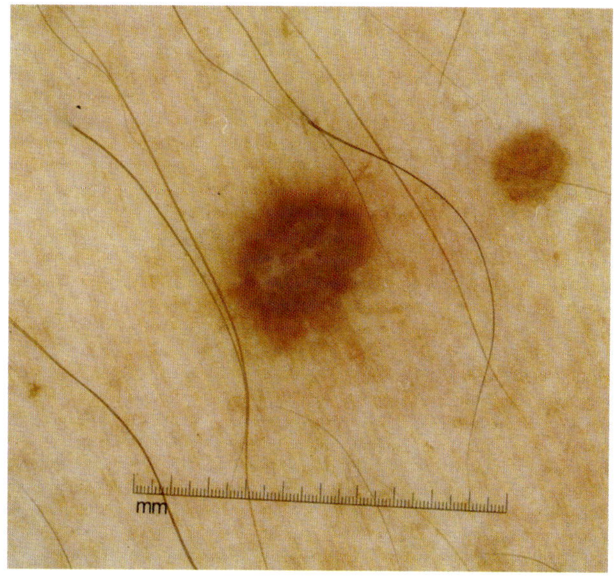

▲ **Figures 5.53, 5.54** Case 4: erythematous, purple-gray nodule on the left arm of a 54-year-old male. Dermoscopy shows a brown pigmented network surrounding a scar-like area. This lesion was not excised.

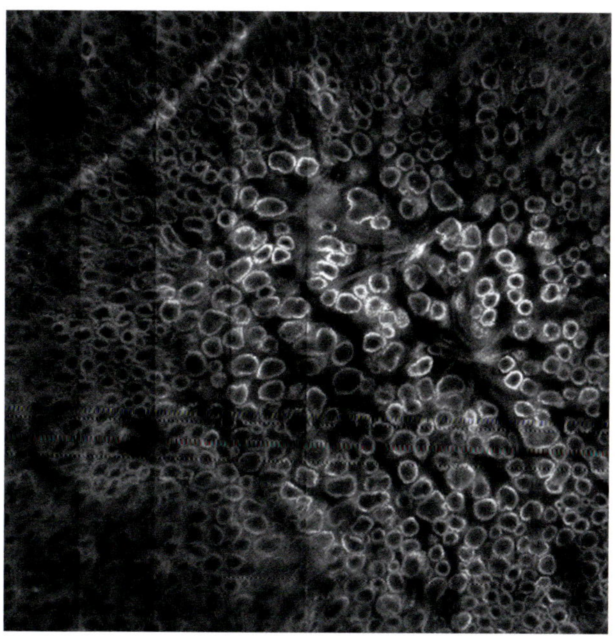

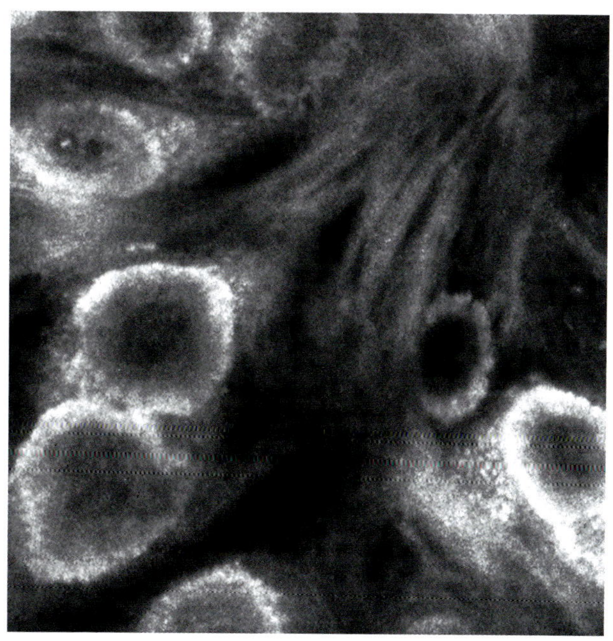

▲ **Figures 5.55, 5.56** Case 4: RCM mosaic (4 mm × 4 mm) at the level of the DEJ reveals an increased density of uniformly sized, homogeneously bright dermal papillary rings. On RCM (0.5 mm × 0.5 mm), bright, thickened collagen bundles appear tethered to the dermal papillary rings.

CHAPTER 5d

Angioma

Melissa Gill, Yogesh G Patel, and Marco Ardigo

Benign vascular lesions represent reactive processes, developmental abnormalities, and benign neoplasms.[1] Although some congenital vascular malformations can cause functional disturbances, most vascular lesions are only cosmetically challenging. Occasionally, vascular lesions, especially those that are deep or thrombosed, may be confused with melanoma and unnecessarily biopsied.[2] More importantly, however, Spitz nevi, Spitzoid melanomas, and amelanotic nodular melanomas may be clinically misdiagnosed as benign vascular lesions, leading to delay in diagnosis or improper biopsy technique.[3,4]

CHERRY HEMANGIOMA

Cherry hemangioma, also called senile hemangioma or Campbell de Morgan spot, is the most common acquired cutaneous vascular neoplasm.[1] Cherry hemangiomas are typically bright red to violaceous, dome-shaped papules, but range from pinpoint macules to large polypoid papules (Figure 5.57). They are most common in adults and tend to increase in number with increasing age. Cherry hemangiomas most frequently develop on the trunk and arms, but can occur anywhere.[5,6] Dermoscopic examination of cherry hemangiomas reveals red, red-blue, blue, blue-black, or maroon colored lacunae, which represent the dilated, blood-filled capillaries that form the tumor (Figure 5.58).[7]

Characteristic features of cherry hemangioma are readily detected by reflectance confocal microscopy (RCM). The normal honeycomb pattern of the stratum spinosum and crisp dermal papillary rings of the stratum basalis are preserved. Within the upper dermis, confocal identifies numerous lobules of variably sized black lumina separated by stromal septa, which correspond to the lobules of dilated capillaries forming the tumor on histology (Figures 5.59, 5.60).[1,8] RCM not only clearly shows the blood cells filling the capillaries (Figures 5.61, 5.62) but also real-time video is able to visualize the cells rapidly coursing through the tumoral lumina. Erythrocytes appear as weakly refractile, round and biconcave structures and granulocytes as round-to-oval structures formed by multiple, brightly refractile granules (Figures 5.63, 5.64).[8–10]

Key RCM features of cherry hemangioma

- Normal epidermis
- Dilated vascular lumina separated by thin septa in the upper dermis
- Blood cells moving briskly through the vascular lumina

ANGIOKERATOMA

Angiokeratoma represents a collection of unrelated, superficial, vascular ectasias associated with overlying hyperkeratosis. Eight clinical variants have been described, both multiple and solitary, inherited syndromic and acquired; solitary acquired angiokeratoma is the most common.[11] The etiology of this subtype is unknown, but it has been suggested that solitary angiokeratomas arise as a result of trauma-induced alteration of microvasculature hemodynamics.[12] Solitary angiokeratoma usually arises in young to middle-aged adults and is mostly commonly found on the lower extremity. The early lesion appears as a soft, dark red, verruciform papule measuring 2–10 mm in diameter. With time, the lesion becomes firm, bluish black, and hyperkeratotic.[11] Especially when thrombotic, solitary angiokeratoma can be confused with nodular melanoma (Figure 5.65).[2] Angiokeratoma may be indistinguishable from cherry hemangioma on dermoscopic examination. Both lesions show red, maroon, blue, or black lacunae in the papillary dermis. The only distinguishing feature of angiokeratoma is hyperkeratosis, which, if present, casts a white-yellow hue over the lesion causing the underlying lacunae to be less well defined. Additionally, angiokeratoma has a tendency to thrombose, which makes the lesion non-blanchable and the lacunae appear blue-black (Figure 5.66).[7]

Confocal microscopic examination of angiokeratoma reveals additional features not seen on dermoscopy. RCM finds a thickened stratum corneum, normal epidermal honeycomb pattern, normal dermal papillary rings, and large, ectatic, superficial dermal, black lumina, abutting the epidermis. These lumina are packed with blood cells (Figure 5.68). Confocal observations parallel the characteristic histologic features of ectatic, congested, thin-walled blood vessels in the papillary dermis underlying a hyperkeratotic epidermis (Figure 5.67).[1]

Key RCM features of angiokeratoma

- Thickened stratum corneum
- Large, ectatic vascular lumina just below the DEJ
- Blood cells packing vascular lumina

REFERENCES

1. Calonje E, Wilson-Jones E. Vascular tumors: tumors and tumor-like conditions of blood vessels and lymphatics. In: Elder DE, Elenitsas R, Johnson BL Jr, Murphy GF, eds. Lever's Histopathology of the Skin, 9th edn. Philadelphia: Lippincott, Williams & Wilkins; 2005: 1015–26.
2. Goldman L, Gibson SH, Richfield DF. Thrombotic angiokeratoma circumscriptum simulating melanoma. Arch Dermatol 1981; 117(3):138–9.
3. Ferrari A, Bono A, Baldi M et al. Does melanoma behave differently in younger children than in adults? A retrospective study of 33 cases of childhood melanoma from a single institution. Pediatrics 2005; 115(3):649–54.
4. Mones JM, Ackerman AB. Melanomas in prepubescent children: review comprehensively, critique historically, criteria diagnostically, and course biologically. Am J Dermatopathol 2003; 25(3):223–38.
5. Odom R, James WD, Berger TG. Dermal and sub-cutaneous tumors: cherry angiomas. In: Burger TG, Odom RB, James WD, eds. Andrew's Diseases of the Skin: Clinical Dermatology, 9th edn. Philadelphia: WB Saunders; 2000:751.
6. Sanchez J, Ackerman AB. Vascular proliferation of skin and subcutaneous tissue. In: Fitzpatrick TB, Austen KF, Wolff R, Eisen A, Freedburg IM, eds. Fitzpatrick's Dermatology in General Medicine 4th edn. New York: McGraw-Hill; 1993:1219–20.
7. Katz B, Rao B, Marghoob A. Vascular lesions, hemangiomas/angiokeratomas. In: Marghoob AA, Braun RP, Kopf AW, eds. Atlas of Dermoscopy. Abingdon, UK: Taylor & Francis; 2005:72.
8. Aghassi D, Anderson RR, Gonzalez S. Time-sequence histologic imaging of laser-treated cherry angiomas with in vivo confocal microscopy. J Am Acad Dermatol 2000; 43(1 Pt 1):37–41.
9. Gonzalez S, Sackstein R, Anderson RR, Rajadhyaksha M. Real-time evidence of in vivo leukocyte trafficking in human skin by reflectance confocal microscopy. J Invest Dermatol 2001; 117(2):384–6.
10. Rajadhyaksha M, Gonzalez S, Zavislan JM, Anderson RR, Webb RH. In vivo confocal scanning laser microscopy of human skin II: advances in instrumentation and comparison with histology. J Invest Dermatol 1999; 113(3):293–303.
11. Schiller PI, Itin PH. Angiokeratomas: an update. Dermatology 1996; 193(4):275–82.
12. Foucar E, Mason WV. Angiokeratoma circumscriptum following damage to underlying vasculature. Arch Dermatol 1986; 122(3):245–6.

CHERRY HEMANGIOMA

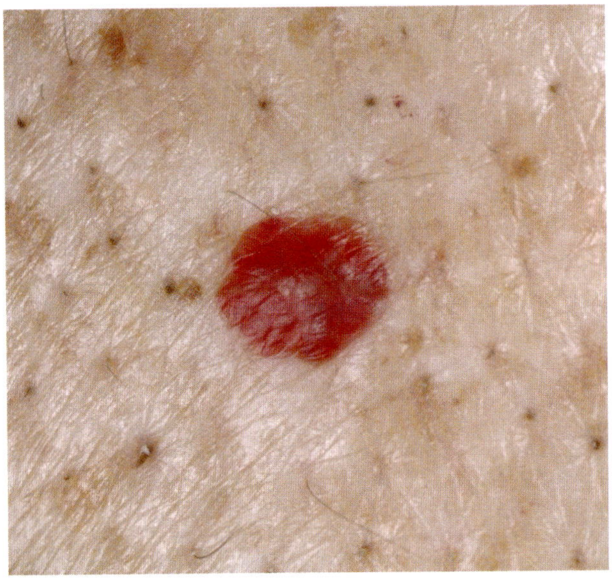

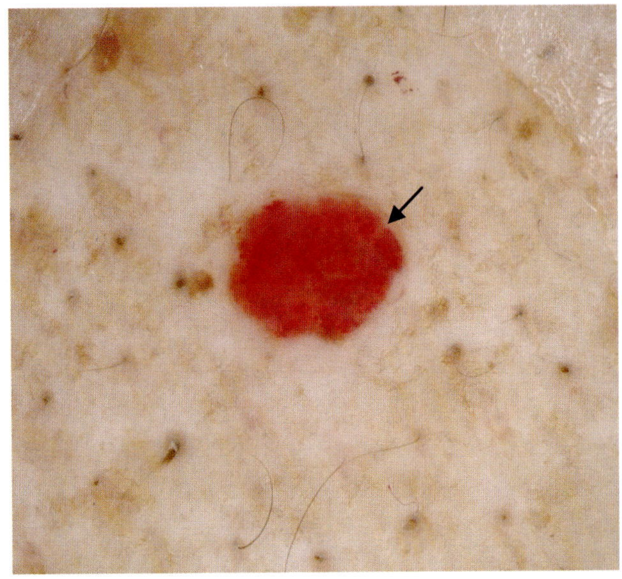

▲ **Figures 5.57, 5.58** Clinical photograph of a 4 mm, bright red, blanchable, dome-shaped papule on the back. Dermoscopic photograph reveals a well-demarcated, round, lobulated tumor composed of tightly clustered, variably sized, round, red lacunae separated by septa (arrow).

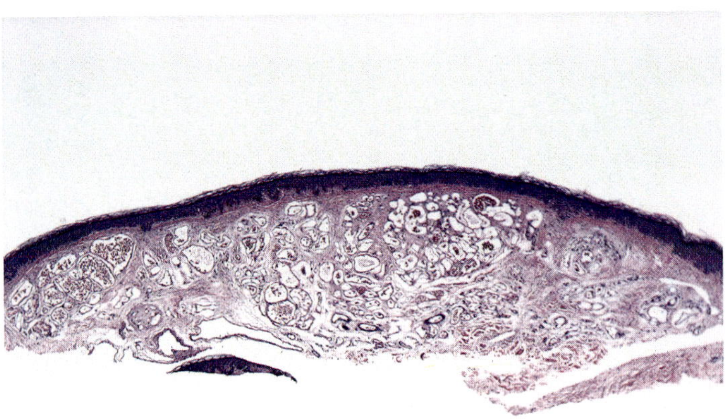

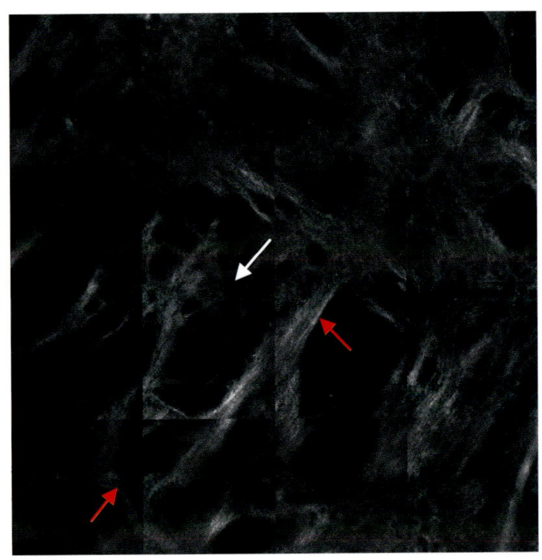

▲ **Figures 5.59, 5.60** Histology (4×) shows normal epidermis and the characteristic lobular proliferation of capillaries within the superficial dermis. Separating some capillary loops and each vascular lobule are bands of fibrous stroma. RCM mosaic (2 mm × 2 mm) at the level of the dermis reveals a Swiss-cheese-like architecture created by multiple black lumina with variably refractile walls (white arrow) that are organized into lobules separated by thick stromal septa (red arrows).

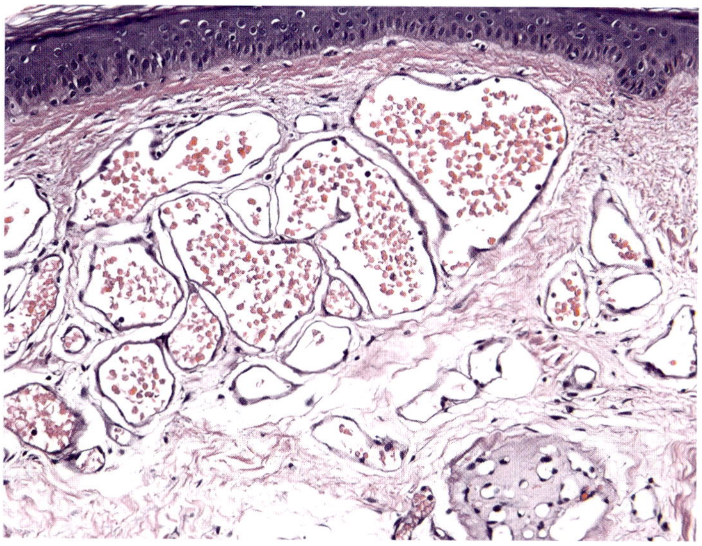

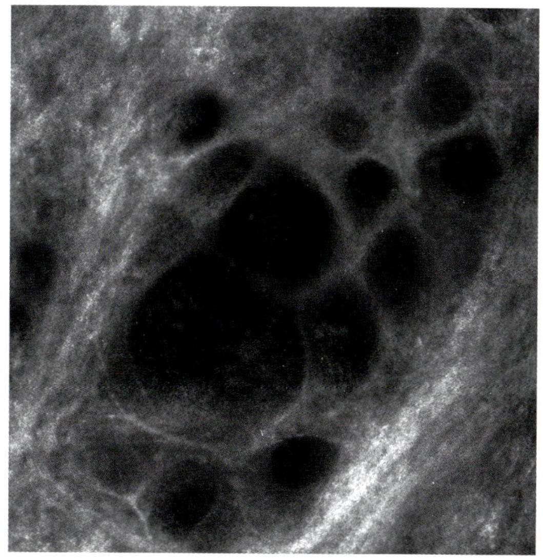

▲ **Figures 5.61, 5.62** At higher magnification, histology (20×) shows that tumoral lobules are composed of variably dilated capillaries containing blood cells. RCM (0.5 mm × 0.5 mm) clearly shows the same lobular arrangement and one can see weakly refractile round and oval structures, corresponding to blood cells, within the black lumina.

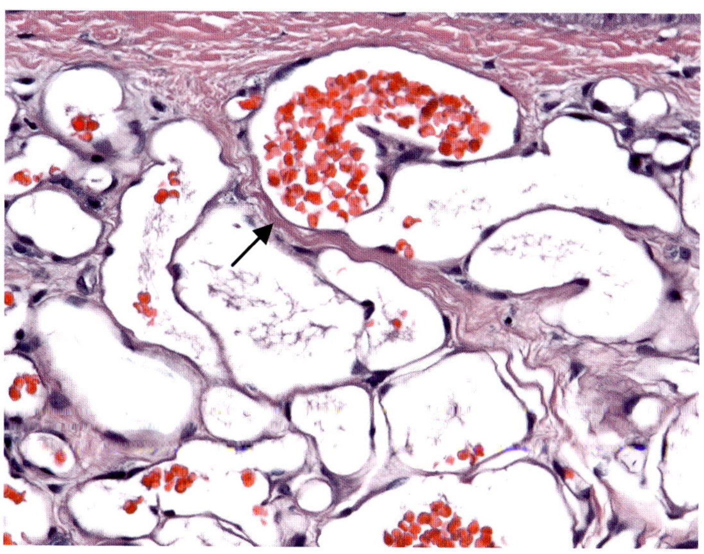

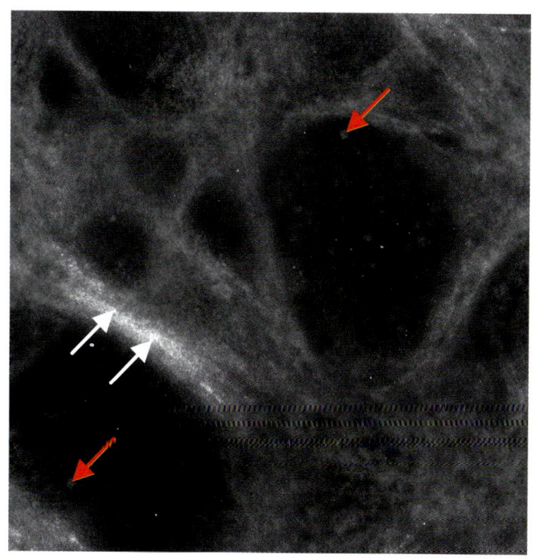

▲ **Figures 5.63, 5.64** At even higher magnification, histology (40×) reveals individual collagen bundles (arrow) forming the fibrous septa, which, on RCM (0.5 mm × 0.5 mm), are brightly refractile streaks (white arrows). Also visible in this RCM optical section are scattered brighter cells (red arrows), which correspond to granulocytes, intermixed with weakly refractile cells, which correspond to erythrocytes, filling the black lumina.

ANGIOKERATOMA

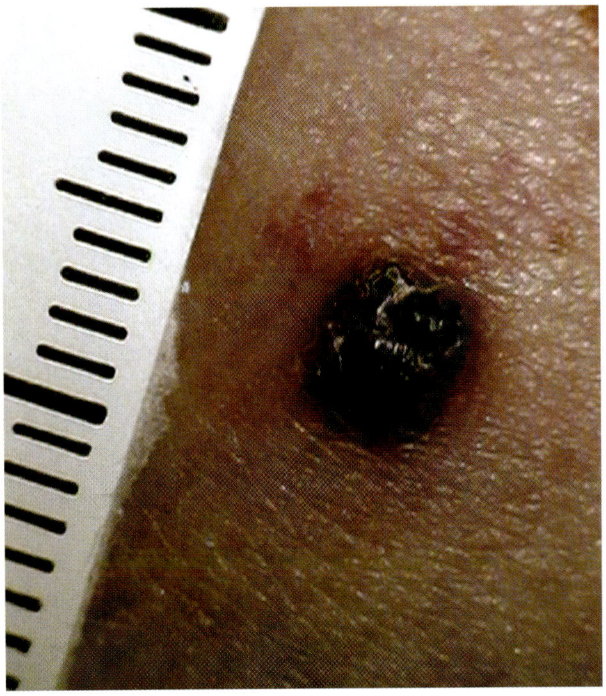
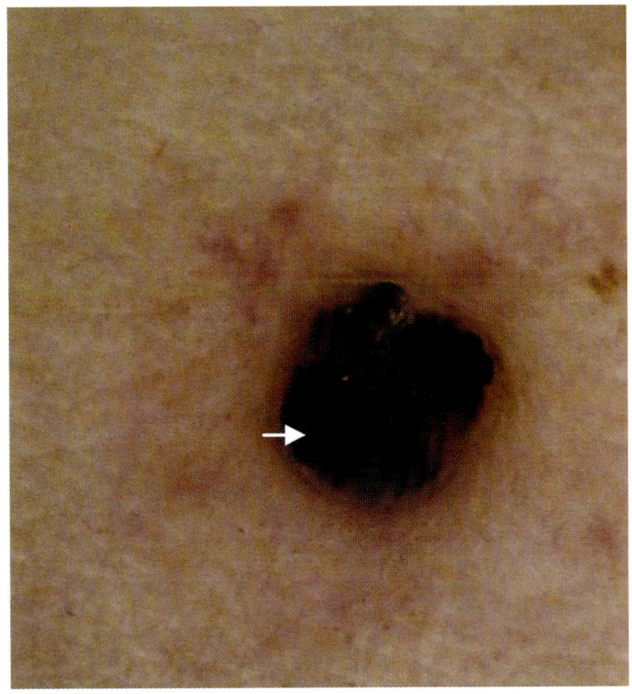

▲ **Figures 5.65, 5.66** Clinical photograph of a 5 mm, black, dome-shaped, keratotic papule on the leg. Dermoscopic photograph reveals a well-demarcated, dark lesion composed of multiple maroon-black lacunae (arrow), consistent with thrombosed angiokeratoma.

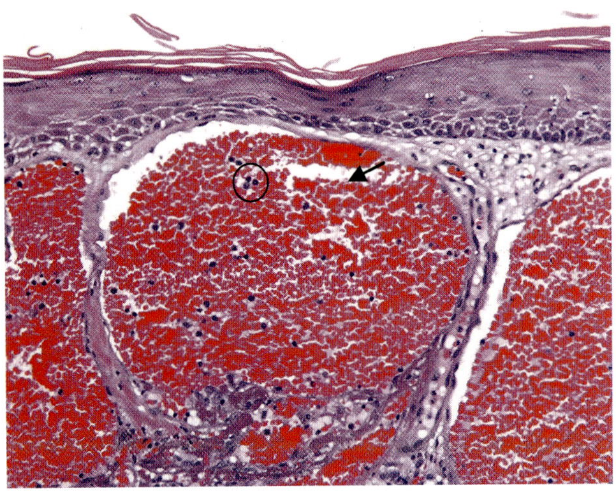
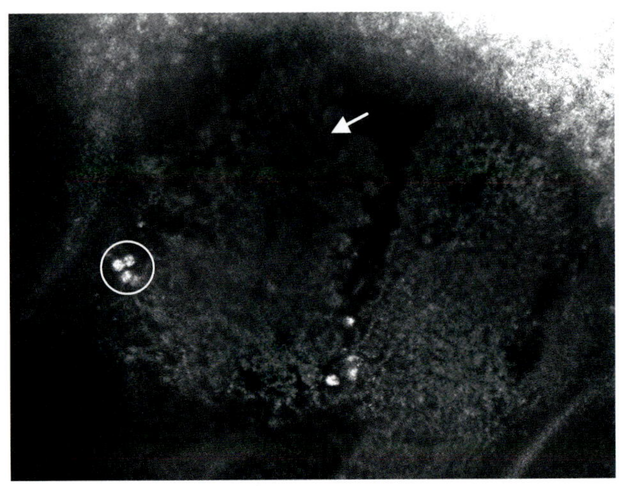

▲ **Figures 5.67, 5.68** Histology (20×) shows dilated and ectatic blood vessels just below the epidermis filled with erythrocytes (black arrow) and scattered granulocytes (circled). RCM (0.45 mm × 0.34 mm) of the superficial dermis shows a large, ectatic, black lumen abutting the epidermis filled with variably refractile cells: rare brightly refractile cells correspond to granulocytes (circled) and numerous less refractile cells correspond to erythrocytes (white arrow).

CHAPTER 5e

Mycosis fungoides

Melissa Gill, Anna Liza C Agero, Marco Ardigo, Patricia Myskowski, and Salvador González

Mycosis fungoides (MF), the most commonly encountered type of cutaneous T-cell lymphoma, is a malignant expansion of skin-homing T cells. It is a low-grade lymphoma with slight male predominance and can occur at any age, but is usually diagnosed in the sixth decade.[1] Usually MF is an indolent disease confined to the skin, characterized by long-standing patches and/or plaques. A minority of cases quickly progresses to an advanced stage, such as tumor or erythroderma, with nodal and/or visceral involvement, or transformation to aggressive large T-cell lymphoma.[1,2] The prognosis of MF is stage-dependent, ranging from 98% 10-year disease-specific survival in patients with limited patch/plaque disease, 20% 10-year disease-specific survival in patients with lymph node involvement, to a 0.9-year median survival in patients with visceral involvement.[1,3]

Correct diagnosis, especially in early skin lesions of MF, is complicated by its diverse and protean clinical expressions, often simulating other inflammatory dermatoses, and frequent non-specific histology.[2,4] Multiple and/or sequential skin biopsies are often needed to establish or confirm the diagnosis of MF.[5,6] In addition, costly ancillary tests, such as T-cell receptor clonality studies and immunohistochemistry to evaluate for down-regulation of pan-T-cell markers, are often employed for lesions with non-definitive histology.[7,8]

More than 25 clinicopathologic variants of MF are recognized; the three most commonly encountered are patch, plaque, and tumor.[2]

PATCH-TYPE MYCOSIS FUNGOIDES

The earliest stage of MF is conventionally characterized by slightly scaling erythematous or light brown flat macules and patches with an asymmetric distribution favoring non-sun-exposed ('bathing suit') areas (Figures 5.69, 5.70). Lesions may be single or multiple, asymptomatic or pruritic.[2,9] Characteristic histologic features of patch-type MF are sparse epidermotropic atypical, sometimes haloed, lymphocytes mainly confined to the basal layer; a superficial, sparse, lichenoid infiltrate of atypical lymphocytes and histiocytes; and wiry bundles of collagen in the papillary dermis (Figure 5.71).[1,4] Pagetoid epidermotropism and the highly characteristic Pautrier's microabscesses are rare.[2]

Reflectance confocal microscopy (RCM) findings of early patch lesions of MF, like histology, can be very subtle. RCM mosaics at the level of the dermal–epidermal junction (DEJ) show hyporefractile dermal papillary rings as compared with normal skin (Figure 5.72). The epidermis may show mild architectural disarray, with focal areas of thickened and blurred intercellular spaces, corresponding to trace-to-mild spongiosis on histology (Figures 5.73, 5.74). Sparse, weakly refractile, round-to-oval cells are scattered within the spinous layer, corresponding to epidermotropic atypical lymphocytes on histology (Figures 5.73, 5.74). These individual round-to-oval cells are sometimes difficult to identify due to similar refractility of intercellular spaces.

At the level of the DEJ, dermal papillary rings appear only faintly refractile and can be difficult to visualize on confocal (Figure 5.76). The hyporefractility of the dermal papillary rings may be due to atypical lymphocytes infiltrating the basal layer, as seen on histology, or possibly melanocyte apoptosis induced by tumor necrosis factor-α (TNF-α), involved in the pathogenesis of MF (Figure 5.75).[10] Normally, the DEJ is characterized by refractile round or oval rings, which is due to pigmented basal cells and interspersed melanocytes arranged circumferentially around dermal papillae (Figures 2.15, 2.16).[11] On RCM, the superficial dermis shows weakly refractile structures, but examination is often limited by a loss of contrast below the DEJ, resulting in difficulty distinguishing among blood flow, inflammatory cells, and collagen bundles (Figure 5.76).[12]

Key RCM features of patch-type mycosis fungoides

- Small weakly refractile round-to-oval cells within the spinous layer
- Hyporefractile dermal papillary rings

PLAQUE-TYPE MYCOSIS FUNGOIDES

Plaques of MF are often observed in concert and sometimes in contiguity with patch-type lesions (Figure 5.77).[2] The lesions appear as variably pruritic, infiltrated, well-demarcated erythematous to reddish-brown plaques with irregular borders and fine scaling (Figure 5.78). Plaques may show central clearing and occasionally are annular or serpiginous in configuration.[2,9,13] The histopathology of plaque-type MF is similar to patch-type MF, but shows much more epidermotropism, more frequent Pautrier's microabscesses (intraepidermal collections of atypical lymphocytes), and a denser dermal lichenoid infiltrate (Figure 5.79).[1,2] Spongiosis is disproportionally mild with respect to the amount of exocytosis.[2]

RCM is most useful for identifying plaque-type MF. Pautrier's microabscesses are readily identified on RCM mosaics at all levels of the epidermis as well-defined, round vesicle- and microvesicle-like dark spaces filled with weakly refractile material (Figure 5.80). Mosaics at the level of the DEJ show hyporefractile dermal papillary rings. RCM optical sections identify small, weakly refractile, round-to-oval cells packing the intraepidermal vesicle-like spaces, corresponding to Pautrier's microabscesses (Figures 5.81, 5.82). Small weakly refractile round-to-oval cells are scattered throughout the epidermis, corresponding to pagetoid epidermotropism on histology. In the surrounding epidermis, minimal-to-mild architectural disarray with thickened and blurred keratinocytic intercellular junctions is also observed; histology shows minimal-to-mild spongiosis and disruption of the epidermal architecture by infiltrating atypical lymphocytes. As with patch-type MF, dermal papillary rings are hyporefractile on RCM, and there is marked loss of contrast in the dermis, resulting in poor visualization of the dense lichenoid infiltrate seen on histology (Figures 5.83, 5.84).[12]

Key RCM features of plaque-type mycosis fungoides

- Small weakly refractile round-to-oval cells scattered within the spinous layer
- Intraepidermal vesicle-like dark spaces filled with small, weakly refractile, round-to-oval cells
- Hyporefractile dermal papillary rings

TUMOR-TYPE MYCOSIS FUNGOIDES

Tumor-type MF represents a more advanced stage of MF. Tumors appear as reddish-violet, commonly ulcerated nodules, which may be localized or generalized and usually occur in concert with MF patches and plaques (Figures 5.85, 5.86).[2,9] Lymph node or visceral involvement is much more common with tumor-type MF as compared with patch or plaque-type MF, with approximately 17% of patients developing extracutaneous disease.[14] Over 50% of patients with tumor-type MF develop large cell transformation, which is associated with a poor prognosis.[1,15] Tumor-type MF is histologically characterized by a diffuse dermal infiltrate of atypical lymphocytes (Figure 5.87). Epidermotropism is diminished and may be lost altogether (Figure 5.89, 5.91).[1,13]

Reflectance confocal microscopy of tumor-type MF may show changes similar to patch-type MF or rarely plaque-type MF. RCM mosaics at the level of the DEJ show hyporefractile dermal papillary rings (Figure 5.88). Optical sections of the epidermis may show slight architectural disarray with thickened intercellular junctions and scattered small, weakly refractile, round-to-oval cells (Figures 5.90, 5.92).

Rarely, intraepidermal vesicle-like dark spaces filled with small, weakly refractile, round-to-oval cells, corresponding to Pautrier's microabscesses, may be seen. As with the other MF lesions, RCM generally finds hyporefractile dermal papillary rings and loss of contrast in the dermis (Figures 5.92–5.94).[12] Lesions with little to no papillary dermal infiltrate may have no abnormal dermal findings on RCM, whereas tumors which abut the epidermis may show small, weakly refractile, round-to-oval cells filling the dermal papillae (Figure 5.92). Some lesions may show minimal discernible changes on confocal. RCM examination of tumor-type MF is mainly helpful in lesions with epidermotropism, where patch- or plaque-type MF confocal features are present. Non-epidermotropic tumor-type MF may be missed entirely on confocal; thus, a 'normal' RCM examination of suspected tumor-type MF should be considered non-diagnostic.

Key RCM features of tumor-type mycosis fungoides

- Variable presence of small, weakly refractile, round-to-oval cells within the spinous layer
- Variable presence of intraepidermal vesicle-like dark spaces filled with small, weakly refractile, round-to-oval cells
- Variable presence of hyporefractile dermal papillary rings
- Variable presence of small, weakly refractile, round-to-oval cells filling the papillary dermis

REFERENCES

1. Willemze R, Jaffe ES, Burg G et al. WHO-EORTC classification for cutaneous lymphomas. Blood 2005; 105(10):3768–85.
2. Cerroni L, Gatter K, Kerl H. Mycosis fungoides. An illustrated guide to skin lymphoma, 2nd edn. Malden, MA: Blackwell; 2004: 9–38.
3. Smith BD, Wilson LD. Management of mycosis fungoides. Part 1. Diagnosis, staging, and prognosis. Oncology (Williston Park) 2003; 17(9):1281–8.
4. Massone C, Kodama K, Kerl H, Cerroni L. Histopathologic features of early (patch) lesions of mycosis fungoides: a morphologic study on 745 biopsy specimens from 427 patients. Am J Surg Pathol 2005; 29(4):550–60.
5. Diamandidou E, Cohen PR, Kurzrock R. Mycosis fungoides and Sezary syndrome. Blood 1996; 88(7): 2385–409.
6. Glass LF, Keller KL, Messina JL et al. Cutaneous T-cell lymphoma. Cancer Control 1998; 5(1):11–8.
7. Florell SR, Cessna M, Lundell RB et al. Usefulness (or lack thereof) of immunophenotyping in atypical cutaneous T-cell infiltrates. Am J Clin Pathol 2006; 125(5):727–36.
8. Ponti R, Quaglino P, Novelli M et al. T-cell receptor gamma gene rearrangement by multiplex polymerase chain reaction/heteroduplex analysis in patients with cutaneous T-cell lymphoma (mycosis fungoides/Sezary syndrome) and benign inflammatory disease: correlation with clinical, histological and immunophenotypical findings. Br J Dermatol 2005; 153(3):565–73.
9. Latkowski J, Heald P. Cutaneous T-cell lymphomas. In: Freedberg IM, Eisen AZ, Wolff K, Austen KF, Goldsmith LA, Katz SI, eds. Fitzpatrick's Dermatology in General Medicine, 6th edn. New York: McGraw-Hill; 2003: 1537–58.
10. Shang J, Eberle J, Geilen CC et al. The role of nuclear factor-kappa B and melanogenesis in tumor necrosis factor-alpha-induced apoptosis of normal human melanocytes. Skin Pharmacol Appl Skin Physiol 2002; 15(5):321–9.
11. Rajadhyaksha M, Gonzalez S, Zavislan JM et al. In vivo confocal scanning laser microscopy of human skin II: advances in instrumentation and comparison with histology. J Invest Dermatol 1999; 113(3):293–303.
12. Agero AL, Gill M, Ardigo M et al. In vivo reflectance confocal microscopy of mycosis fungoides: a preliminary study. J Am Acad Dermatol 2007; 57(3): 435–41.
13. Murphy G, Schwarting R. Cutaneous lymphomas and leukemias. In: Elder D, Elenitsas R, Johnson BL, Murphy GF, eds. Lever's Histopathology of the Skin, 9th edn. Philadelphia: Lippincott-Raven; 2005: 950–6.
14. van Doorn R, Van Haselen CW, van Voorst Vader PC et al. Mycosis fungoides: disease evolution and prognosis of 309 Dutch patients. Arch Dermatol 2000; 136(4):504–10.
15. Cerroni L, Rieger E, Hodl S, Kerl H. Clinicopathologic and immunologic features associated with transformation of mycosis fungoides to large-cell lymphoma. Am J Surg Pathol 1992; 16(6):543–52.

PATCH-TYPE MYCOSIS FUNGOIDES

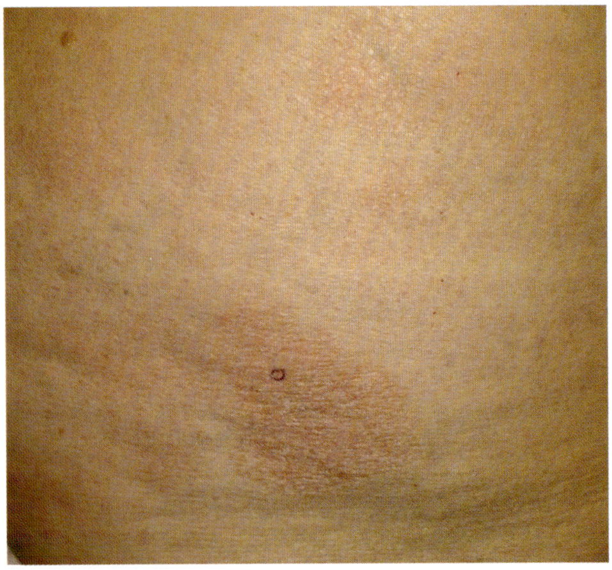

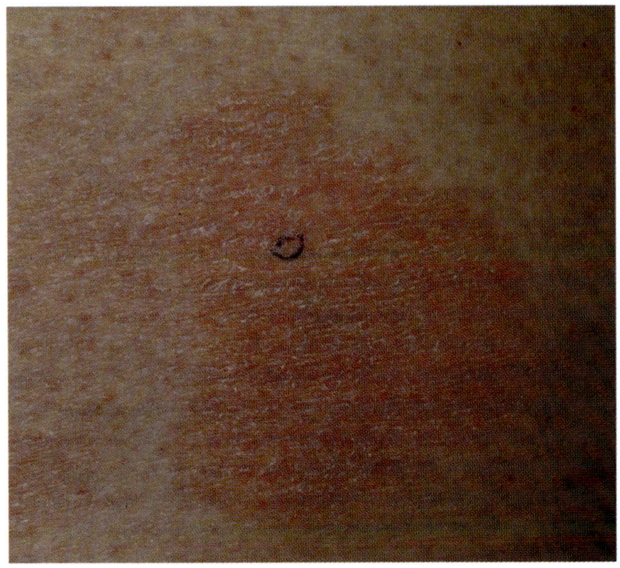

▲ **Figures 5.69, 5.70** Clinical photograph of the right hip of a 61-year-old female with multiple erythematous (pink to orange) finely scaling patches. The patient had a 6-year history of similar patches on the trunk. A close-up photograph of one patch; the circle marks the area where confocal followed by punch biopsy was performed.

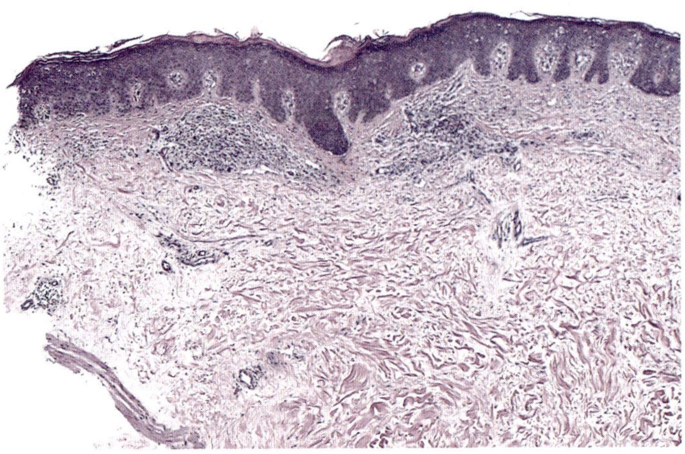

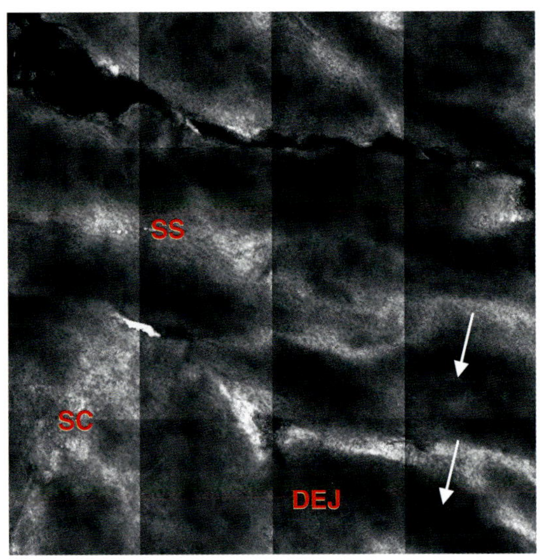

▲ **Figures 5.71, 5.72** Histology (4×) shows hyperkeratotic stratum corneum, mild acanthosis, and a patchy lichenoid infiltrate within the superficial dermis. The surface contour shows an irregular undulating pattern. Due to this undulation, RCM mosaic (2 mm × 2 mm) shows several epidermal layers simultaneously: stratum corneum (SC), stratum spinosum (SS), and dermal–epidermal junction (DEJ). Dermal papillary rings are notably hyporefractile (arrows).

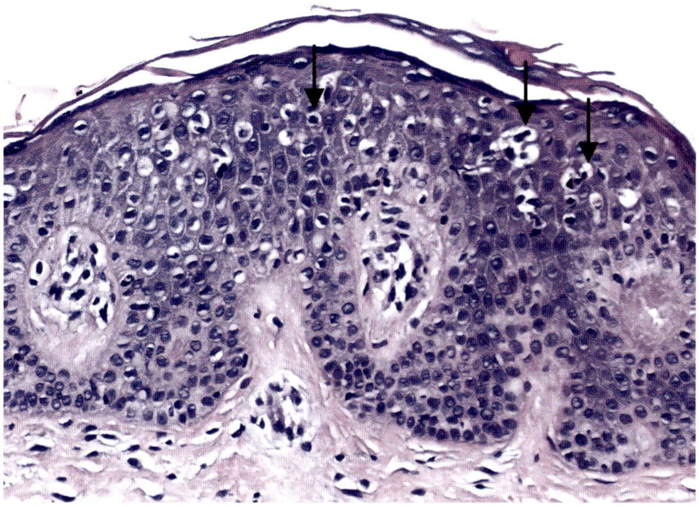

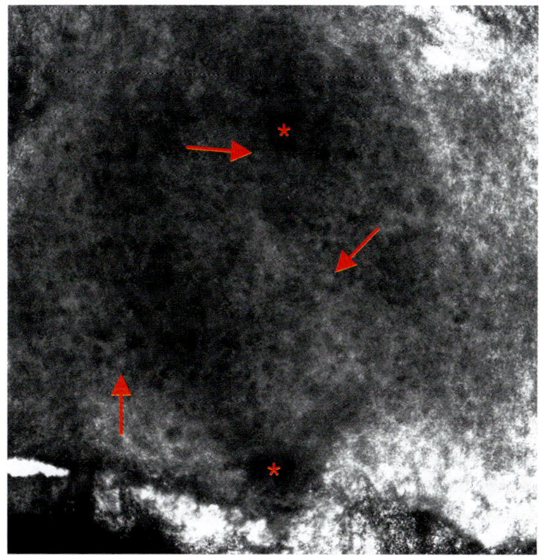

▲ **Figures 5.73, 5.74** Histology (20×) shows disproportionate exocytosis: the presence of many epidermotropic haloed lymphocytes (black arrows) with only minimal associated spongiosis. RCM (0.5 mm × 0.5 mm) of the spinous layer shows many small weakly refractile round-to-oval cells (red arrows) scattered among the keratinocytes and mild epidermal disarray, characterized by thickened, hazy keratinocytic intercellular junctions and focal loss of intercellular junctions (asterisks).

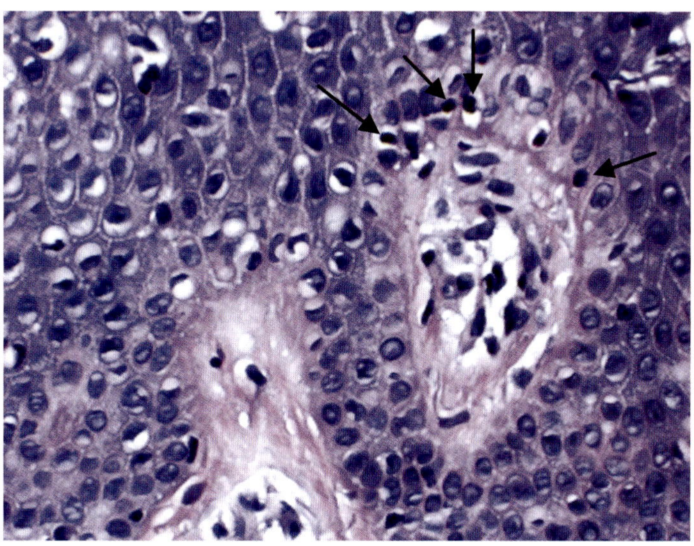

▲ **Figures 5.75, 5.76** Histology (40×) shows atypical lymphocytes in the papillary dermis and within the basal layer of the epidermis (arrows). RCM (0.5 mm × 0.5 mm) at the level of the DEJ shows hyporefractile dermal papillary rings.

PLAQUE-TYPE MYCOSIS FUNGOIDES

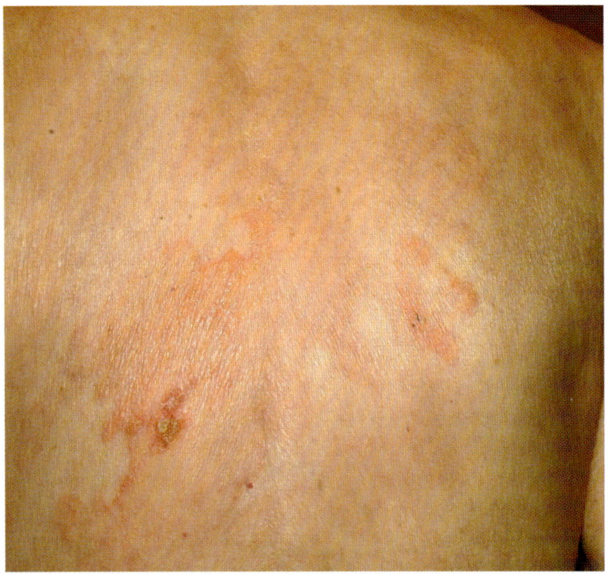
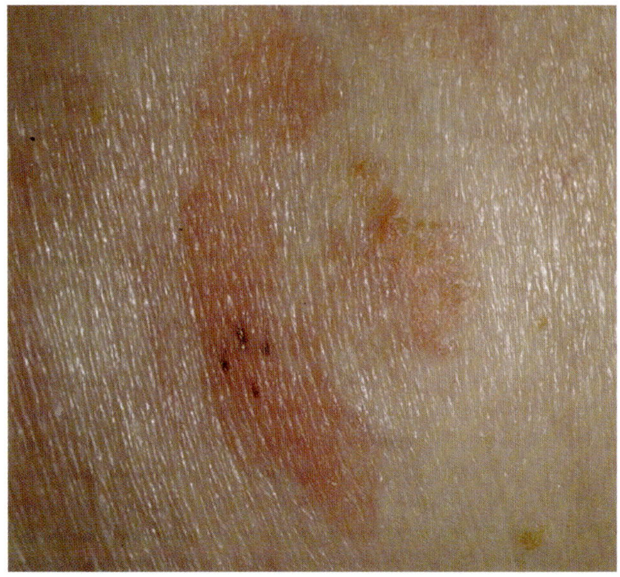

▲ **Figures 5.77, 5.78** Clinical photograph of the back of a 79-year-old woman with erythematous patches and plaques on her posterior trunk for 6 months. The patient recently developed similar lesions on her thighs and hips. A close-up photograph of a plaque on her right upper back; the four purple dots mark the area where confocal followed by punch biopsy was performed.

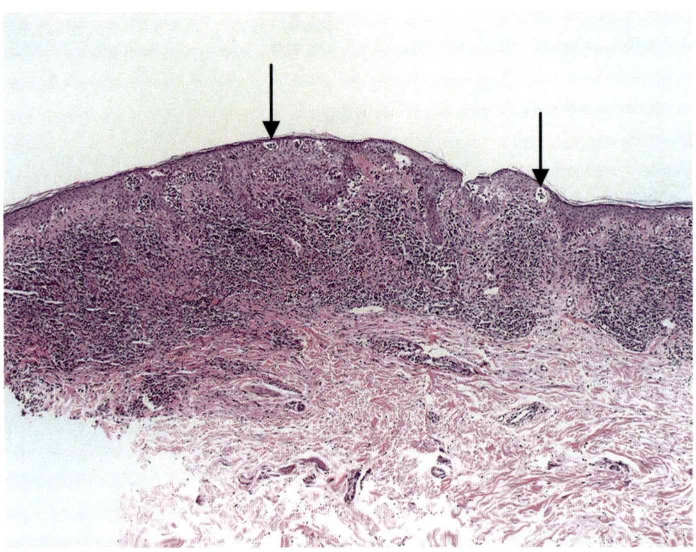
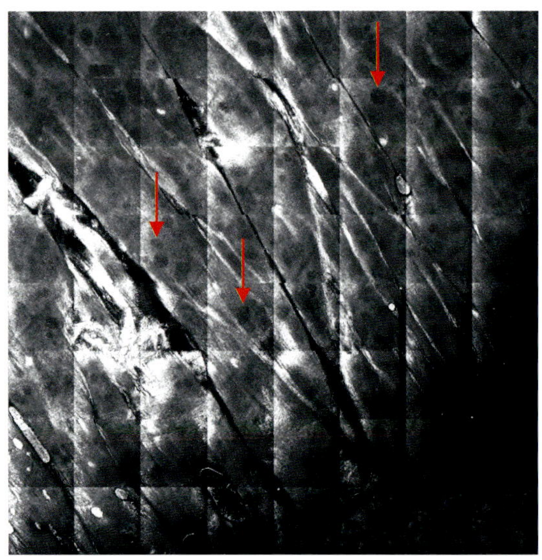

▲ **Figures 5.79, 5.80** Histology (4×) shows intraepidermal collections (black arrows) of lymphocytes and a dense, band-like infiltrate in the superficial dermis. Corresponding RCM mosaic (4 mm × 4 mm) reveals multiple vesicle-like dark spaces in the epidermis (red arrows).

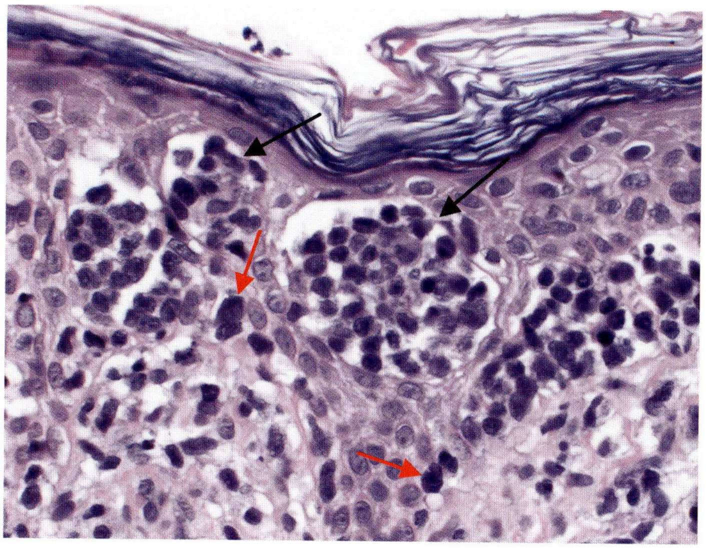

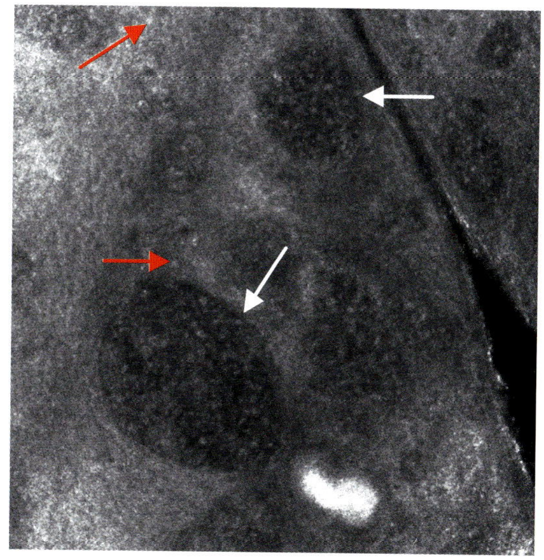

▲ **Figures 5.81, 5.82** Histology (40×) shows intraepidermal collections of atypical lymphocytes (Pautrier's microabscess) (black arrows) and scattered epidermotropic atypical lymphocytes (red arrows). RCM (0.5 mm × 0.5 mm) at the level of the stratum spinosum shows weakly refractile round-to-oval cells, both within vesicle-like dark spaces (white arrows) and scattered among keratinocytes (red arrows).

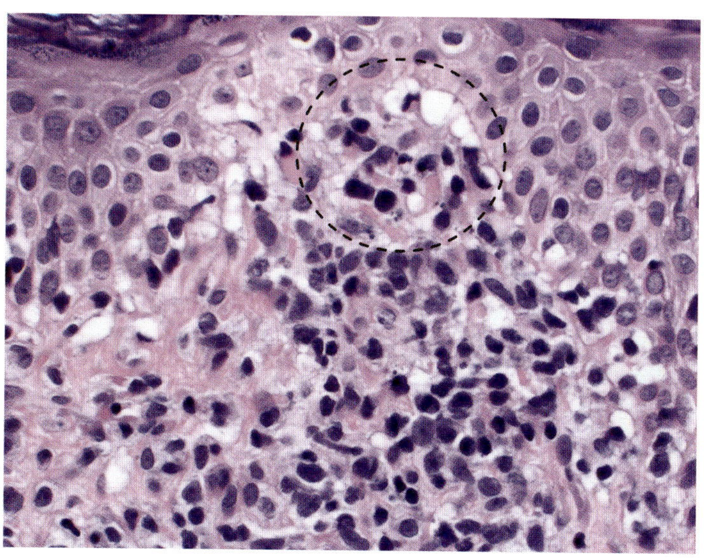

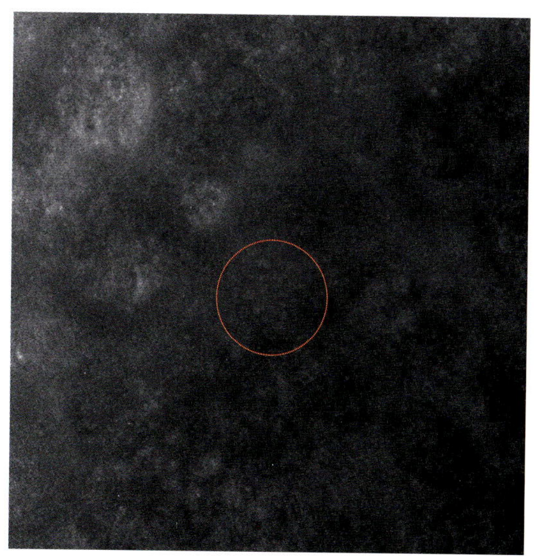

▲ **Figures 5.83, 5.84** Histopathology (40×) shows the presence of atypical lymphocytes obscuring the DEJ (circled) and filling the dermal papilla. Hyporefractile dermal papillary rings are almost impossible to discern on RCM (0.5 mm × 0.5 mm). Within the papillary dermis, several weakly refractile oval-to-round cells are seen (circled).

TUMOR-TYPE MYCOSIS FUNGOIDES

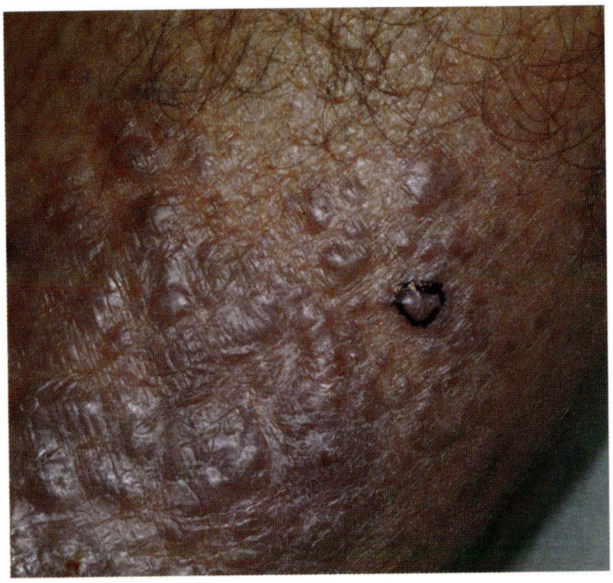
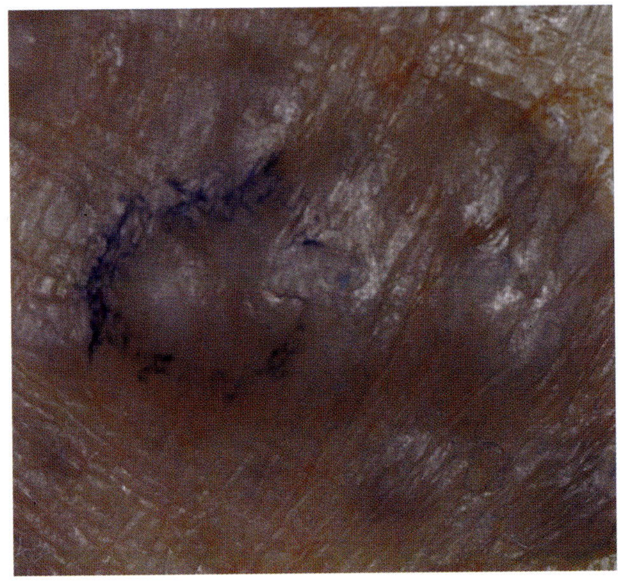

▲ **Figures 5.85, 5.86** Clinical photograph of coalescing violaceous nodules on the lower leg of a 66-year-old man. This patient also had erythematous patches and plaques on his arms and trunk. A close-up photograph of a nodule; the circle marks the area where confocal followed by punch biopsy was performed.

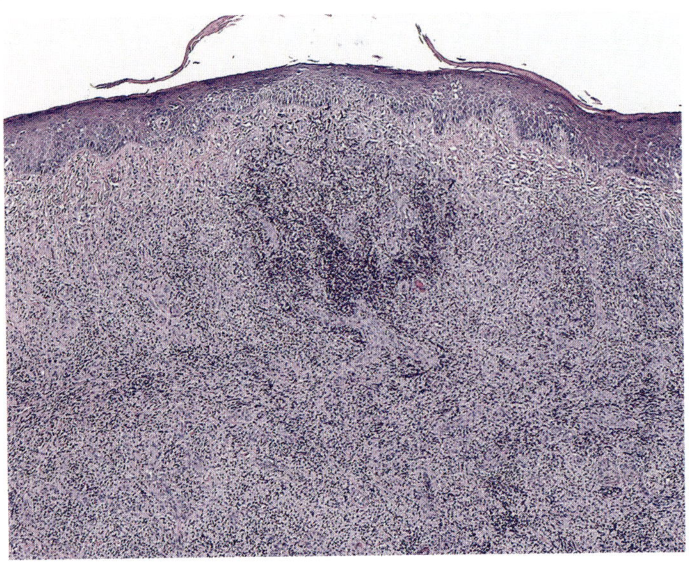
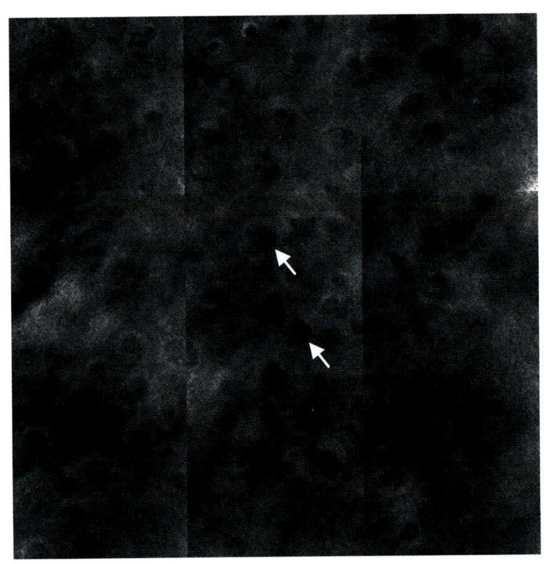

▲ **Figures 5.87, 5.88** Histopathology (4×) shows a dense dermal infiltrate. There is a relative paucity of lymphocytes in the very superficial dermis and only mild epidermotropism is seen. Corresponding RCM mosaic (1.5 mm × 1.5 mm) at the level of the DEJ reveals hyporefractile dermal papillary rings (white arrows).

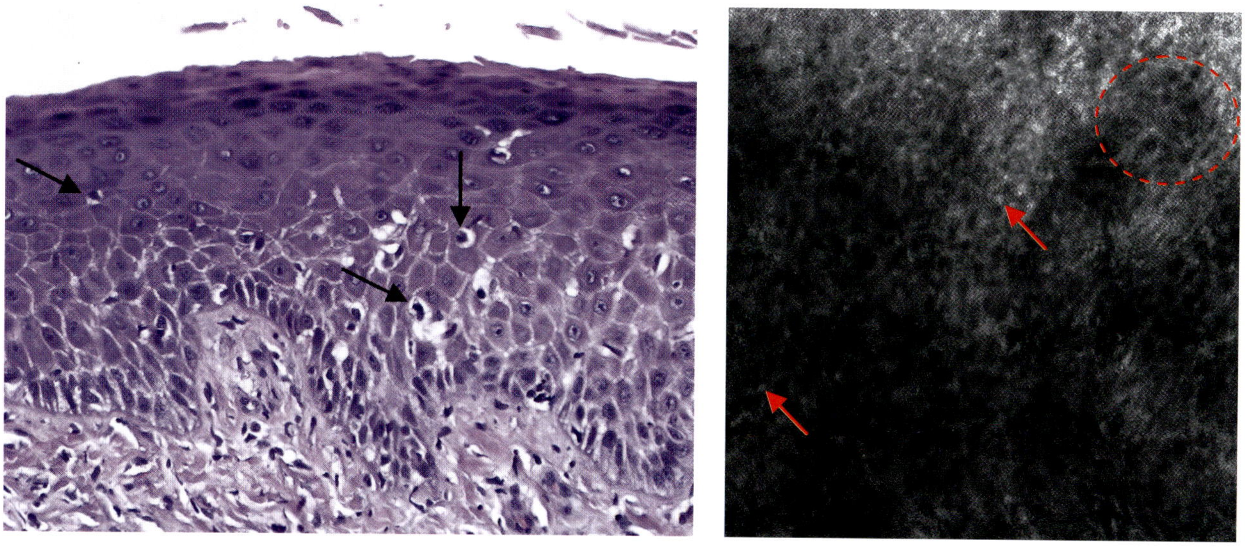

▲ **Figures 5.89, 5.90** Histology (20×) shows sparse intraepidermal atypical lymphocytes (arrows) and mild spongiosis. RCM (0.5 mm × 0.5 mm) at the level of the stratum spinosum shows a few small weakly refractile round-to-oval cells scattered among the keratinocytes (arrows). Also seen are variably thickened keratinocytic intercellular junctions (circle). Reproduced with permission of J Am Acad Dermatol from Agero AL, Gill M, Ardigo M et al. In vivo reflectance confocal microscopy of mycosis fungoides: a preliminary study. 57(3): 435–41.

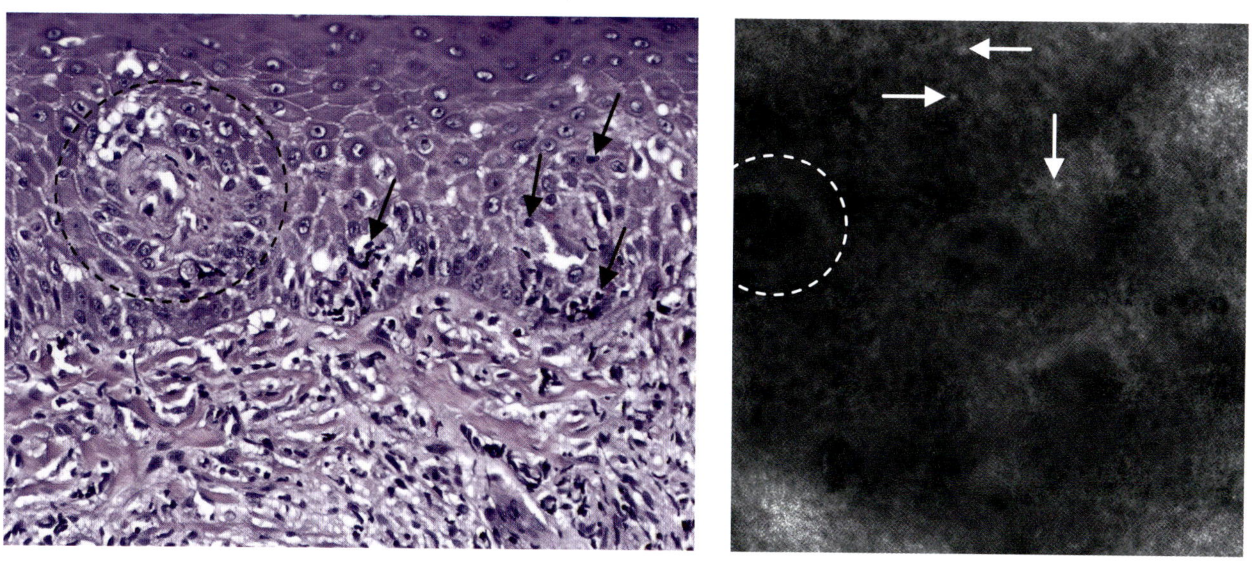

▲ **Figures 5.91, 5.92** Histology (20×) shows atypical lymphocytes in the stratum spinosum and infiltrating the stratum basalis (arrows) with associated mild spongiosis. Within the dermal papilla (circled) and the superficial dermis, scattered atypical lymphocytes and coarse collagen bundles are seen. RCM (0.5 mm × 0.5 mm) at the level of the superficial DEJ shows weakly refractile round cells scattered among keratinocytes (arrows). Dermal papillary rings are hyporefractile (circled) and contain weakly refractile round-to-oval structures.

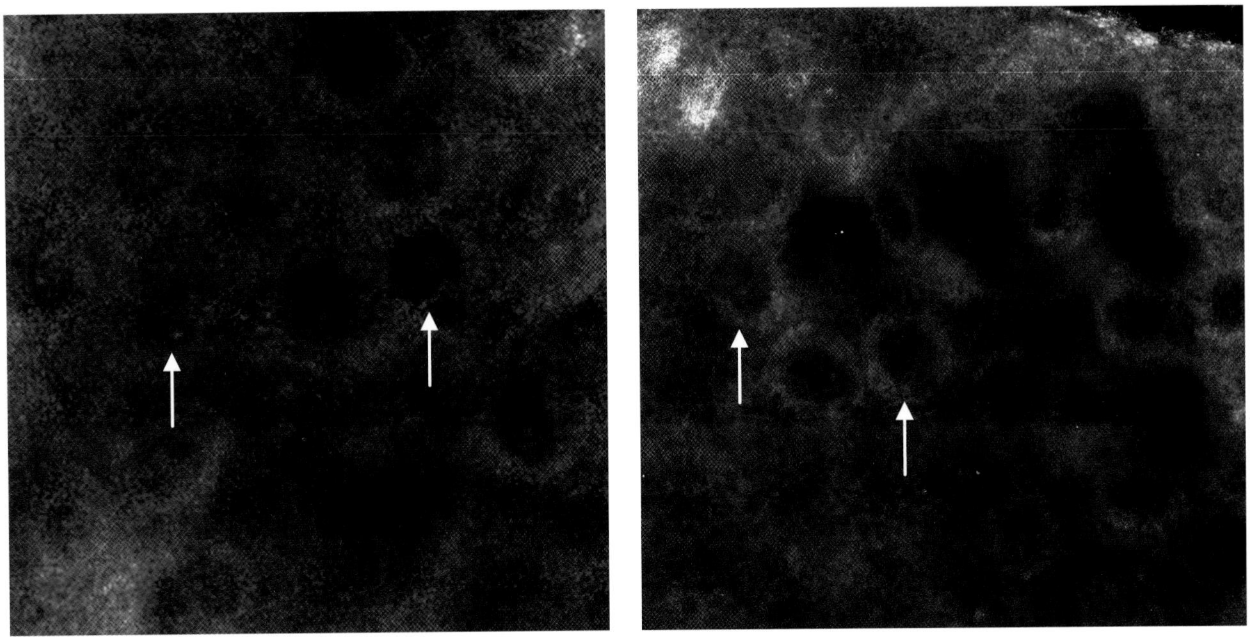

▲ **Figures 5.93, 5.94** RCM (0.5 mm × 0.5 mm) of lesional skin (left) from the level of the DEJ shows dermal papillary rings (arrows) which are hyporefractile in comparison to contralateral non-lesional skin (right).

CHAPTER 6a

Adjunct to clinical diagnosis

Alon Scope, Allan C Halpern, Melissa Gill, Salvador González, and Ashfaq A Marghoob

Recognition of the primary morphology of skin disease is the foundation on which dermatologic diagnosis is based. To better identify and understand primary morphology requires that dermatologists attain knowledge in skin pathology. Thus, it stands to reason that in-vivo visualization of the deeper layers of the skin – those layers that are beyond the reach of examination with the unaided eye – has the potential to improve the clinician's diagnostic accuracy.[1] This, in part, has fueled the development of various bedside optical instruments, which are designed to enhance the in-vivo visual examination of skin lesions and diseases.[2] These devices range from plain surface magnification by a handheld lens, through contrast augmentation by Wood's lamp, to subsurface visualization by dermoscopy. However, the ability to image the skin in-vivo at the microscopic and cellular level may herald a new era for clinicians. Reflectance confocal microscopy (RCM) is making important inroads at becoming a tool that increases diagnostic acumen by allowing clinicians to better appreciate skin pathology at the bedside.[3–5] Potential benefits of RCM as an adjunct to clinical diagnosis include identification of skin cancers at an earlier stage and avoiding unnecessary biopsies of benign lesions. In this chapter, we present examples of cases in which RCM was utilized as a clinical adjunct to diagnosis.

CASE PRESENTATIONS

Case 1

This case demonstrates how RCM increased the clinician's diagnostic acumen beyond clinical and dermoscopic examination for a nondescript pink lesion, correctly identifying the lesion as a melanoma.

A 43-year-old female patient with a history of extensive childhood sun-exposure presented to the pigmented lesion clinic for dermatologic cancer screening. She was not aware of any new or changed lesions. During the physical examination, the dermatologist noted a 7 mm nondescript pink-to-brown papule on the patient's posterior leg, within a background of multiple solar lentigines (Figures 6.1, 6.2). Under dermoscopy (Figure 6.3), most of the lesion was found to harbor structureless areas with faint tan-to-pink pigmentation. At one pole of the lesion, a 2 mm ill-defined brown-gray area with faint peripheral streaks and globules was observed, suggesting a suspicious melanocytic lesion with asymmetric distribution of dermoscopic colors and structures. The dermatologist decided to further assess the lesion using RCM.

RCM examination of the pigmented pole revealed architectural disarray of the dermal–epidermal junction (DEJ) with a thickened rete meshwork and poorly delineated aggregates of bright cells (Figure 6.4).

Furthermore, RCM examination of the area that was structureless on dermoscopy revealed numerous, bright, large atypical cells both in aggregates and individually at the DEJ (Figure 6.6). An additional observation was the presence of bright, nucleated roundish cells in the stratum spinosum with focal loss of the honeycomb pattern, suggesting pagetoid spread (Figure 6.8). Given the architectural disarray and cellular atypia (Figure 6.10), the lesion was considered suspicious for melanoma. The clinician performed an excisional biopsy with 2 mm margins. Histopathologic analysis revealed melanoma, focally invasive to a Breslow thickness of 0.4 mm with features of regression (Figures 6.5, 6.7, 6.9, 6.11).

Case 2

This case demonstrates how RCM increased the clinician's suspicion for melanoma beyond equivocal clinical and dermoscopic examination for a small pigmented macule. The clinician's confidence in the diagnosis contributed to his decision to perform a biopsy in a cosmetically sensitive area.

A 79-year-old male patient without any history of skin cancer, but with multiple atypical nevi, presented for routine total cutaneous examination. The patient did not bring to attention new or changed lesions. The dermatologist noted a 5 mm nondescript brown macule on the tip of the nose (Figure 6.12) that, according to the patient's history, had been present for over 5 years and had been treated with liquid nitrogen several years previously to no avail. On dermoscopic examination (Figure 6.13), the lesion had equivocal focal findings of asymmetric follicular openings and perifollicular annular–granular pattern that raised concern of an early lentigo maligna. Given the cosmetic implications of a biopsy on the tip of the nose in a long-standing small lesion with inconclusive dermoscopic findings, the dermatologist decided to further assess the lesion with RCM.

RCM examination revealed perifollicular bright dendritic cells in the basal layer of the epidermis with focal follicular extension (Figures 6.14, 6.17). Bright dendritic cells were also focally seen extending up to the stratum granulosum, suspicious for upward migration of melanocytes (Figure 6.20). Multiple plump bright cells, compatible with melanophages, were observed in the superficial dermis (Figure 6.23). The RCM findings, suspicious for lentigo maligna, increased the clinician's confidence that a biopsy was needed. The lesion was removed by a deep shave biopsy and histopathologic analysis confirmed the diagnosis of malignant melanoma in situ, lentigo maligna type (Figures 6.15, 6.16, 6.18, 6.19, 6.21, 6.22, 6.24).

Case 3

This case demonstrates how RCM analysis increased the clinician's confidence that a lesion was benign and could be conservatively monitored. The decision *not* to perform a biopsy has greater cosmetic implications on the face.

A 64-year-old female patient with an unremarkable medical history has been followed over 4 years for a pigmented lesion on the forehead, which darkened compared with baseline photography. Clinically, this was a 5 mm brown macule, and, dermoscopically, it showed fine reticulation and gray peppering, compatible with a solar lentigo with features of lichen planus-like keratosis (Figures 6.25, 6.26). The clinical assessment was that of a benign lesion, but the patient remained skeptical. The dermatologist decided to perform an RCM examination with the notion that, if RCM showed only banal findings, the lesion would be rendered to short-term monitoring and, if suspicious findings were observed, the lesion would be biopsied.

RCM examination revealed an organized rete meshwork outlined by monomorphic round, bright keratinocytes in the basal layer of the epidermis (Figures 6.27–6.30). In addition, plump bright cells and small bright cells, compatible with melanophages and other inflammatory cells, were seen in the upper dermis (Figures 6.31, 6.32). The lesion did not show any RCM findings suspicious for malignancy. The patient was reassured by the dermatologist, and further photographically assisted follow-up over the next 4 months did not identify any worrisome clinical or dermoscopic changes. At 1-year follow-up, the lesion had undergone near complete resolution.

Case 4

This case demonstrates how RCM helped clinch the correct diagnosis of two new pink lesions with nonspecific clinical and dermoscopic characteristics.

A 62-year-old male patient, with history of two primary invasive melanomas in the past year, presented for interval dermatologic follow-up. He was not aware of any new or changed lesions. During the physical examination, the dermatologist noted two new concerning erythematous lesions (Figure 6.33). The first lesion was a 1 cm, ill-marginated, erythematous papule on the mid back (Figure 6.34, inset). On dermoscopy, this lesion was mostly nondescript, with few short, branching blood vessels (Figure 6.34). The clinical differential diagnosis was between a basal cell carcinoma (BCC) and an amelanotic melanoma. The other lesion was a 1 cm, pink-brown papule on the right shoulder (Figure 6.35, inset). On dermoscopy, this lesion showed multiple milia-like cysts, comedo-like openings, pigmented globules, and an area with clustered comma-shaped blood vessels (Figure 6.35). Diagnosis was uncertain since this lesion was complex, showing dermoscopic features of both a seborrheic keratosis and a melanocytic lesion.

RCM of the lesion on the mid back revealed areas at the level of the basal epidermis and upper dermis that were less refractile than surrounding tissue (Figures 6.36, 6.38). In addition, one was able to observe aggregates of elongated ill-demarcated cells and increased capillary blood flow within the lesion (Figure 6.40). These RCM findings were suggestive of BCC, and this lesion was removed by shave biopsy. The final histologic diagnosis was indeed superficial BCC (Figures 6.37, 6.39, 6.41). RCM of the lesion on the right shoulder revealed DEJ disarray with focal loss of the dermal papillae architecture, and multiple cystic inclusions containing highly refractile material (keratin) in the epidermis (Figure 6.42). In addition, increased capillary blood flow was seen in the superficial dermis during real-time examination (Figure 6.44). Dense nests and sparse aggregates of refractile nucleated cells at the DEJ and in the papillary dermis (Figures 6.42, 6.44, 6.46) confirmed the presence of a melanocytic lesion. Melanocytes in suprabasal layers of the epidermis and atypical melanocytes were not observed on RCM. However, given the unusual dermoscopic findings in a lesion that was confirmed to be melanocytic by RCM, the lesion was completely excised. The final diagnosis was compound melanocytic nevus focally inflamed and with epidermal seborrheic keratosis-like changes (Figures 6.43, 6.45, 6.47).

Key points for the use of RCM as an adjunct to clinical diagnosis

- RCM examination can increase the clinician's suspicion that a clinically and dermoscopically equivocal lesion is indeed skin cancer (i.e. increased sensitivity)
- RCM examination can increase the clinician's confidence that a lesion that appears clinically and dermoscopically banal is indeed benign (i.e. increased specificity)
- RCM may provide complementary information on nondescript lesions, resulting in an increased diagnostic accuracy and also impacting management

REFERENCES

1. Marghoob AA, Halpern AC. Confocal scanning laser reflectance microscopy: why bother? Arch Dermatol 2005; 141(2):212–15.

2. Marghoob AA, Swindle LD, Moricz CZ et al. Instruments and new technologies for the in vivo diagnosis of melanoma. J Am Acad Dermatol 2003; 49(5):777–97; quiz 798–9.

3. Gerger A, Koller S, Weger W et al. Sensitivity and specificity of confocal laser-scanning microscopy for in vivo diagnosis of malignant skin tumors. Cancer 2006; 107(1):193–200.

4. Nori S, Rius-Diaz F, Cuevas J et al. Sensitivity and specificity of reflectance-mode confocal microscopy for in vivo diagnosis of basal cell carcinoma: a multicenter study. J Am Acad Dermatol 2004; 51(6): 923–30.

5. Pellacani G, Cesinaro AM, Seidenari S. Reflectance-mode confocal microscopy of pigmented skin lesions – improvement in melanoma diagnostic specificity. J Am Acad Dermatol 2005; 53(6):979–85.

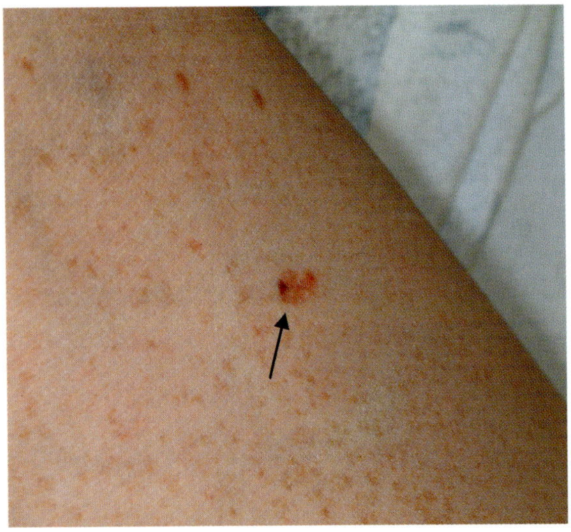

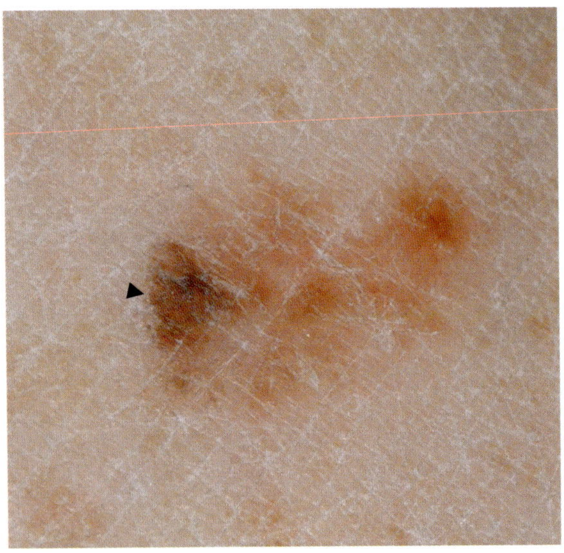

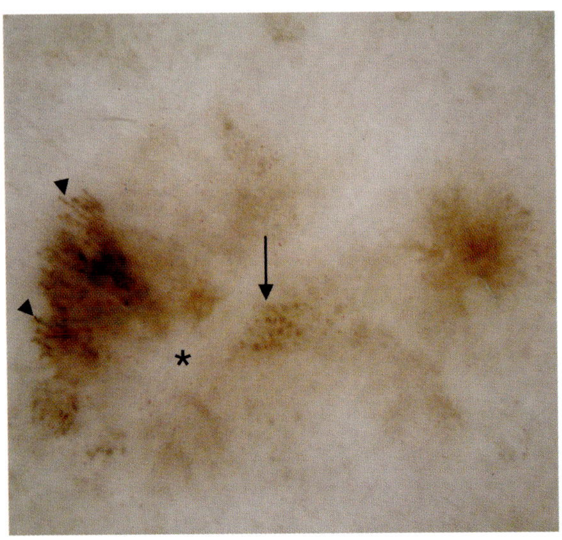

◀ **Figures 6.1–6.3**

Case 1: clinical overview photograph of a small nondescript lesion (arrow) arising in a background of multiple lentigines on the posterior leg of a 43-year-old woman. Close-up clinical inspection reveals a 7 mm irregularly pigmented pink-red macule with a darker brown pole (arrowhead). Dermoscopic image shows a multicomponent lesion with central globules (arrow), regression area (asterisk), and an ill-defined brown-bluish blotch from which peripheral streaks and irregular globules emanate (arrowheads).

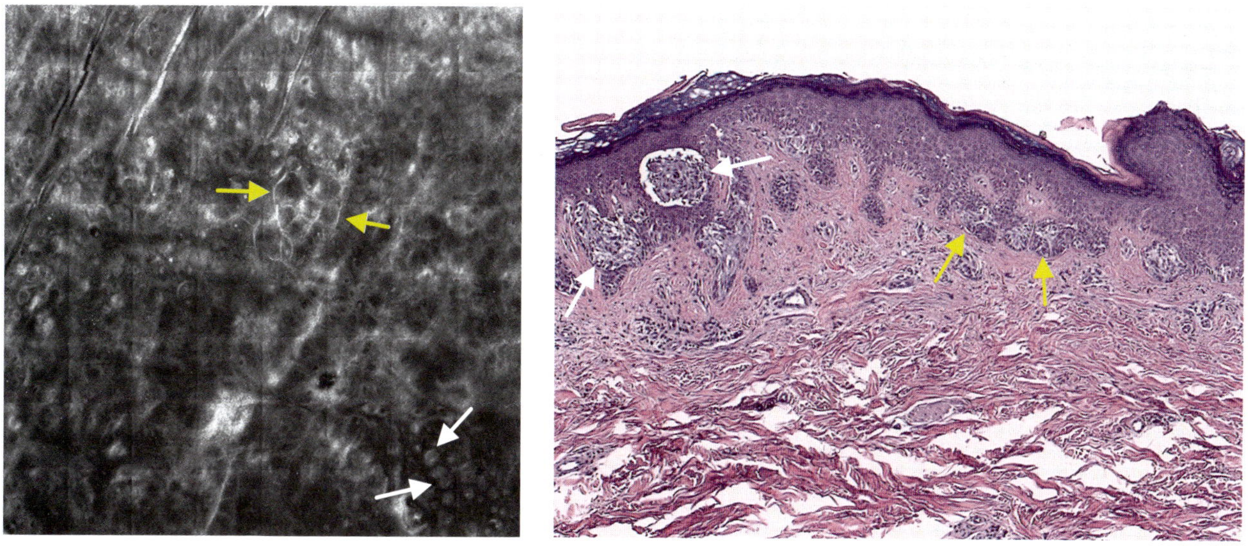

▲ **Figures 6.4, 6.5** Case 1: RCM mosaic (4 mm × 4 mm) at the level of the DEJ obtained at the pigmented pole of the lesion demonstrates an asymmetrical lesion with non-edged papillae showing bright, prominent interlacing rete (yellow arrows) in one area and aggregated cell clusters (white arrows) in another area. Corresponding histology (4×) shows focally discohesive (white arrows) junctional nests of melanocytes, which vary in size and bridge adjacent rete (yellow arrows).

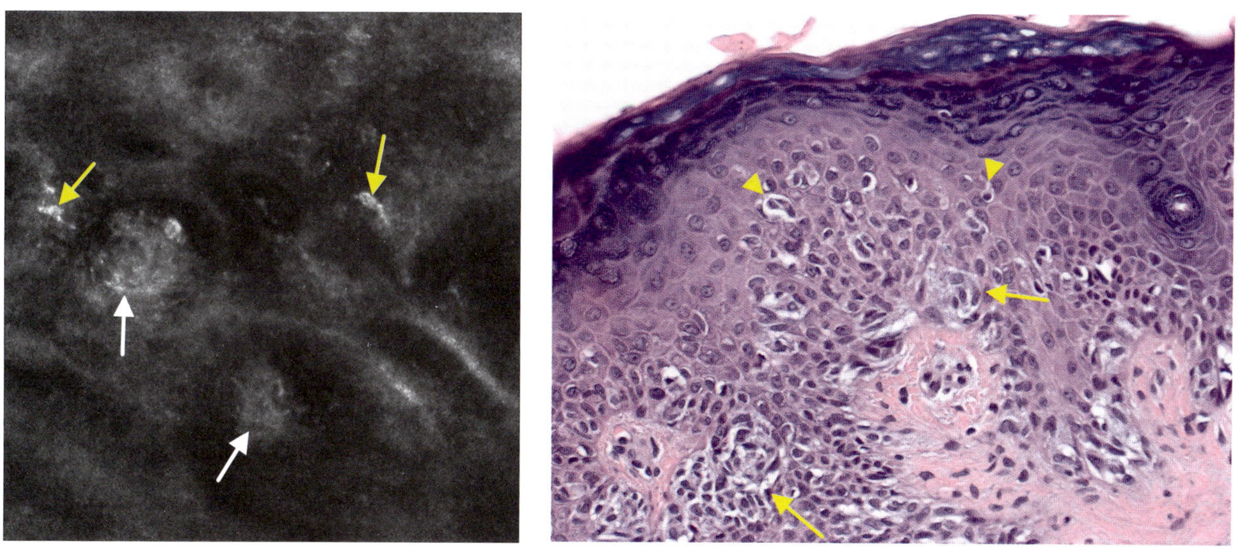

▲ **Figures 6.6, 6.7** Case 1: RCM (0.5 mm × 0.5 mm) at the level of the lower stratum spinosum/upper DEJ demonstrates near total loss of the normal honeycomb pattern, non-edged papillae, and the presence of ill-formed, dishomogeneous cell clusters, (white arrows) containing dendritic cells and large, atypical bright, round nucleated cells. Solitary atypical cells (yellow arrows), refractile particles, and dendritic structures are also seen. Corresponding histology (20×) shows a haphazard proliferation of enlarged, solitary and nested (arrows) melanocytes at the DEJ and scattered within the stratum spinosum (arrowheads). Focal junctional confluence is seen.

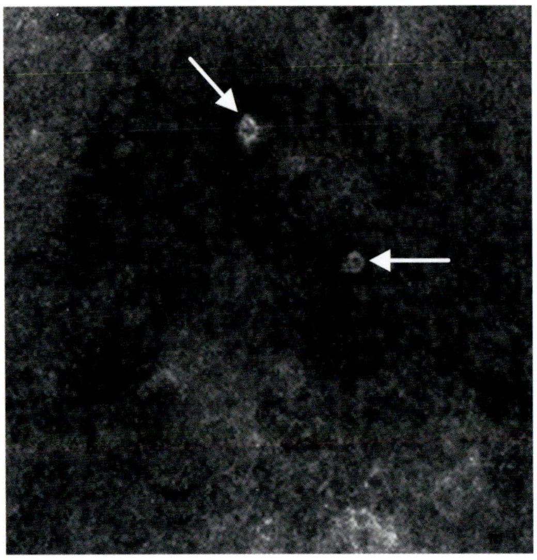
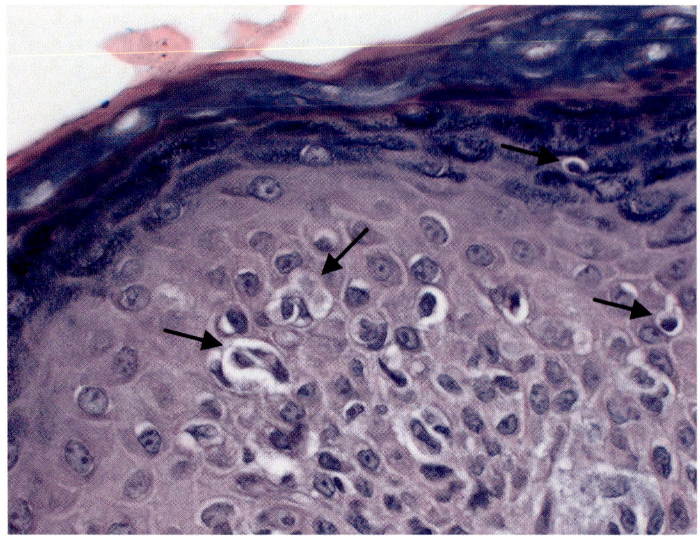

▲ **Figures 6.8, 6.9** Case 1: RCM (0.5 mm × 0.5 mm) at the level of the stratum granulosum/upper stratum spinosum shows bright, round nucleated cells (white arrows), compatible with melanocytes, in an area with loss of the normal honeycomb pattern. Corresponding histology (40×) shows pagetoid upward migration of melanocytes (black arrows) in the epidermis.

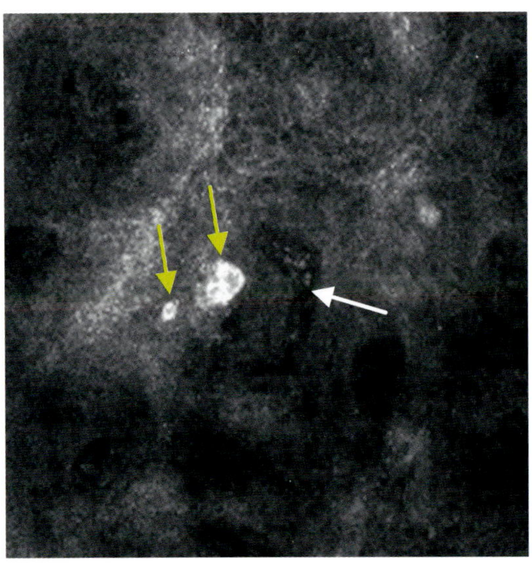
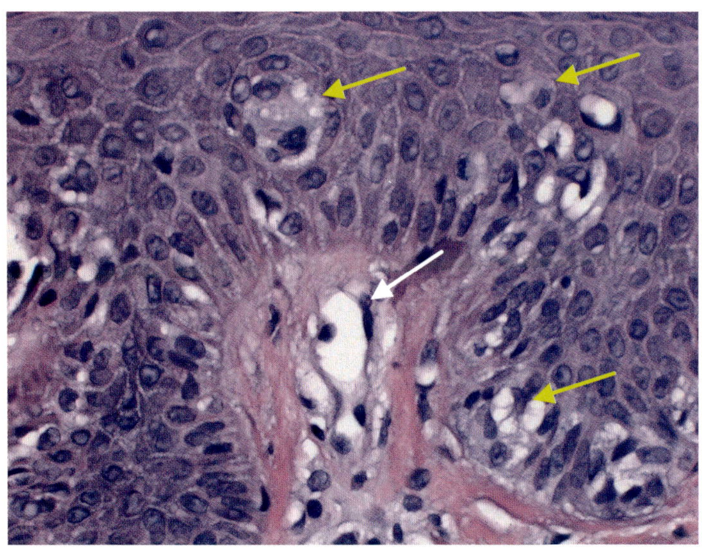

▲ **Figures 6.10, 6.11** Case 1: RCM (0.5 mm × 0.5 mm) at the level of the lower stratum spinosum/DEJ shows the presence of variably sized, refractile, polygonal, nucleated cells singly and in small clusters, compatible with atypical melanocytes (yellow arrows), non-edged papillae, and a dilated vessel in the superficial dermis (white arrow). Histology (40×) shows enlarged, atypical melanocytes as solitary units and small clusters within the stratum basalis and stratum spinosum (yellow arrows) and a dilated vessel in the papillary dermis (white arrow).

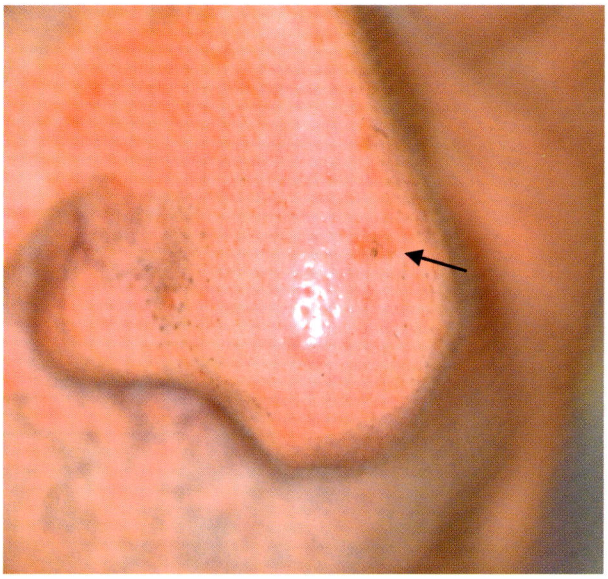

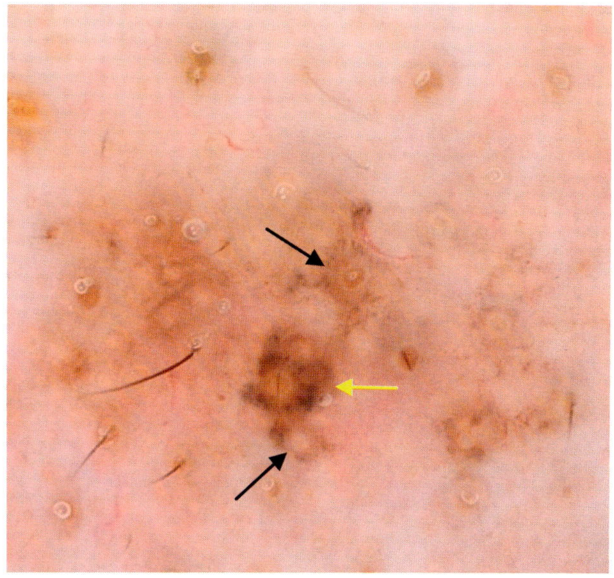

▲ **Figures 6.12, 6.13** Case 2: clinical photograph of a 5 mm light-brown macule (arrow) on the tip of the nose of a 79-year-old man. Dermoscopy reveals a perifollicular annular–granular pattern (black arrows), coalescing in one area into a rhomboidal structure (yellow arrow). These dermoscopic findings are suggestive of an early lentigo maligna.

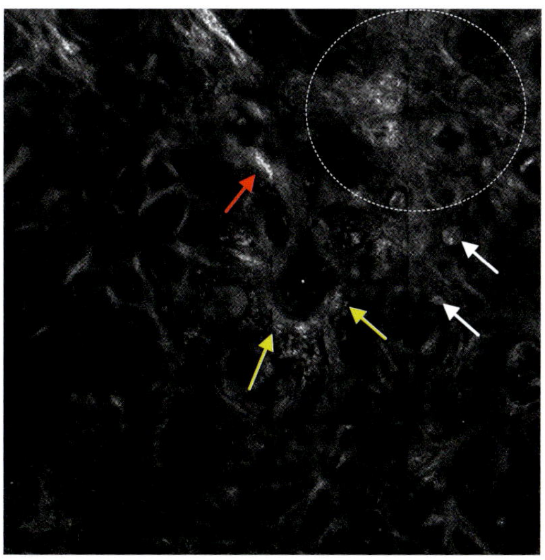

◀ **Figures 6.14–6.16**

Case 2: RCM mosaic (2 mm × 2 mm) at the level of the DEJ reveals perifollicular, irregular aggregates of bright cells (yellow arrows), junctional cell clusters (white arrows), junctional thickening (red arrow), and areas with effacement of the normal architecture (circled). Corresponding conventional (10×) and Melan-A immunohistochemically stained histology (10×) show a high density of melanocytes as single units and nests along the DEJ and extending down follicular epithelium (yellow arrows). Rare melanocytes can be seen scattered at all levels of the epidermis (black arrows).

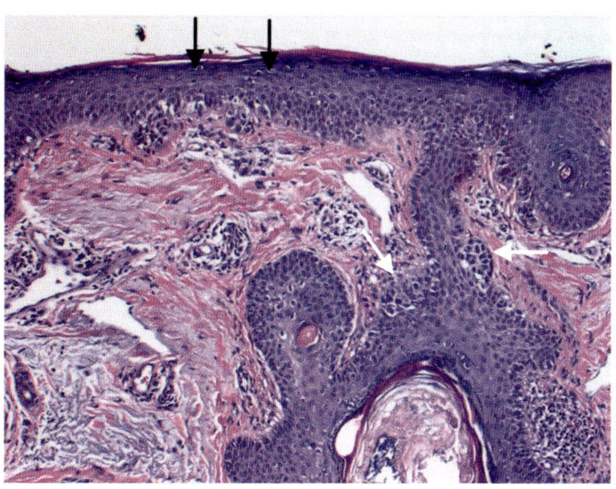

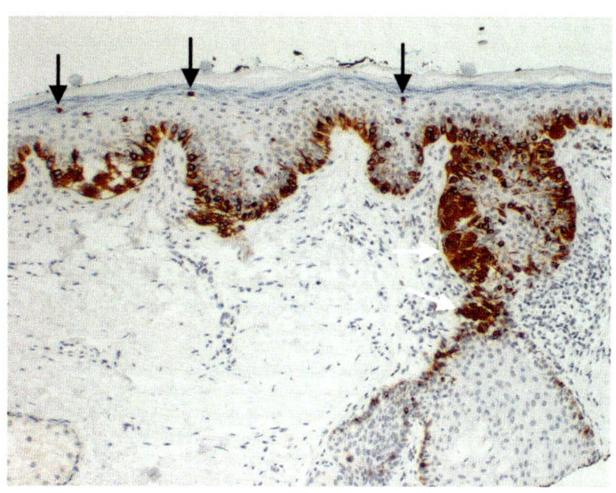

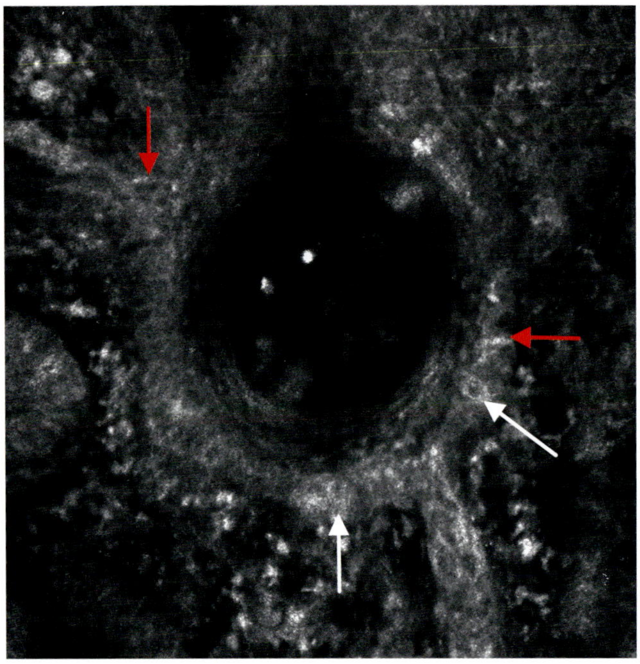

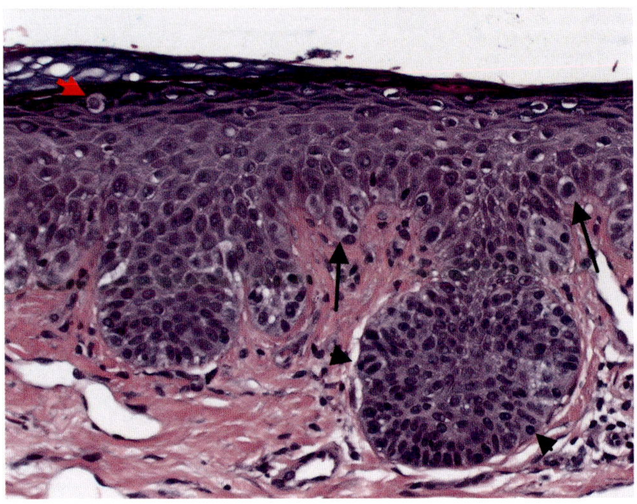

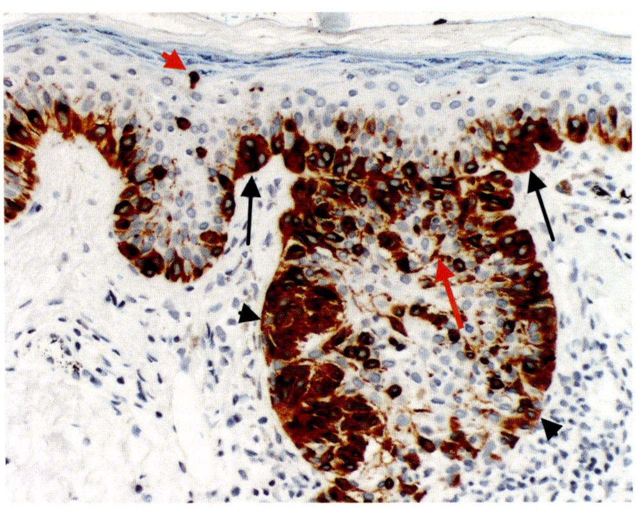

◀ **Figures 6.17–6.19**

Case 2: RCM (0.5 mm × 0.5 mm) at the level of the DEJ shows bright nucleated cells (white arrows) and coarse, bright dendritic structures (red arrows) within the follicular epithelium. Conventional (20×) and Melan-A immunohistochemically stained histology (20×) show a proliferation of atypical melanocytes at the DEJ (black arrows) with extension down adnexal epithelium (black arrowheads) and upward scatter of rare melanocytes (red arrowheads). Many of the melanocytes have prominent, thickened dendrites (red arrow).

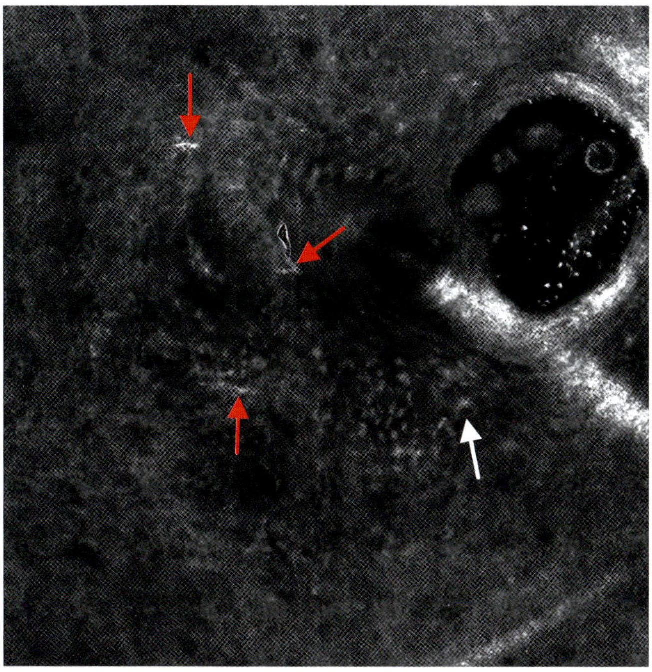

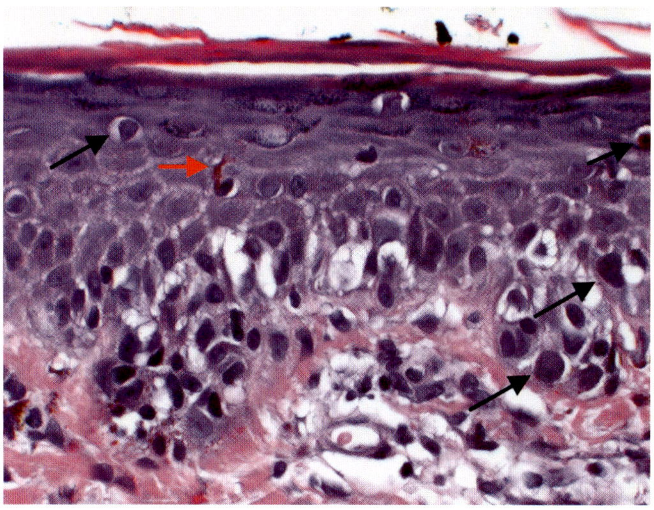

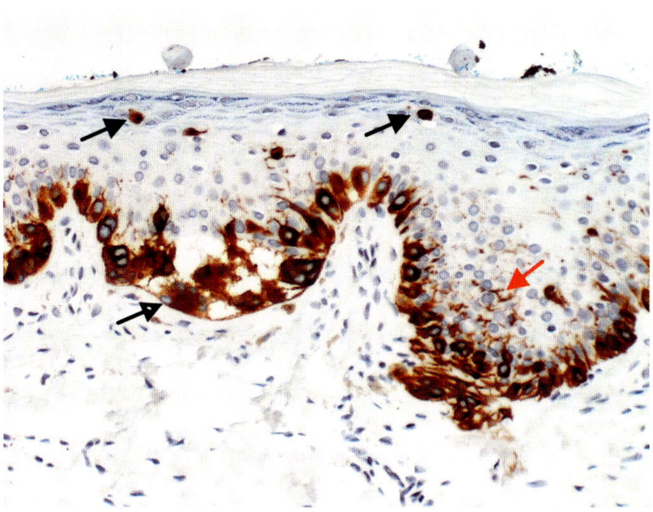

Figures 6.20–6.22

Case 2: RCM (0.5 mm × 0.5 mm) at the level of the stratum granulosum/upper stratum spinosum reveals distortion with focal loss of the normal honeycomb pattern, bright dendritic structures (red arrows) and rare refractile nucleated cells (white arrow) among keratinocytes. Corresponding conventional (40×) and Melan-A immunohistochemically stained histology (20×) show melanocytes (black arrows) and coarse melanocytic dendrites (red arrows) at all levels of the epidermis.

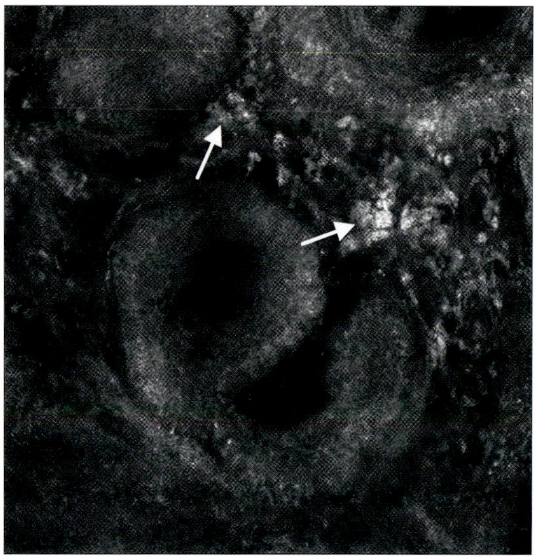

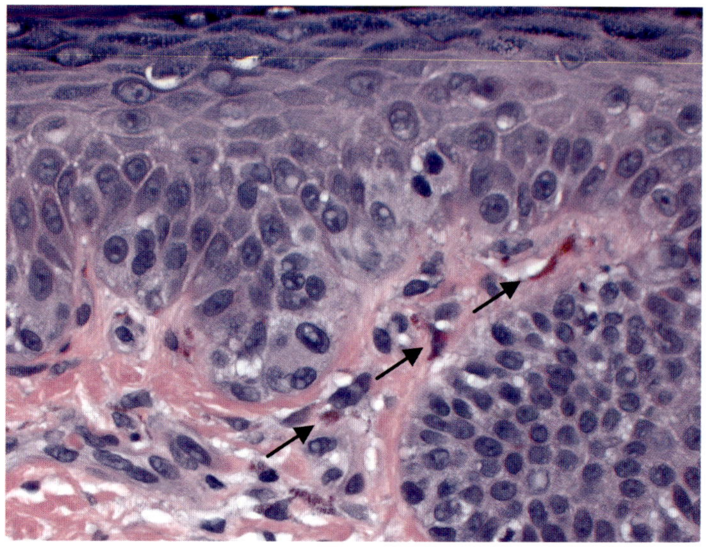

▲ **Figures 6.23, 6.24** Case 2: bright plump polygonal cells (white arrows) in the upper dermis on RCM examination (0.5 mm × 0.5 mm) correspond to melanophages (black arrows) in the superficial dermis seen on histology (40×).

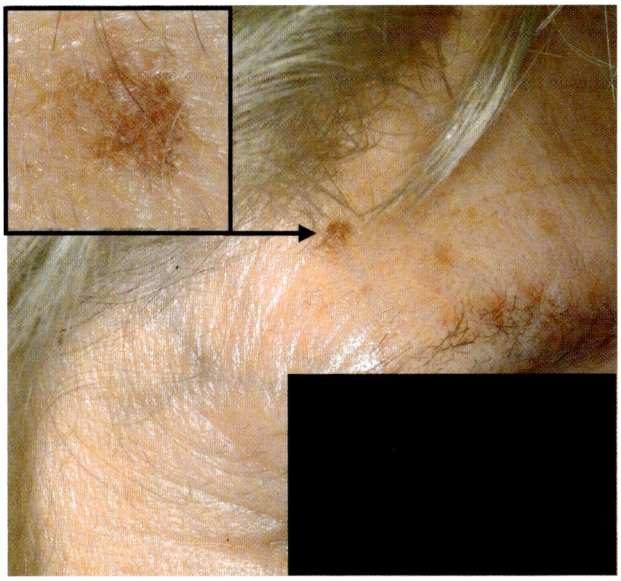
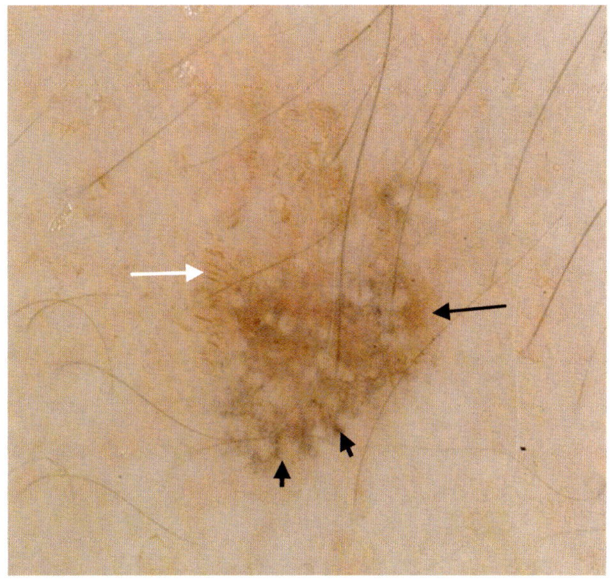

▲ **Figures 6.25, 6.26** Case 3: clinical photograph of a 5 mm, irregular brown macule (arrow, the inset shows the clinical close-up image) on the lateral forehead of a 64-year-old woman. Dermoscopy reveals fine reticulation (black arrow), grayish peppering (arrowheads), and fingerprint-like structures (white arrow).

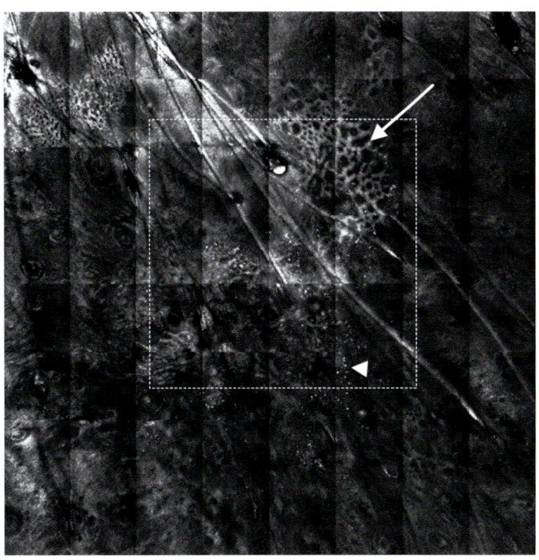
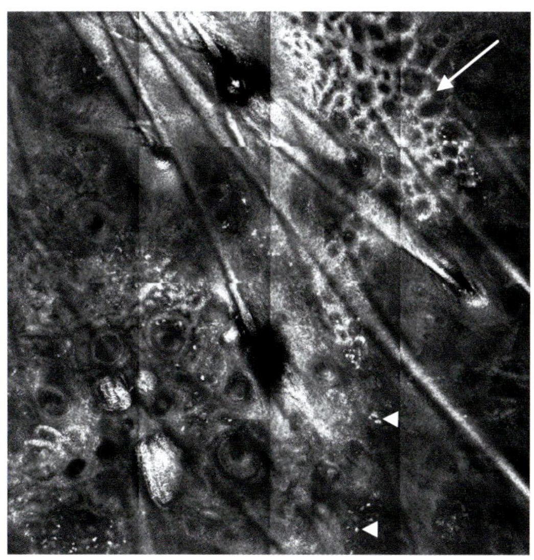

▲ **Figures 6.27, 6.28** Case 3: RCM mosaic (left: 4 mm × 4 mm) and submosaic (right: 2 mm × 2 mm), corresponding to the boxed area taken at slightly different levels of the DEJ, show a bright rete meshwork (arrows), and multiple small refractive structures (arrowheads), which correspond with the dermoscopic features of fine reticulation and grayish peppering, respectively.

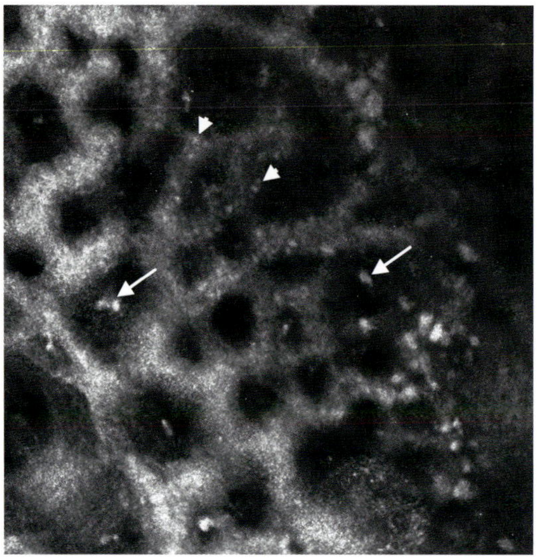
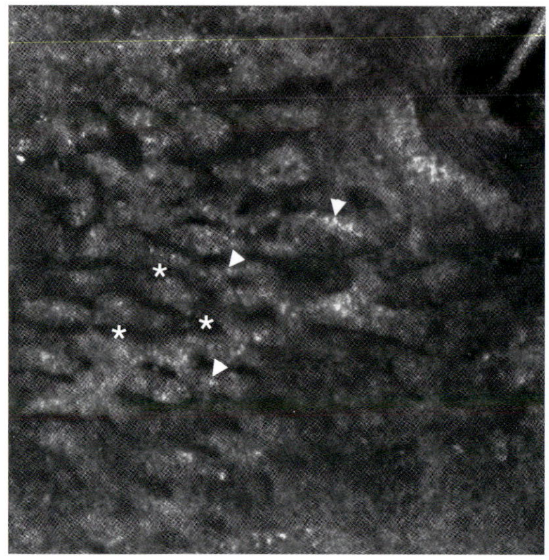

▲ **Figures 6.29, 6.30** Case 3: RCM (left, 0.5 mm × 0.5 mm) obtained from the dermoscopically identified reticulated area at the level of the DEJ shows a bright rete meshwork composed of uniform small round cells (arrowheads) in a carpet-like distribution, variably sized and shaped dermal papillae, and plump bright cells in the superficial dermis (arrows). RCM (right, 0.5 mm × 0.5 mm) obtained from the center of the lesion at the level of the DEJ, shows somewhat cerebriform architecture of the epidermis and narrow, polycyclic dermal papillae (asterisks). Multiple small, round refractile cells (arrowheads), corresponding to pigmented keratinocytes, can be seen within the stratum spinosum of the rete. These images, taken together, are compatible with solar lentigo.

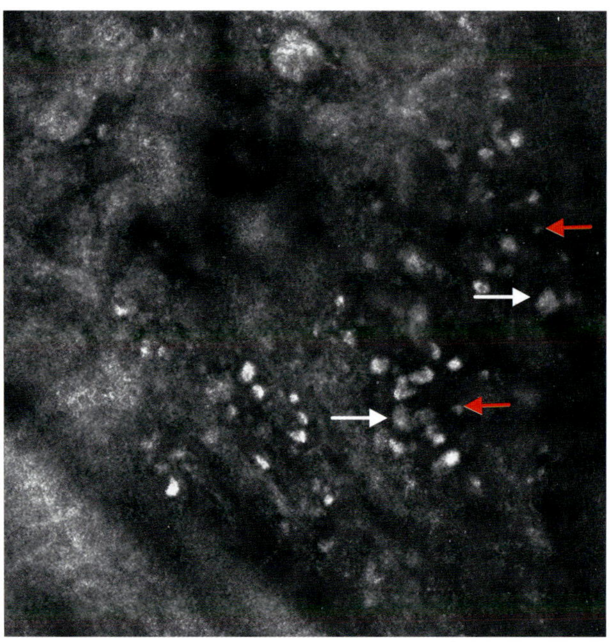
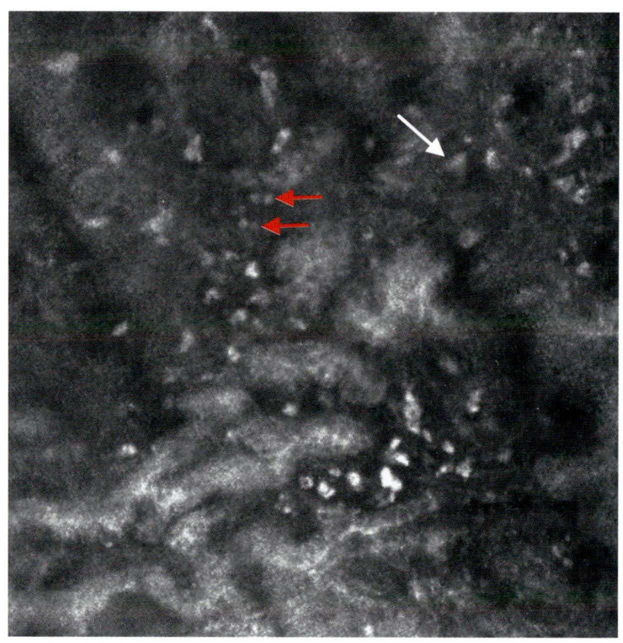

▲ **Figures 6.31, 6.32** Case 3: RCM (0.5 mm × 0.5 mm) obtained from the dermoscopically identified peppering area at the level of the lower stratum spinosum/upper DEJ shows focal loss of the rete meshwork, multiple oval-to-polygonal, plump bright cells with fuzzy outlines (white arrows) compatible with melanophages, and several small round bright cells (red arrows) compatible with inflammatory cells, highly suggestive of lichenoid inflammation.

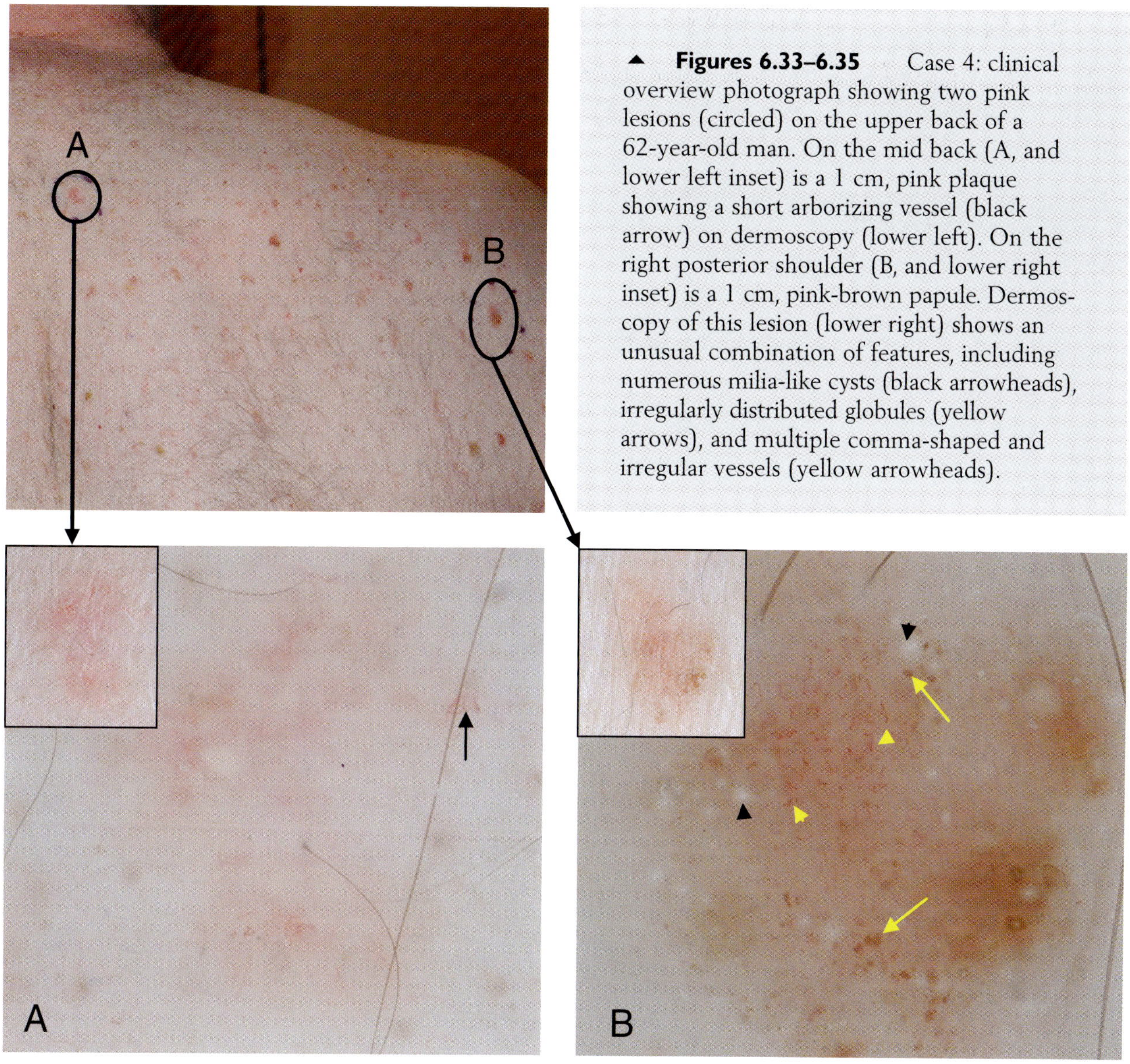

▲ **Figures 6.33–6.35** Case 4: clinical overview photograph showing two pink lesions (circled) on the upper back of a 62-year-old man. On the mid back (A, and lower left inset) is a 1 cm, pink plaque showing a short arborizing vessel (black arrow) on dermoscopy (lower left). On the right posterior shoulder (B, and lower right inset) is a 1 cm, pink-brown papule. Dermoscopy of this lesion (lower right) shows an unusual combination of features, including numerous milia-like cysts (black arrowheads), irregularly distributed globules (yellow arrows), and multiple comma-shaped and irregular vessels (yellow arrowheads).

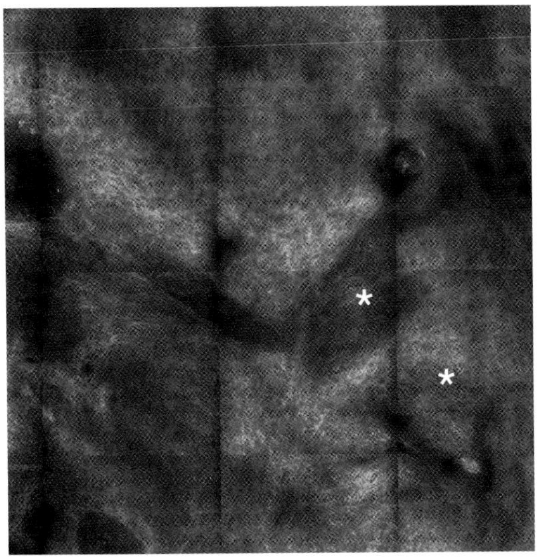

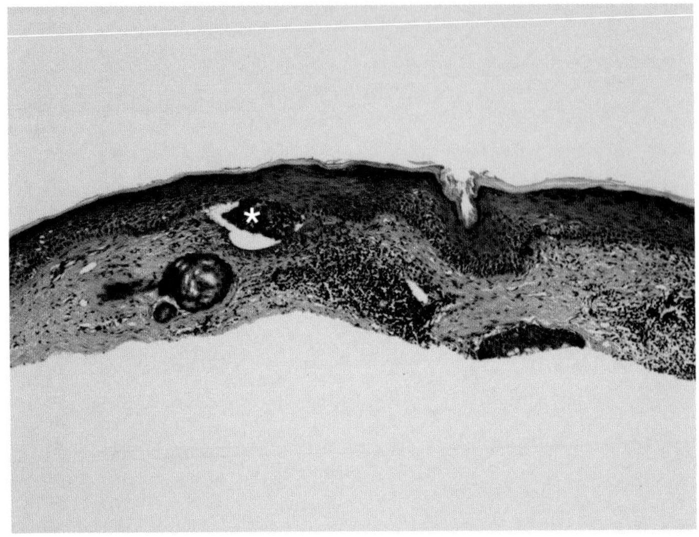

▲ **Figures 6.36, 6.37** Case 4A: RCM mosaic (1.5 mm × 1.5 mm) at the level of the lower epidermis demonstrates areas that are less refractile than the surrounding epidermis and show nuclear streaming (asterisks). Corresponding histology (10×) shows a flattened DEJ, an aggregate of basaloid cells (asterisk) in the lower epidermis with peritumoral clefting, and a dense inflammatory infiltrate in the superficial dermis.

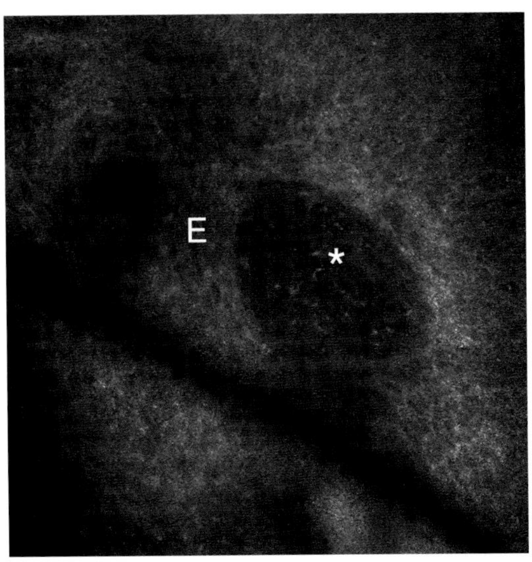

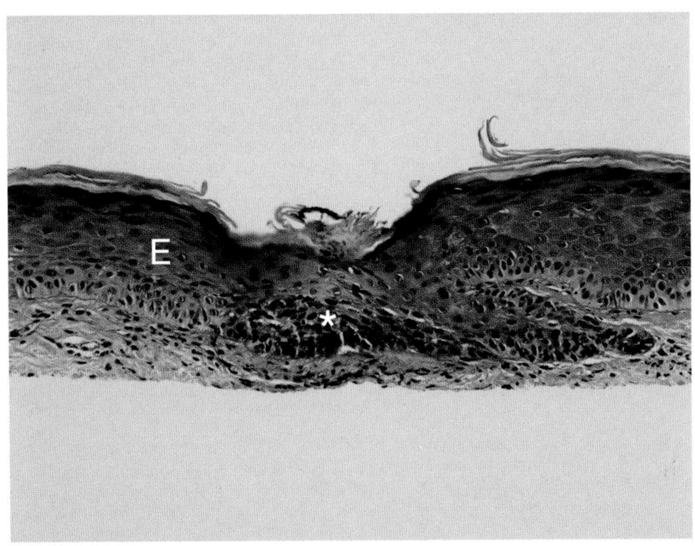

▲ **Figures 6.38, 6.39** Case 4A: RCM (0.5 mm × 0.5 mm) at the level of the lower epidermis demonstrates a tumor island (asterisk) that was less refractile than the surrounding epidermis (E). Corresponding histology (20×) shows a basaloid tumor island (asterisk) within the lower epidermis (E).

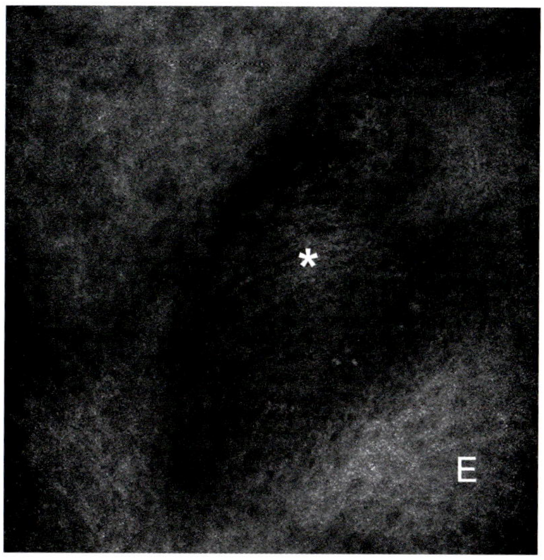

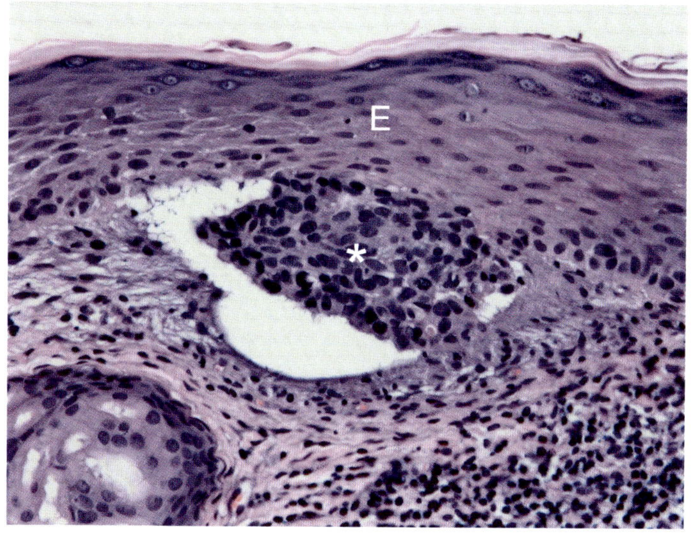

▲ **Figures 6.40, 6.41** Case 4A: RCM (0.5 mm × 0.5 mm) at the level of the lower epidermis (E) demonstrates a darker area (asterisk) that contains cells with elongated nuclei polarized along the same axis, or nuclear streaming. Corresponding histology (40×) shows at higher magnification the basaloid tumor island (asterisk), which bulges from the lower epidermis (E) into the superficial dermis, where peritumoral clefting and a dense inflammatory infiltrate are seen.

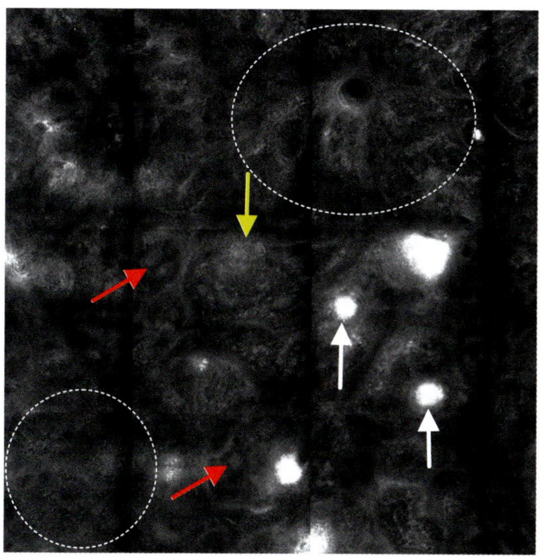

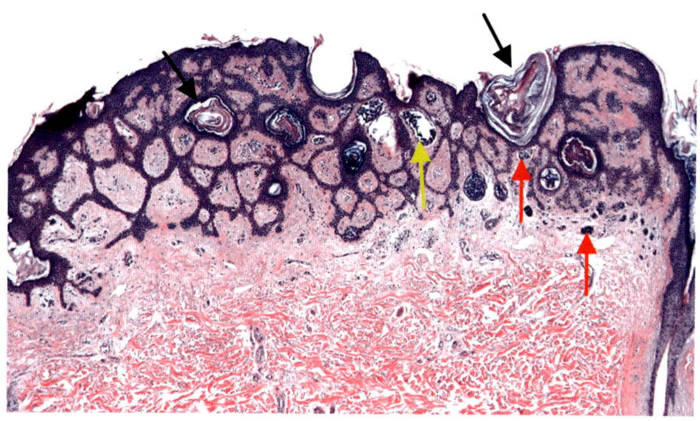

▲ **Figures 6.42, 6.43** Case 4B: RCM mosaic (1.5 mm × 1.5 mm) at the level of the lower DEJ shows multiple highly refractile round structures (white arrows), compatible with the horn pseudocysts. Junctional and dermal, small dense cell clusters (red arrows) and larger loose cell clusters (yellow arrow) can be seen. There is disarray of the DEJ with patchy loss of its normal architecture (circles). Corresponding histology (4×) shows reticulated epidermal hyperplasia with multiple horn pseudocysts (black arrows) and junctional and dermal melanocytic nests, many of which are cohesive (red arrows) and a few of which are discohesive (yellow arrow). The overall pattern suggests a compound melanocytic nevus with seborrheic keratosis-like features.

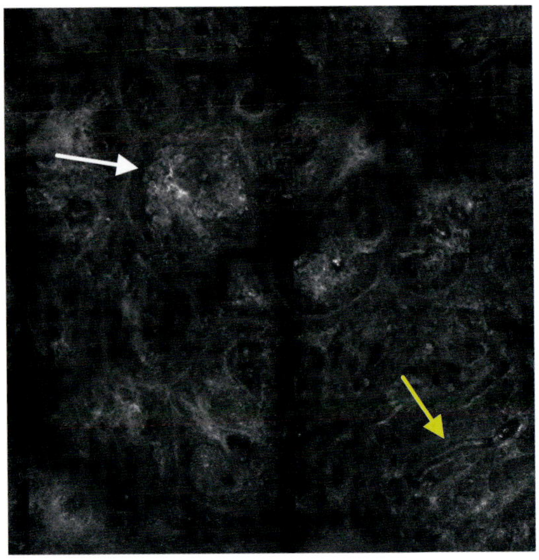
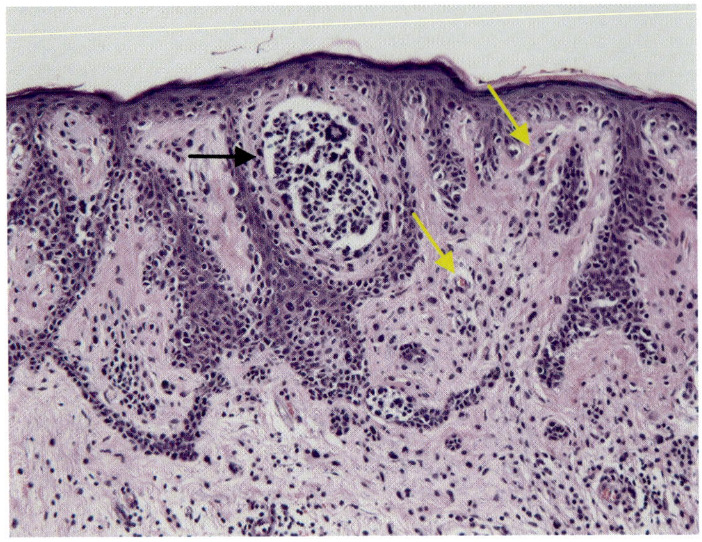

▲ **Figures 6.44, 6.45** Case 4B: RCM mosaic (1 mm × 1 mm) at the level of the DEJ shows a large, loose cell cluster in a dermal papilla (white arrow). Corresponding histology (20×) shows a large discohesive nest in the papillary dermis (black arrow). Notably, the increased capillary blood flow (yellow arrow) seen in the papillary dermis during real-time RCM examination, is not well appreciated on histology (yellow arrows).

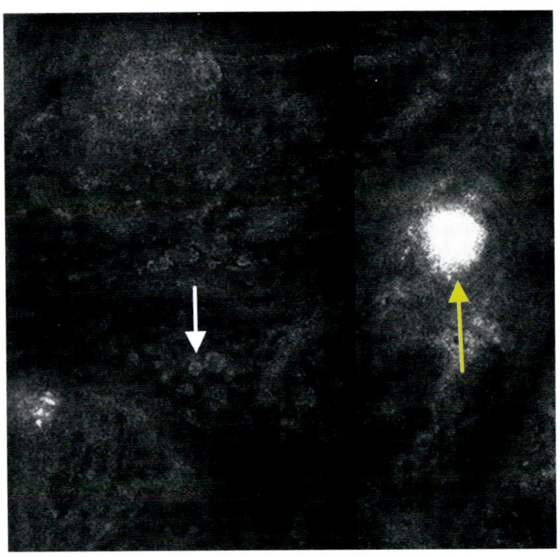
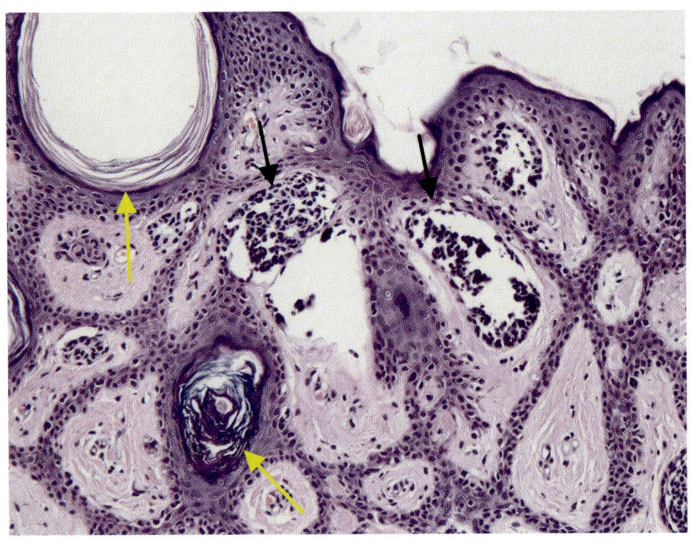

▲ **Figures 6.46, 6.47** Case 4B: RCM (0.5 mm × 0.5 mm) at the level of the DEJ shows a loose aggregate of refractile nucleated cells in a dermal papilla (white arrow) and a large highly refractile round structure (yellow arrow), corresponding to discohesive nests of melanocytes (black arrows) and horn pseudocysts (yellow arrows), respectively, on histology (20×).

CHAPTER 6b

RCM-guided biopsy site selection

Melissa Gill, Anna Liza C Agero, Marco Ardigo, Ashfaq A Marghoob, and Patricia Myskowski

Skin biopsies for histopathologic examination are generally expected to provide definitive diagnoses for cutaneous lesions. Histopathology is currently accepted as the gold standard; however, it can be an imperfect system, with limitations that may reduce diagnostic accuracy. These limitations include errors in histopathologic interpretation, discordance among histopathologists on the microscopic diagnosis, and sampling errors.[1,2] Sampling errors include the clinician biopsying a non-diagnostic lesion/site, the grossing technician/pathologist macroscopically not sampling through the diagnostic area, and the histopathologist not step-sectioning through the diagnostic area.[1,3]

As histopathologic examination is currently the primary means of confirming a presumptive clinical diagnosis, it is important to reduce limitations that negatively impact on accurate diagnosis. Attempts to help reduce these limitations start with the clinician, who needs to decide how to provide the most appropriate lesion sample for histopathologic study. Depending on the size, body location, and clinical differential diagnosis of a lesion, the clinician chooses the most appropriate biopsy method (i.e. shave, saucerization, punch, incisional, or excisional biopsy) in order to (a) obtain the most representative sample and (b) provide an adequate tissue sample for accurate microscopic diagnosis.

Although the decision on when, where, what, and how to biopsy is usually straightforward, some conditions may present challenges for the clinician. For example, the diagnosis of mycosis fungoides (MF) can be frustratingly difficult, owing to its diverse clinical presentations and non-specific or non-definitive findings on histopathology.[4,5] Frequently, multiple and/or sequential skin biopsies are necessary before the diagnosis of MF is established or confirmed.[6,7] Small congenital melanocytic nevi (CMN) pose yet another potential problem. These lesions require close monitoring with the aim of detecting any changes that may be indicative of melanoma.[8] However, it is not uncommon for small benign CMN to undergo changes over time; thus, many of these lesions are excised unnecessarily, with biopsy specimens showing no evidence of melanoma.[9] Large lesions on cosmetically sensitive areas, such as the face, also present a management challenge. In some such lesions, the clinical differential diagnosis includes benign solar lentigo or malignant melanoma (lentigo maligna or lentigo maligna melanoma). As the latter often contains areas resembling solar lentigo on histology, adequate sampling is critical, but excisional biopsy is not desirable as it would provide an unnecessary disfiguring scar if the lesion proved to be solar lentigo.[10]

An in-vivo instrument that can non-invasively sample multiple areas within one lesion and/or multiple lesions to help 'predict' the biopsy site that will yield the most definitive histopathologic diagnosis may help solve the aforementioned problems. Furthermore, such an instrument may not only allow for early definitive diagnosis in difficult cases but also significantly minimize the number of non-diagnostic or unnecessary biopsies performed. Reflectance confocal microscopy (RCM) can be performed in real time and is non-invasive; it permits both repeated assessment of multiple suspicious lesions and/or the evaluation of different areas within a large lesion for key RCM features that have already been described for several benign and malignant skin conditions.[11–19] For example, RCM may help identify the most 'appropriate' lesion or area within a lesion to biopsy when a diagnosis of MF is considered by pinpointing areas with the most significant epidermal changes, preferably including Pautrier's microabscesses, which are easily identified on RCM mosaics.[19] RCM may also aid in the evaluation of small CMN for the presence or absence of atypical features, helping the clinician determine which lesions require a biopsy and which can be followed clinically. Similarly, for large lesions on cosmetically sensitive areas, RCM allows for non-invasive evaluation of the entire lesion at the cellular level, and may help the clinician pinpoint the most suspicious area for biopsy. In cases where biopsy indicates a benign lesion, such as solar lentigo or congenital nevus, RCM could be used to evaluate the entire lesion over time and, combined with clinical and dermoscopic examination, may be able to reduce the number of subsequent biopsies needed. Moreover, when a diagnosis of melanoma is established, RCM may help delineate the lesion's borders, which may be difficult to discern clinically, allowing for more efficient surgical excision.[20–22]

In certain settings, the clinical diagnosis is quite clear, but for reasons such as cosmesis, the extent of the lesion, or complicating medical conditions, physical removal of a lesion (either by excision or curette) is not desirable or feasible. In such cases, non-invasive treatment, such as topical imiquimod therapy, topical 5-fluorouracil (5-FU), or photodynamic therapy, may be preferable. In the future, non-invasive diagnosis by RCM may be acceptable, but at present biopsy diagnosis remains the gold standard. Therefore, in this setting, the smallest diagnostic biopsy possible is paramount. RCM may assist the clinician in choosing the most diagnostic area of the lesion to allow for definitive histopathologic diagnosis with minimal sampling. RCM has already been used to monitor non-invasive treatment of basal cell carcinoma, actinic keratosis, and lentigo maligna.[21,23–25]

The reflectance confocal microscopic features of a variety of benign and malignant cutaneous tumors have been described and shown to have good correlation with histologic findings.[11–19] Notably, several of the key RCM features of basal cell carcinoma and melanoma have been reported to have good sensitivity and specificity in the research setting; similar studies for MF are still in progress.[17,18,26] Further investigations are certainly needed to verify the applicability of RCM as a screening or diagnostic tool, but these studies may enable the application of this technology as an adjunct to histopathologic diagnosis by assisting in optimal biopsy site selection.

CASE PRESENTATIONS

Examples in which RCM was used to guide biopsy site selection in the setting of non-invasive therapy and in the setting of margin mapping before Mohs' surgery can be found in the RCM-assisted assessment of treatment response and RCM-assisted in-vivo margin mapping chapters, respectively. The following are examples of cases wherein RCM was able to provide sufficient information to serve as a guide for optimal biopsy site selection in the setting of mycosis fungoides and small congenital melanocytic nevus.

Case I

A 32-year-old man with a 5-year history of stage 1A mycosis fungoides, responsive to low-dose topical nitrogen mustard, presented with a 6-month history of several new, larger lesions, not responsive to therapy. Examination found several patches and early plaques on the trunk and proximal extremities, covering approximately 15% of his total body surface area. The clinical impression was progression to stage 1B disease, and the possibility of large cell transformation was also considered. To help determine appropriate therapy, the attending physician sought to confirm that these new lesions were indeed MF and to determine the presence or absence of large cell transformation.

RCM was performed on a large patch with focal early plaque formation (Figures 6.48, 6.49) and was able to identify an area with marked epidermal changes suggestive of MF.[19] Small round vesicle- and microvesicle-like dark spaces were visible on 3 mm × 3 mm mosaics at all levels of the epidermis (Figure 6.50). These round dark spaces were filled with monomorphous mildly refractile oval-to-round cells (Figure 6.52). Surrounding areas showed architectural disarray, with focal loss of intercellular demarcations and focally thickened intercellular junctions (Figure 6.52). RCM at the level of the dermal–epidermal junction

(DEJ) showed marked loss of contrast in lesional skin as compared to non-lesional skin (Figures 6.54, 6.55). A 4 mm punch biopsy was performed on the area pinpointed by RCM; histopathology showed Pautrier's microabscesses and a lichenoid and superficial perivascular infiltrate of small-to-intermediate-sized atypical lymphocytes, compatible with plaque type MF (Figures 6.51, 6.53). Only a few CD30-positive larger lymphocytes were present.

Case 2

A 70-year-old man presented with a 1.4 cm melanocytic lesion on the left chest near the areola (Figure 6.56). The patient stated that the lesion was present at birth, and the lesion was documented on a photograph taken when he was 2 years old. Over the past 3 years, the patient noted an increase in pigmentation on the medial aspect of the nevus, together with an increase in size and change in contour. On dermoscopy, the lesion showed asymmetry and sharp borders; the lateral lightly pigmented part of the lesion showed cobblestone-like globules, while the hyperpigmented medial area had multiple colors (light brown, dark brown, blue-gray, and black) with reticulation, a few globules, and atypical black dots which were not associated with the network and haphazardly placed (Figure 6.57).

RCM was performed on both the lightly and darkly pigmented areas of the nevus. On the lightly pigmented lateral side of the nevus, dense cell clusters composed of oval-shaped, uniformly-sized, nucleated cells with refractile cytoplasms, which decrease in brightness with increasing depth, were seen extending from just below the epidermis to the maximal depth of light penetration (Figures 6.58A–D), consistent with a benign melanocytic nevus.[16–18] RCM examination of the medial darkly pigmented area showed loss of the normal honeycomb pattern in the granular and spinous layers and a pleomorphic 'pagetoid' infiltrate composed of several bright, round-to-oval nucleated cells and scattered refractile dendritic cells (Figures 6.59A–C). At the basal layer/DEJ, junctional thickening, or a bright broadened rete meshwork, and non-edged papillae were seen (Figure 6.59D). Numerous refractile dendrites and particles were also seen in the epidermis (Figures 6.59C, D). These findings strongly suggested melanoma in situ, and excision of the lesion was performed.[16–18] Histopathologic analysis of the lesion confirmed the presence of melanoma in situ arising within a congenital melanocytic nevus (Figures 6.58E, F, 6.59E, F, 6.60).[9]

Interestingly, our institution performed RCM examination on other cases of CMN that were concerning for malignant transformation, either clinically or dermoscopically, and/or had a history of change. RCM did not identify features suggestive of melanoma in these cases, and all six were subsequently proven benign by histopathologic examination.[9]

Key RCM features of RCM-guided biopsy site selection

- RCM allows one to screen several lesions at the cellular level for features that may be diagnostic histologically, increasing the likelihood of achieving a diagnostic and representative biopsy.
- RCM enables one to examine the entirety of a single large lesion at the cellular level for features that may be diagnostic histologically, helping to ensure that a small biopsy is representative of the lesion as a whole.
- RCM-guided biopsy may achieve specific diagnoses with fewer biopsies and thus enable earlier diagnosis and treatment.

REFERENCES

1. Swanson NA, Lee KK, Gorman A et al. Biopsy techniques. Diagnosis of melanoma. Dermatol Clin 2002; 20:677–80.
2. Brochez L, Verhaeghe E, Grosshans E et al. Inter-observer variation in the histopathological diagnosis of clinically suspicious pigmented skin lesions. J Pathol 2002; 196:459–66.
3. Crowson AN. Medicolegal aspects of neoplastic dermatology. Mod Pathol 2006; 19(Suppl 2):S148–54.
4. Hoppe RT, Wood GS, Abel EA. Mycosis fungoides and the Sézary syndrome: pathology, staging, and treatment. Current Probl Cancer 1990; 14:293–371.
5. Santucci M, Biggeri A, Feller AC et al. Efficacy of histologic criteria for diagnosing early mycosis fungoides: an EORTC cutaneous lymphoma study group investigation. European Organization for Research and Treatment of Cancer. Am J Surg Pathol 2000; 24:40–50.
6. Diamandidou E, Cohen PR, Kurzrock R. Mycosis fungoides and Sezary syndrome. Blood 1996; 88: 2385–409.
7. Glass LF, Keller KL, Messina JL et al. Cutaneous T-cell lymphoma. Cancer Control 1998; 5:11–18.

8. Tromberg J, Bauer B, Benvenuto-Andrade C et al. Congenital melanocytic nevi needing treatment. Dermatol Ther 2005; 18:136–50.

9. Marghoob AA, Charles CA, Busam KJ et al. In vivo confocal scanning laser microscopy of a series of congenital melanocytic nevi suggestive of having developed malignant melanoma. Arch Dermatol 2005; 141:1401–12.

10. Dalton SR, Gardner TL, Libow LF et al. Contiguous lesions in lentigo maligna. J Am Acad Dermatol 2005; 52:859–62.

11. Aghassi D, Anderson RR, Gonzalez S. Confocal laser microscopic imaging of actinic keratoses in vivo: a preliminary report. J Am Acad Dermatol 2000; 43:42–8.

12. Langley RG, Rajadhyaksha M, Dwyer PJ et al. Confocal scanning laser microscopy of benign and malignant melanocytic skin lesions in vivo. J Am Acad Dermatol 2001; 45:365–76.

13. Langley RG, Burton E, Walsh N et al. In vivo confocal scanning laser microscopy of benign lentigines: comparison to conventional histology and in vivo characteristics of lentigo maligna. J Am Acad Dermatol 2006; 55:88–97.

14. Tannous ZS, Mihm MC, Flotte TJ et al. In vivo examination of lentigo maligna and malignant melanoma in situ, lentigo maligna type by near-infrared reflectance confocal microscopy: comparison of in vivo confocal images with histologic sections. J Am Acad Dermatol 2002; 46:260–3.

15. Nori S, Rius-Diaz F, Cuevas J et al. Sensitivity and specificity of reflectance-mode confocal microscopy for in vivo diagnosis of basal cell carcinoma: a multicenter study. J Am Acad Dermatol 2004; 51:923–30.

16. Gerger A, Koller S, Kern T et al. Diagnostic applicability of in vivo confocal laser scanning microscopy in melanocytic skin tumors. J Invest Dermatol 2005; 124:493–8.

17. Pellacani G, Cesinaro AM, Seidenari S. Reflectance-mode confocal microscopy of pigmented skin lesions – improvement in melanoma diagnostic specificity. J Am Acad Dermatol 2005; 53:979–85.

18. Pellacani G, Guitera P, Longo C et al. The impact of in vivo reflectance confocal microscopy for the diagnostic accuracy of melanoma and equivocal melanocytic lesions. J Invest Dermatol 2007; July 26 [Epub ahead of print].

19. Agero AL, Gill M, Ardigo M et al. In vivo reflectance confocal microscopy of mycosis fungoides: a preliminary study. J Am Acad Dermatol 2007; 57(3):435–41.

20. Busam KJ, Hester K, Charles C et al. Detection of clinically amelanotic malignant melanoma and assessment of its margins by in vivo confocal scanning laser microscopy. Arch Dermatol 2001; 137:923–9.

21. Curiel-Lewandrowski C, Williams CM, Swindells KJ et al. Use of in vivo confocal microscopy in malignant melanoma: an aid in diagnosis and assessment of surgical and nonsurgical therapeutic approaches. Arch Dermatology 2004; 140:1127–32.

22. Chen CS, Elias M, Busam K et al. Multimodal in vivo optical imaging, including confocal microscopy, facilitates presurgical margin mapping for clinically complex lentigo maligna melanoma. Br J Dermatol 2005; 153:1031–6.

23. Goldgeier M, Fox CA, Zavislan JM et al. Noninvasive imaging, treatment, and microscopic confirmation of clearance of basal cell carcinoma. Dermatol Surg 2003; 29:205–10.

24. Torres A, Niemeyer A, Berkes B et al. 5% imiquimod cream and reflectance-mode confocal microscopy as adjunct modalities to Mohs micrographic surgery for treatment of basal cell carcinoma. Dermatol Surg 2004; 30:1462–9.

25. Trehan M, Swindells KJ, Taylor CR et al. Confocal microscopy imaging of actinic keratoses post-photodynamic therapy with 5-ALA. In: 20th World Congress of Dermatology, Paris, 2003.

26. Gerger A, Koller S, Weger W et al. Sensitivity and specificity of confocal laser-scanning microscopy for in vivo diagnosis of malignant skin tumors. Cancer 2006; 107:193–200.

RCM-GUIDED BIOPSY SITE SELECTION

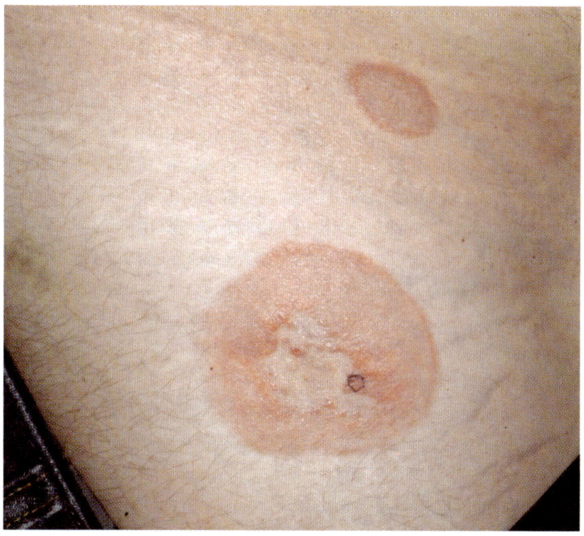
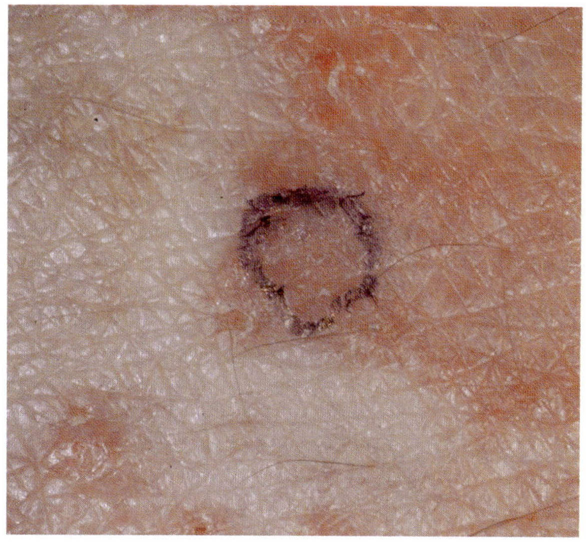

▲ **Figures 6.48, 6.49** Case 1: clinical photographs show the hip of a 32-year-old man with two smaller patches and a larger, somewhat annular patch with some central clearing and early plaque formation. Note the salmon-colored hue of the lesions. A close-up view of the large lesion shows a small raised edge with fine scale and central clearing.

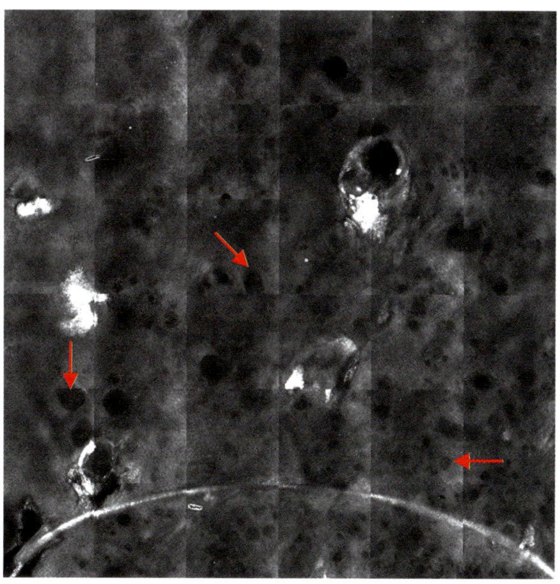
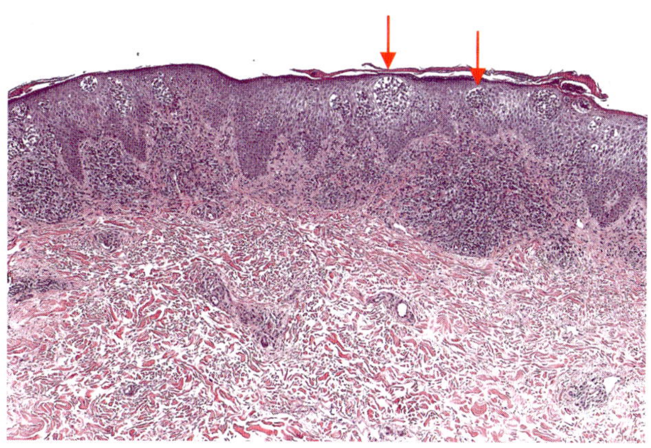

▲ **Figures 6.50, 6.51** Case 1: RCM mosaic (3 mm × 3 mm) at the level of the spinous layer shows numerous dark, variably sized, vesicle-like dark spaces (arrows) filled with weakly refractile cells. Corresponding low-power histology (4×) shows numerous round collections of lymphocytes (Pautrier's microabscesses) throughout the epidermis, a lichenoid lymphocytic infiltrate expanding the papillary dermis, and only slight epidermal reaction, including patchy parakeratosis and mild spongiosis.

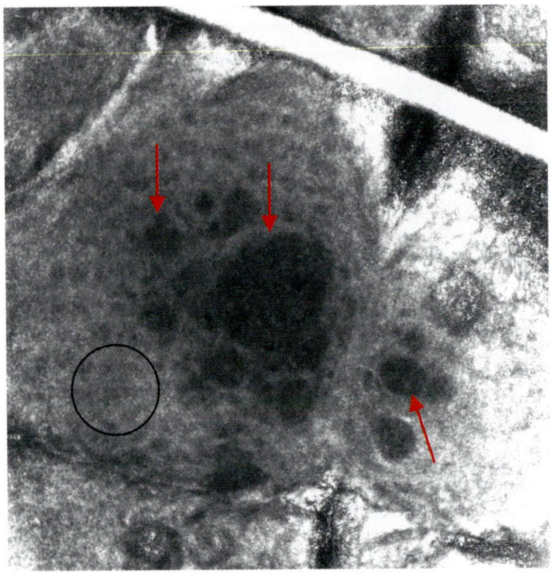

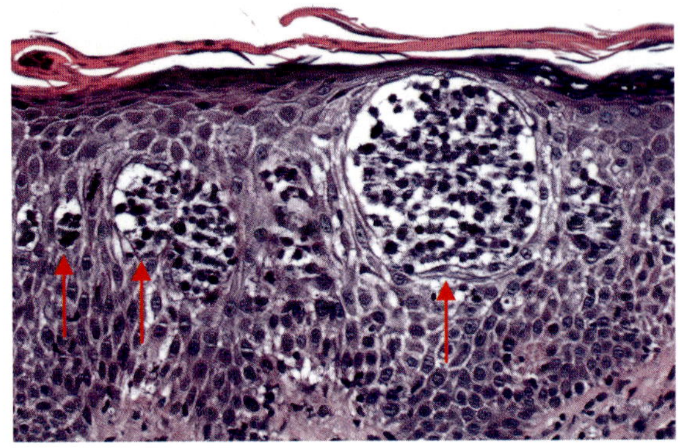

▲ **Figures 6.52, 6.53** Case 1: RCM (0.5 mm × 0.5 mm) at the level of the stratum spinosum shows numerous, variably sized, dark, round vesicle-like spaces filled with weakly refractile round cells (arrows) and adjacent focal loss of intercellular demarcations (circled) with surrounding widening of intercellular spaces. Corresponding histology (20×) shows several Pautrier's microabscesses (arrows) of varying size within the spinous layer with mild associated spongiosis and overlying fine parakeratotic scale. Reproduced with permission by J Am Acad Dermatol from Agero AL, Gill M, Ardigo M et al. In vivo reluctance confocal microscopy of mycosis fungoides: a preliminary study. 2007; 57(3): 435–41.

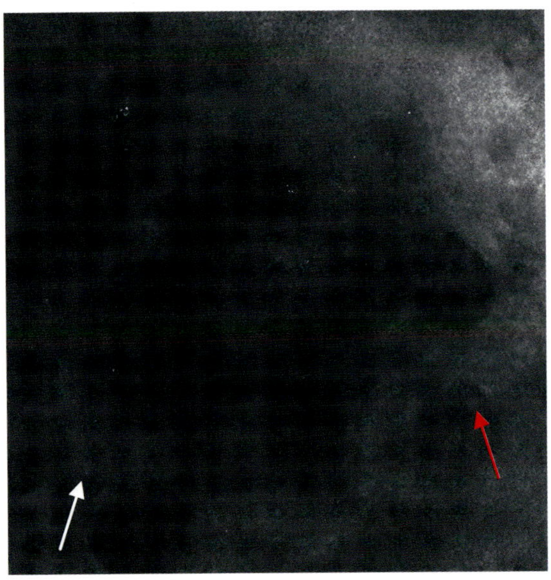

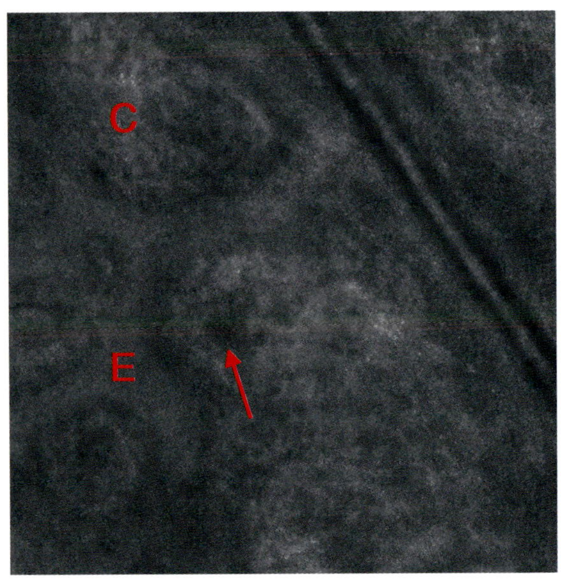

▲ **Figures 6.54, 6.55** Case 1: RCM (left, 0.5 mm × 0.5 mm) of the MF plaque at the level of the DEJ shows loss of contrast with poor light penetration. Subtle, round weakly refractile cells within the epidermis (white arrow) and the dermal papillae (red arrow) are barely visible. Corresponding RCM (right, 0.5 mm × 0.5 mm) of non-lesional skin clearly visualizes dermal papillae containing reticulated collagen (C) and capillary loops (red arrow) surrounded by epidermis (E). Note, as this patient has very fair skin, the papillary dermal collagen appears relatively more refractile than the surrounding basal layer epidermis.

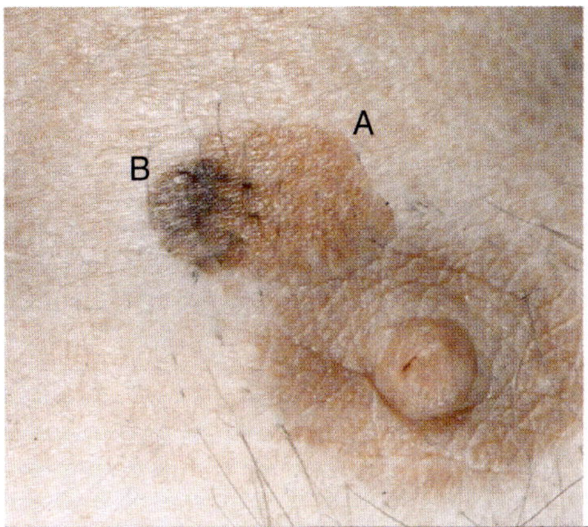

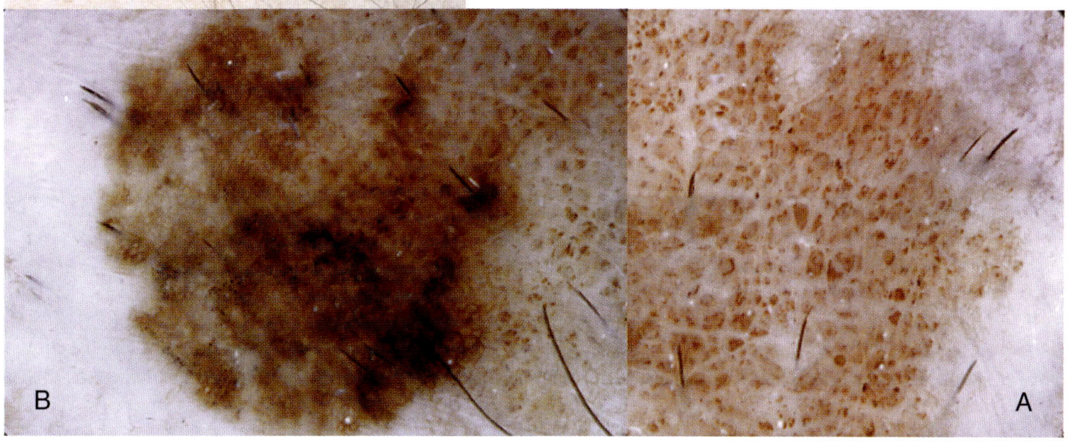

▲ **Figures 6.56, 6.57** Case 2: clinical photograph of a small (1.4 cm) congenital melanocytic nevus (A) on the left chest near the areola of a 70-year-old man. The lesion had recently increased in size and developed a darkly pigmented area in its medial aspect (B). Dermoscopy revealed uniform light-brown pigmented cobblestone-like globules on the lateral aspect (A), and variegated colors, pigment network, globules, and atypical black dots (i.e. dots not associated with the network and located away from the center of the lesion) on the medial aspect (B). Reproduced with permission of Arch Dermotol from Marghoob AA, Charles CA, Busam KJ et al. In vivo confocal scanning laser microscopy of a series of congenital melanocytic nevi suggestive of having developed malignant melanoma. 2005; 141: 1401–12.

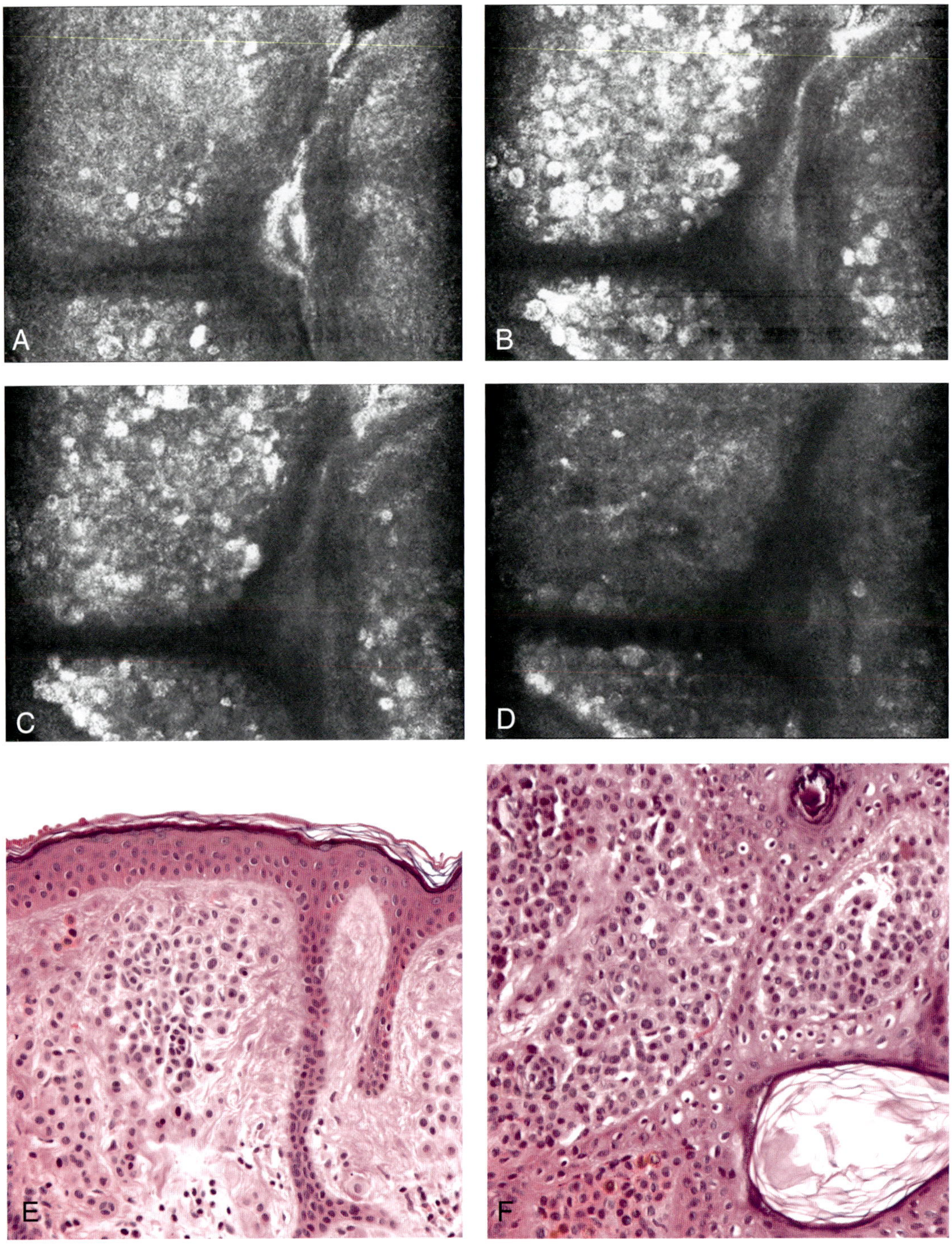

▲ **Figure 6.58** Case 2: RCM (0.245 mm × 0.175 mm) of area A revealed a normal honeycomb pattern of the epidermis. At the transition from stratum basalis to papillary dermis (A), clusters of oval nucleated cells can be seen just below the epidermis. With deeper progression into the dermis (B–D), dense cell clusters composed of uniformly sized cells, which decrease in brightness with increasing depth, can be seen. Representative vertical (E) and horizontal (F) histology (40×) from area A showed a congenital pattern nevus composed of nests and cords of bland, uniform melanocytes. Nevus cells show loss of cytoplasmic melanin with descent on histology, which corresponds to decreasing refractility with descent on RCM, a feature of maturation.

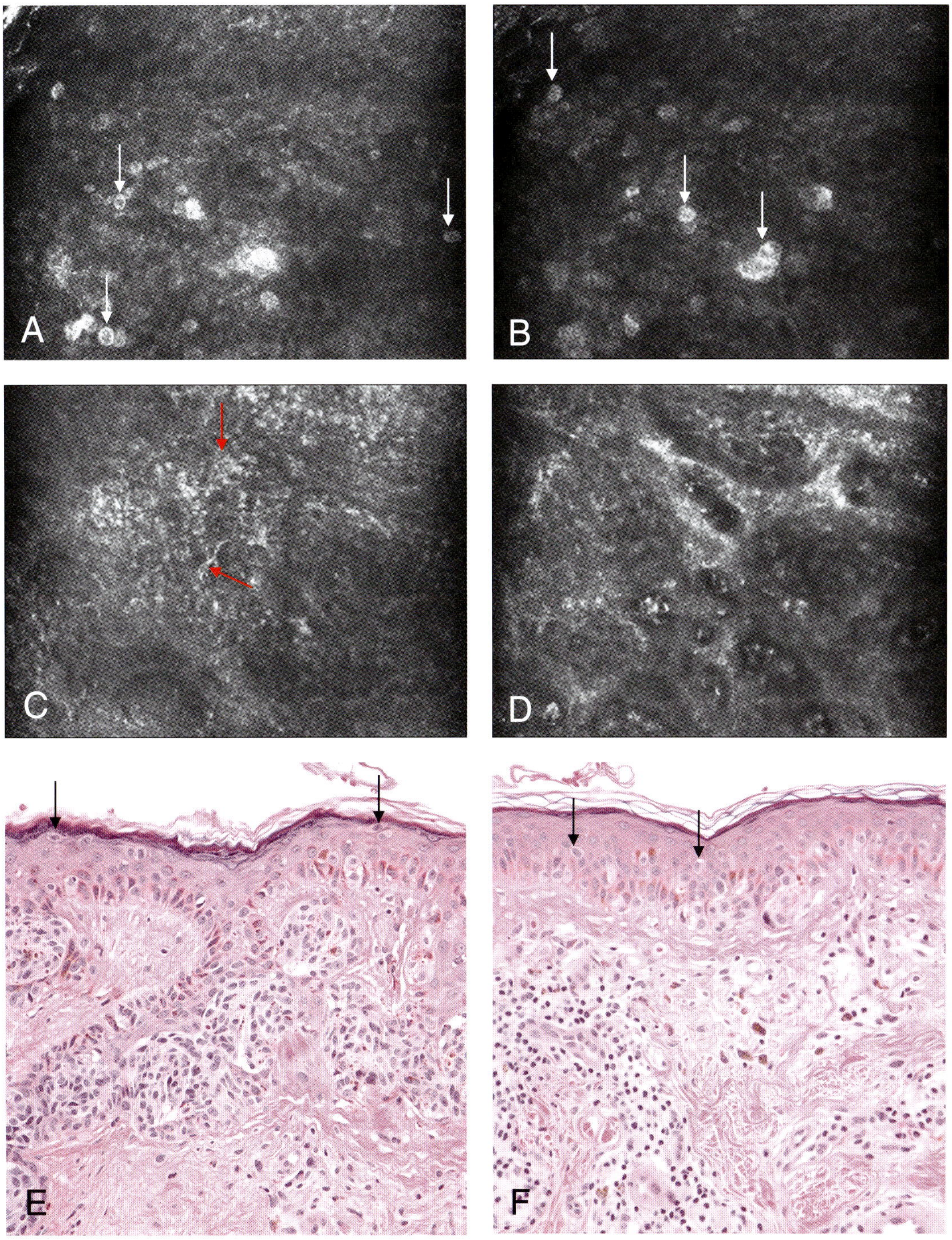

▲ **Figure 6.59** Case 2: RCM (0.245 mm × 0.175 mm) of area B shows loss of the normal honeycomb pattern in the granular (A) and spinous layers (B, C) and a pleomorphic 'pagetoid' infiltrate composed of several bright, round-to-oval nucleated cells (white arrows) and scattered refractile dendritic cells (red arrows). At the basal layer/DEJ (D), junctional thickening, or a bright broadened rete meshwork, and non-edged papillae are seen. Numerous refractile dendrites and particles are also present in the epidermis (C, D). Histology (40×) shows scatter of melanocytes at all levels of the epidermis (black arrows) and confluent nests of melanocytes at the DEJ (E, F).

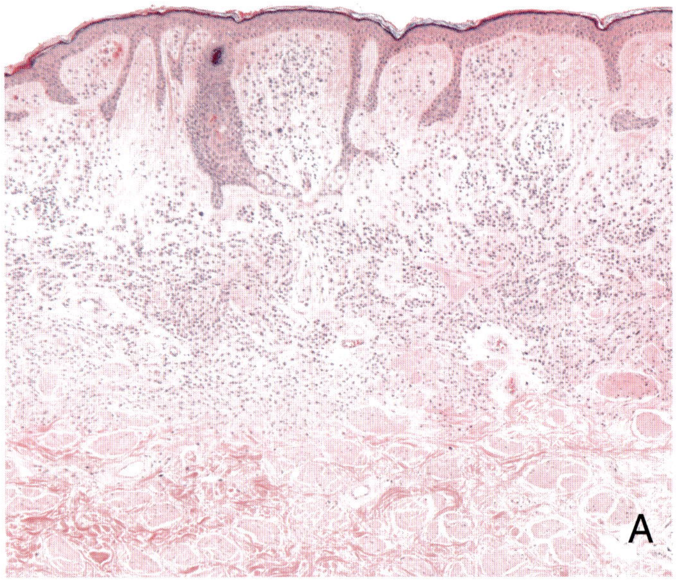

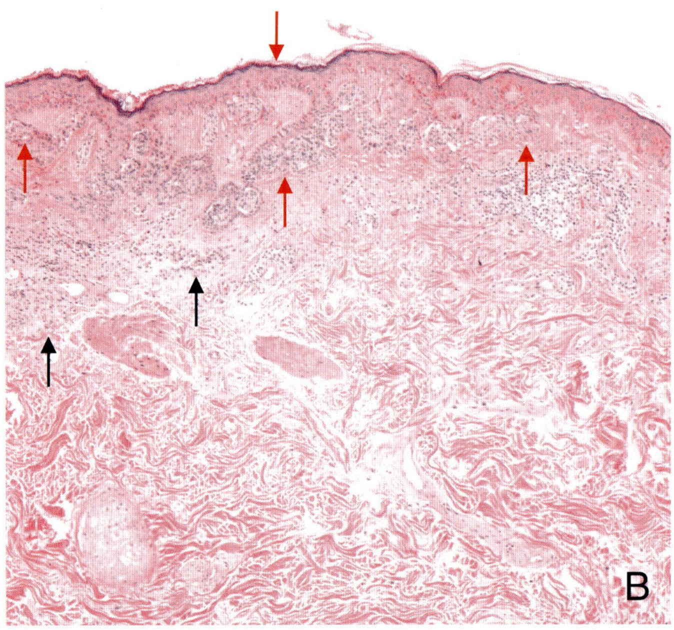

▲ **Figure 6.60** Case 2: histology (10×) of the excision specimen showed a dermal population of small, uniform melanocytes which mature with descent in the dermis, corresponding to area A. Area B showed a dermal population of small, uniform melanocytes which mature with descent in the dermis (black arrows) in addition to a second population of enlarged atypical melanocytes (red arrows) in variably confluent nests at the DEJ and as solitary cells scattered at all levels of the epidermis, compatible with melanoma in situ arising within a congenital melanocytic nevus. The melanoma in situ extended laterally beyond the dermal nevus component.

CHAPTER 6c

RCM-assisted assessment of treatment response

Susanne Astner and Salvador González

Routine histopathology is the gold standard for diagnosis of skin cancer. By obtaining biopsies from representative skin sites, however, the tissue under investigation is irreversibly altered; in addition, the process is associated with considerable pain and obligatory scar formation. While excisional biopsies aim at complete removal of the cancerous tissue, incisional biopsies aim at establishing or confirming a clinically suspected diagnosis before any decision on the therapeutic management can be obtained. To avoid repeated invasive surgical procedures, efforts have been made to develop non-invasive therapies for skin cancer. However, at the present time, treatment efficacy can only be determined by re-biopsing the tissue upon completion of therapy. In that regard, the establishment of non-invasive therapies for skin cancers has prompted the development of non-invasive high-resolution imaging devices to monitor treatment response and evaluate therapeutic efficacy. In-vivo reflectance confocal microscopy (RCM) has previously been used to analyze non-melanoma skin cancer (NMSC) and melanoma non-invasively, and diagnostic RCM evaluation criteria have been published previously.[1–6]

The investigational use of RCM for non-invasive monitoring of topical treatments for skin cancers has been reported. In a recent study performed by Torres and his co-workers, in-vivo RCM was performed on a series of 72 patients with biopsy-proven basal cell carcinoma to evaluate the therapeutic efficacy of topical imiquimod as an adjunctive treatment to Mohs' micrographic surgery. This study showed high concordance between routine histology and RCM, and results indicated higher positive predictive values than clinical assessment alone, suggesting that RCM as an adjunct optical tool may permit a more accurate clinical diagnosis.[7]

Similarly, the current gold standard for diagnosis of melanoma is excisional biopsy. Yet, with amelanotic or impalpable melanocytic skin lesions, the extent of atypical melanocytic proliferation is often difficult to assess by clinical examination and other non-invasive tools, such as Wood's lamp and dermatoscope alone.[8,9] Standard of care for the treatment of malignant melanoma is surgical excision, with surgical margins determined by visual examination prior to the procedure.[10] However, these recommendations may not be feasible for melanocytic proliferations with ill-defined margins, such as lentigo maligna melanoma, amelanotic melanoma, and lesions with lentiginous extension. In an attempt to offer non-invasive treatment alternatives for selected patients, topical therapy with imiquimod as an immune-response modifier has been used for treatment of melanoma in situ, lentigo maligna type.[11,12]

CASE PRESENTATIONS

Herein two examples are given: the first example (Case 1) illustrates the non-invasive therapeutic monitoring of actinic keratoses (AKs) treated with photodynamic therapy using aminolevulinic acid (ALA-PDT); the second example (Case 2) describes a patient with amelanotic malignant melanoma treated with topical imiquimod, whose therapeutic response was successfully monitored by RCM.

Case 1: non-invasive monitoring of actinic keratoses treated with photodynamic therapy

Photodynamic therapy using ALA or methyl-ALA has emerged as a promising, non-invasive treatment for AKs and superficial basal cell carcinomas.[13] However, to date, there have been no means for monitoring the efficacy of these treatment modalities, other than by obtaining skin biopsies. We performed a preliminary study that included six patients with actinic keratoses. Each subject was treated with ALA-PDT under occlusion for 3 hours, followed by irradiation with a blue light source (417 nm) at a dose of 10 J/cm^2.

We report the case of an otherwise healthy, 63-year-old male patient with multiple clinically uniform AKs on the scalp and temple region (Figure 6.61). The patient received numerous treatments for skin cancer prior to presentation to our clinic, including liquid nitrogen, curettage, and surgical excision. PDT was chosen due to the widespread involvement of the scalp region and lack of long-lasting remissions after previous therapies. Serial RCM evaluations were performed at selected time intervals and each evaluation included the systematic grading of cellular atypia, keratinocyte disarray, and inflammatory skin response following PDT.[14] RCM imaging at baseline revealed epidermal disarray, marked keratinocyte atypia, and pleomorphism (Figures 6.62, 6.64A–D); the diagnosis of actinic keratosis was confirmed by histology (Figures 6.63, 6.64). Immediately post-treatment, evaluated skin sites were erythematous (Figure 6.65), and RCM revealed marked inflammation and intraepidermal necrosis leading to architectural disruption (Figures 6.66–6.68). Similarly, 24 hours post PDT follow-up, evaluated skin sites showed clinical erythema (Figure 6.69) and a prominent dermal and epidermal inflammatory infiltrate and spongiosis on RCM (Figures 6.70–6.72). At 4 and 6 weeks after PDT treatment, the area showed only faint erythema on clinical examination (Figure 6.73), and RCM showed increased normalization of epidermal architecture with no residual atypia or inflammation (Figures 6.74, 6.75).

Case 2: non-invasive monitoring of melanoma in situ, lentigo maligna type treated with topical imiquimod

A 58-year-old male presented with a 1 mm discrete flesh-colored macule on his right distal nasal wall that was extending onto the site of a skin flap taken from his right cheek to repair a melanoma (0.3 mm in Breslow thickness, Clark level III) excision defect 12 years previously (Figure 6.76). Eight weeks prior to his current presentation, an invasive, non-ulcerated, primary amelanotic malignant melanoma (1.25 mm Breslow thickness, Clark level IV) was surgically excised with 1 cm margins from his right cheek. Sentinel lymph node biopsy was without evidence of metastasis. Review of systems and physical examination were negative for evidence of extracutaneous disease.

RCM examination of the new flesh-colored macule on the nose revealed findings suspicious for amelanotic melanoma, including loss of the normal honeycomb pattern of the epidermis and clusters of atypical cells with weakly refractile granular cytoplasms and dendrites in addition to rare more brightly refractile oval cells at all levels of the epidermis (Figures 6.77–6.79). Biopsy of the area most suspicious on RCM examination was performed and showed melanoma in situ, lentigo maligna type, with extension down adnexal epithelium (Figure 6.80). The patient underwent Mohs' micrographic surgery; yet, after four stages of Mohs' surgery, surgical margins remained positive for melanoma in situ (Figures 6.81, 6.82). Since the risk of deformity with further surgery was considerable, less-invasive treatment options such as radiotherapy and topical imiquimod were considered.

Treatment with topical imiquimod with close follow-up and serial RCM examinations for therapeutic monitoring was employed. Imiquimod was applied three times weekly, for a total of 6 weeks. Clinical evaluations were performed at regular weekly intervals and RCM was performed at baseline, upon completion of therapy (week 6) and 6 weeks after cessation of therapy (week 12). Upon initial examination, RCM was able to visualize confocal features consistent with malignant melanoma and these findings correlated with routine histology (Figures 6.77–6.84). Upon completion of 6 weeks of therapy, clinical evaluation revealed circumscribed inflammation, erythema, edema, and significant crusting (Figure 6.85). RCM evaluation was able to visualize parakeratosis and dendritic cells in the stratum granulosum (Figures 6.86, 6.87). In the superficial dermis, a prominent inflammatory infiltrate and marked blood vessel dilatation was detected (Figures 6.88, 6.89). At 6 weeks after cessation of therapy, the inflammation had subsided (Figure 6.90). RCM was performed on all skin sites previously evaluated, revealing a normalization of the epidermal architecture, with no atypical dendritic cells and no residual inflammation (Figures 6.91–6.94). Selected skin sites were excised for confirmation by routine hematoxylin and eosin (H&E) histology, and findings correlated well with RCM.

In summary, longitudinal evaluations using RCM permit new insights into the dynamic pathophysiologic events of diseased skin in vivo. Preliminary investigations indicate that RCM may be a promising tool for the non-invasive evaluation, diagnosis, and monitoring of melanoma and NMSC, and, in well-defined indications, RCM may be a feasible alternative to routine histology.

Key RCM features of RCM to monitor treatment response

- RCM allows for in vivo monitoring of cutaneous disease longitudinally over time.
- RCM can assist in the management of skin cancer with either large extent (i.e. actinic field cancerization), or where the full extent of the lesion cannot be delineated easily (i.e. amelanotic melanoma).
- Indications for the use of RCM to monitor treatment response:
  - When non-invasive therapies are a viable alternative to surgical or other invasive treatments.
  - When residual or recurrent disease is not amenable to surgical resection.

REFERENCES

1. Aghassi D, Anderson RR, Gonzalez S. Confocal laser microscopic imaging of actinic keratoses in vivo: a preliminary report. J Am Acad Dermatol 2000; 43:42–8.
2. Busam KJ, Hester K, Charles C et al. Detection of clinically amelanotic malignant melanoma and assessment of its margins by in vivo confocal scanning laser microscopy. Arch Dermatol 2001; 137:923–9.
3. Langley RG, Rajadhyaksha M, Dwyer PJ et al. Confocal scanning laser microscopy of benign and malignant melanocytic skin lesions in vivo. J Am Acad Dermatol 2001; 45:365–76.
4. Pellacani G, Cesinaro AM, Seidenari S. Reflectance-mode confocal microscopy of pigmented skin lesions – improvement in melanoma diagnostic specificity. J Am Acad Dermatol 2005; 53:979–85.
5. Pellacani G, Guitera P, Longo C et al. The impact of in vivo reflectance confocal microscopy for the diagnostic accuracy of melanoma and equivocal melanocytic lesions. J Invest Dermatol 2007; July 26 [Epub ahead of print].
6. Tannous ZS, Mihm MC, Flotte TJ et al. In vivo examination of lentigo maligna and malignant melanoma in situ, lentigo maligna type by near-infrared reflectance confocal microscopy: comparison of in vivo confocal images with histologic sections. J Am Acad Dermatol 2002; 46:260–3.
7. Torres A, Niemeyer A, Berkes B et al. 5% imiquimod cream and reflectance-mode confocal microscopy as adjunct modalities to Mohs micrographic surgery for treatment of basal cell carcinoma. Dermatol Surg 2004; 30:1462–9.
8. Koch SE, Lange JR. Amelanotic melanoma: the great masquerader. J Am Acad Dermatol 2000; 42:731–4.
9. Osborne JE, Hutchinson PE. A follow-up study to investigate the efficacy of initial treatment of lentigo maligna with surgical excision. Br J Plast Surg 2002; 55:611–5.
10. Sober AJ, Chuang TY, Duvic M et al. Guidelines of care for primary cutaneous melanoma. J Am Acad Dermatol 2001; 45:579–86.
11. Ahmed I, Berth-Jones J. Imiquimod: a novel treatment for lentigo maligna. Br J Dermatol 2000; 143:843–5.
12. Curiel-Lewandrowski C, Williams CM, Swindells KJ et al. Use of in vivo confocal microscopy in malignant melanoma: an aid in diagnosis and assessment of surgical and nonsurgical therapeutic approaches. Arch Dermatol 2004; 140:1127–32.
13. Blume JE, Oseroff AR. Aminolevulinic acid photodynamic therapy for skin cancers. Dermatol Clin 2007; 25(1):5–14.
14. Trehan M, Swindells KJ, Taylor CR et al. Confocal microscopy imaging of actinic keratoses post-photodynamic therapy with 5-ALA. In: 20th World Congress of Dermatology, Paris, 2003.

RCM-ASSISTED ASSESSMENT OF TREATMENT RESPONSE

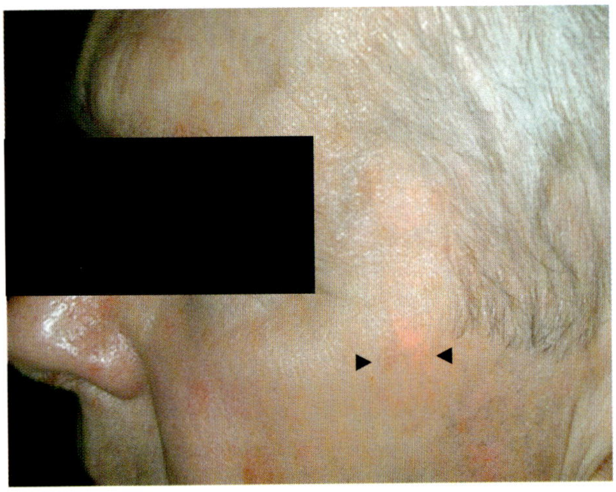

Figure 6.61

Case 1: clinical photograph obtained at baseline, illustrating numerous erythematous macules with fine hyperkeratotic scale, marked dyspigmentation, and skin atrophy, consistent with multiple actinic keratoses. A 12 mm × 15 mm lesion on the left temple region (arrowheads) was selected for imaging.

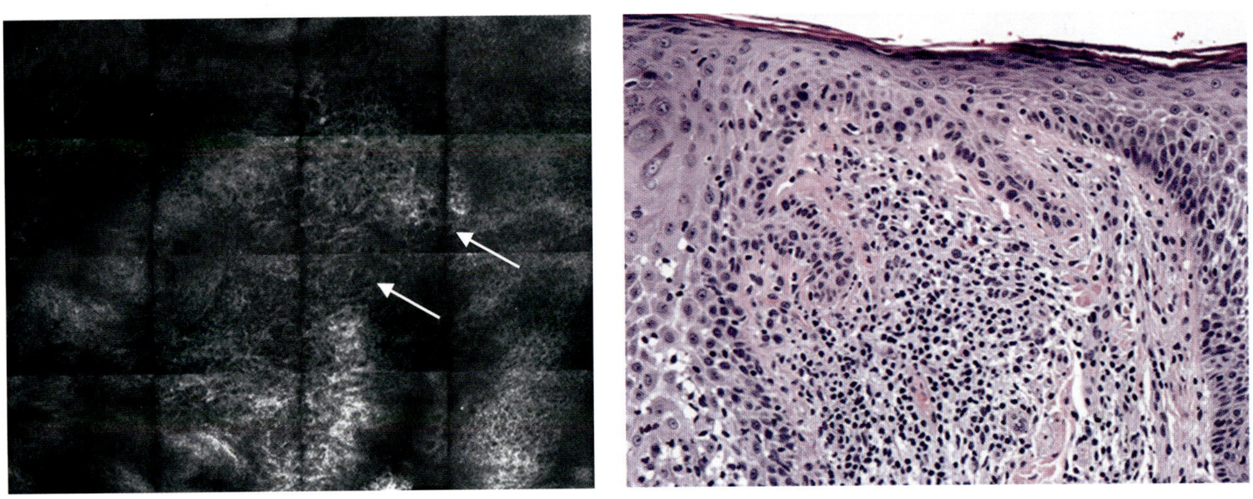

Figures 6.62, 6.63 Case 1: RCM mosaic (1.900 mm × 1.360 mm) at the level of the stratum spinosum reveals epidermal disarray with cellular and nuclear pleomorphism. Arrows indicate groups of atypical keratinocytes. Corresponding histology (10×) illustrates focal parakeratosis, keratinocytic atypia in the lower levels of the epidermis, and chronic inflammation.

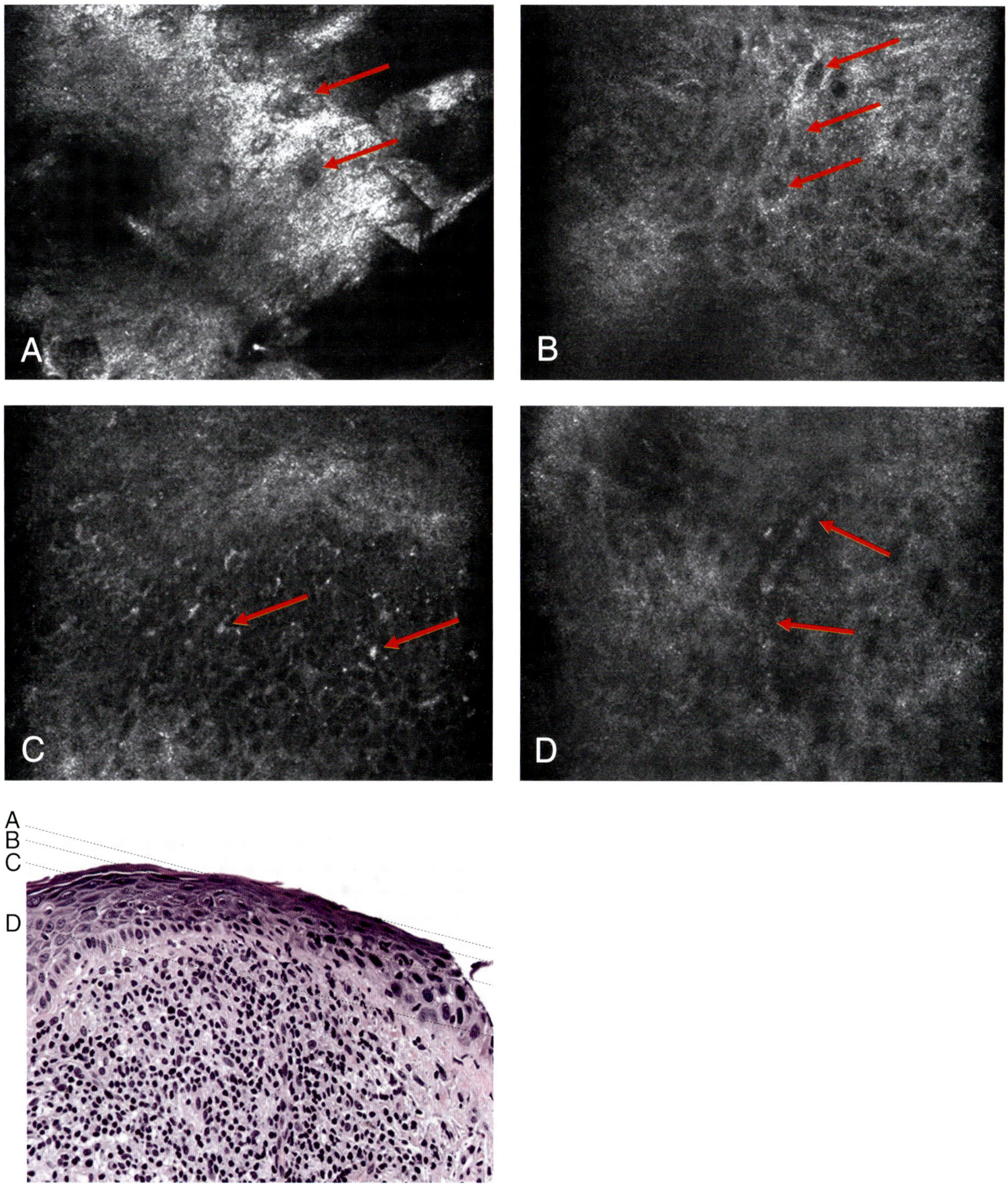

▲ **Figure 6.64** Case 1: histology (20×) shows another area within the actinic keratosis; transverse lines labeled A–D indicate from where each confocal image (0.475 mm × 0.340 mm) is captured. RCM at the level of the stratum corneum (A) identifies retention of nuclei (arrows), indicating parakeratosis. The upper stratum spinosum (B) shows alteration of the normal honeycomb pattern and keratinocyte atypia evidenced by variation in cell and nuclear size (arrows). The lower stratum spinosum (C) shows small refractile inflammatory cells (arrows) among the atypical keratinocytes. In the dermis (D), elongated canalicular structures containing refractile cells (arrows), corresponding to prominent blood vessels, are seen.

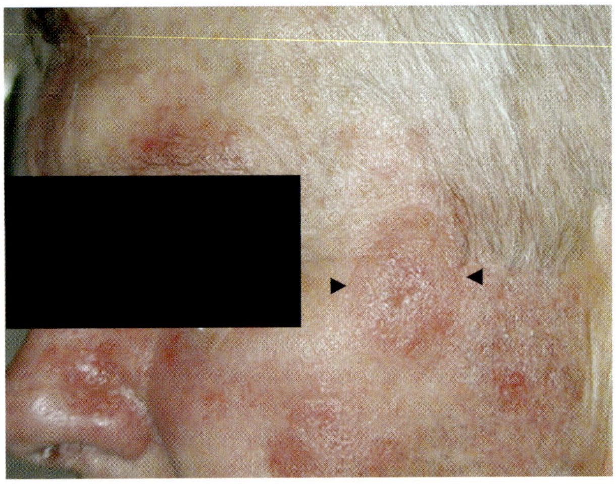

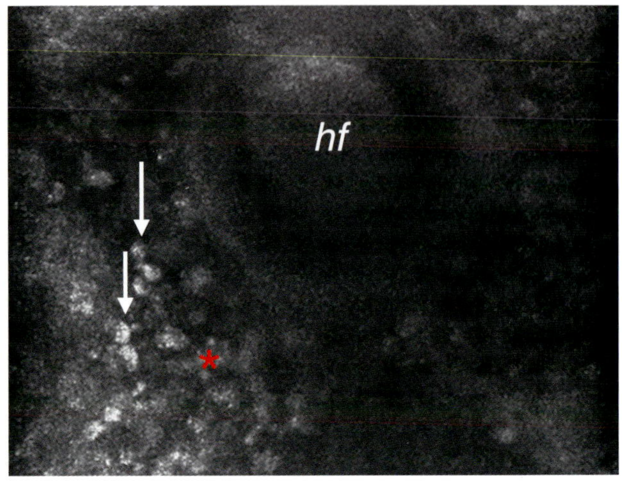

▲ **Figures 6.65, 6.66** Case 1: clinical image immediately after ALA-PDT. Note erythema and edema of the irradiated skin sites (arrowheads) and the presence of erythema in skin sites that previously appeared normal on clinical examination. Corresponding RCM (0.475 mm × 0.340 mm) at the level of the upper epidermis of the actinic keratosis immediately after ALA-PDT, illustrates marked infiltration by refractile inflammatory cells (arrows) and necrosis near a hair follicle (hf).

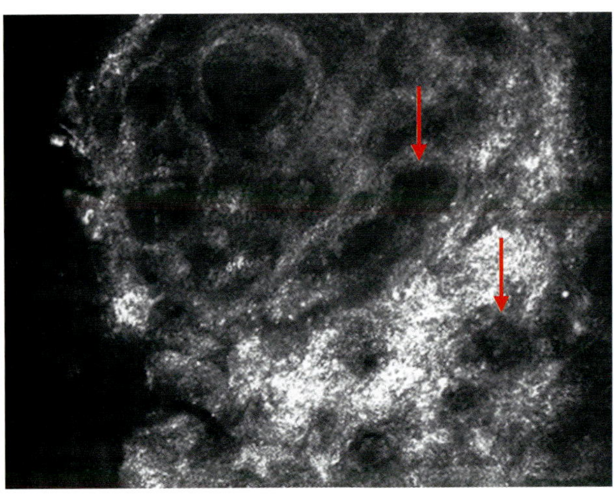

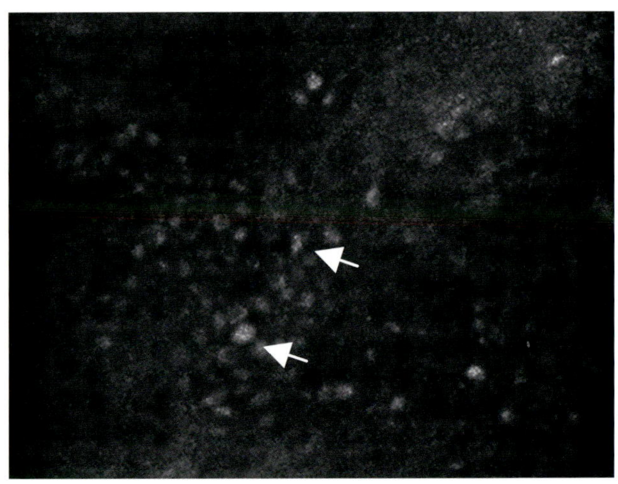

▲ **Figures 6.67, 6.68** Case 1: RCM (0.475 mm × 0.340 mm) obtained immediately after ALA-PDT at the level of the stratum corneum (left) shows retention of nuclei (arrows) or parakeratosis. At the level of the stratum spinosum (right) reveals near total loss of the normal honeycomb pattern, a prominent infiltrate of numerous round to oval, highly refractile cells (arrows) and dark areas, corresponding to the acute response to therapy including inflammatory exocytosis and epidermal necrosis.

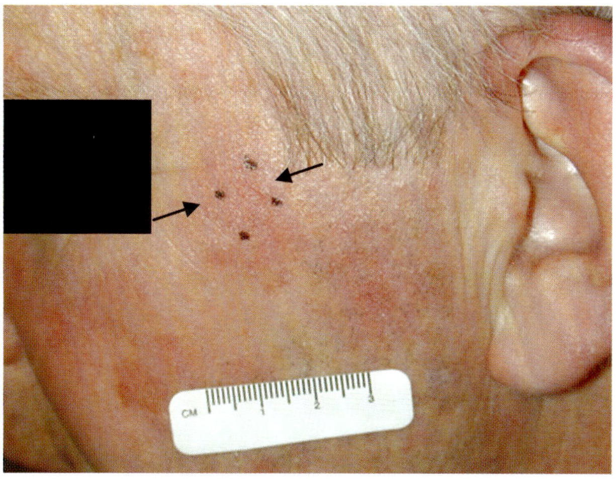
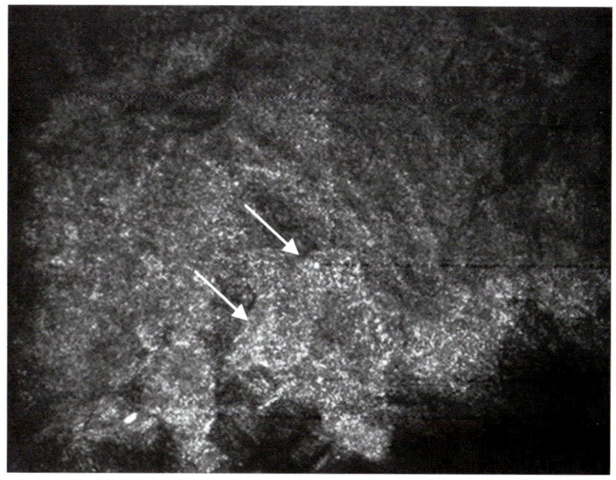

▲ **Figures 6.69, 6.70** Case 1: clinical image obtained 24 hours after completion of ALA-PDT illustrating persistent erythema and somewhat diminished edema of irradiated skin sites (arrows) and, to a lesser extent, of clinically normal areas which showed reaction (see Figure 6.65). Corresponding RCM (0.475 mm × 0.340 mm) obtained at the level of the superficial stratum corneum illustrates detached corneocytes (white arrows).

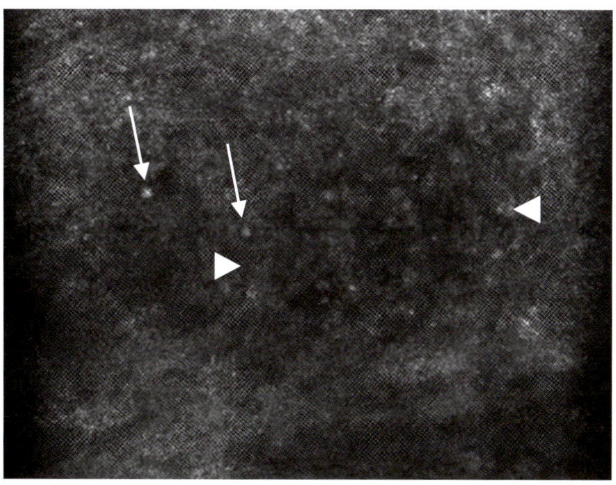
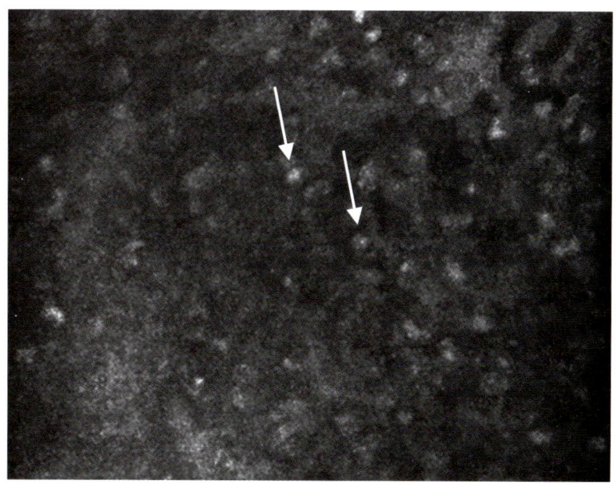

▲ **Figures 6.71, 6.72** Case 1: RCM (0.475 mm × 0.340 mm) obtained 24 hours after completion of ALA-PDT at the level of the deep stratum corneum (left) illustrates sparse refractile round inflammatory cells (arrows) and circumscribed dark mottled areas (arrowheads) composed of discohesive keratinocytes with ill-defined nuclear and cytoplasmic borders admixed with round, refractile cells, corresponding to necrotic keratinocytes, cellular debris, and inflammatory cells. At the level of the stratum spinosum (right) shows a marked epidermal inflammatory infiltrate (arrows) and necrosis.

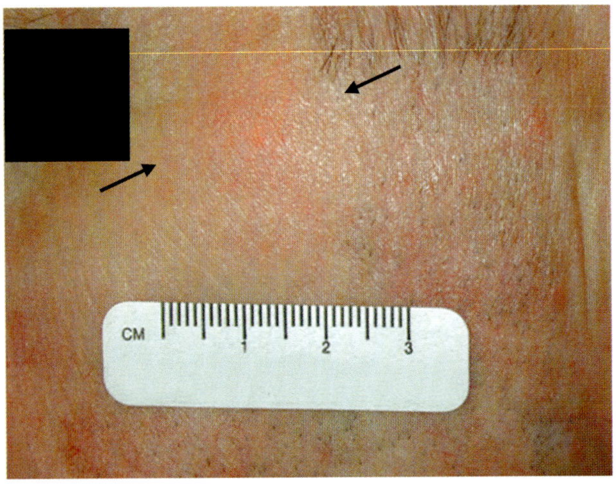

◀ **Figure 6.73**

Case 1: clinical image obtained 6 weeks after cessation of ALA-PDT illustrates only faint residual erythema (arrows) at the treatment site. No scaling is present.

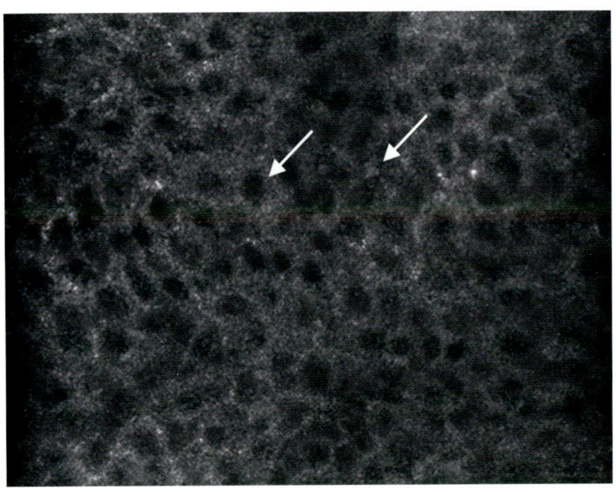

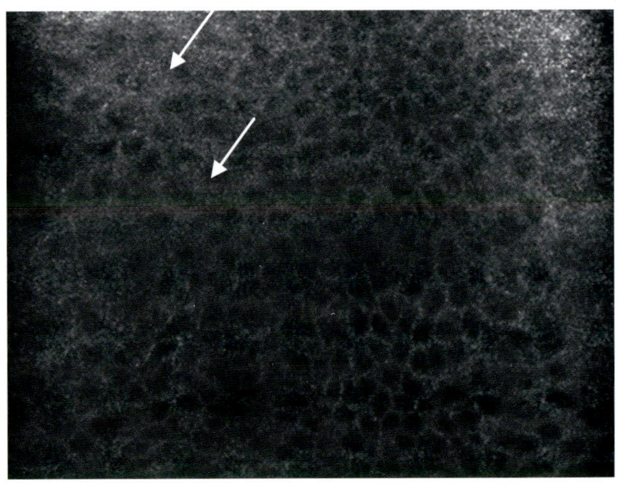

▲ **Figures 6.74, 6.75** Case 1: RCM images (0.475 mm × 0.340 mm) obtained 6 weeks after cessation of ALA-PDT. Left image obtained at the level of the stratum granulosum reveals further normalization of the epidermal architecture with return of the honeycomb pattern; thickened intercellular demarcations (arrows), corresponding to residual spongiosis, are noted. Right image obtained at the level of stratum spinosum shows a more normal honeycomb pattern with only focal residual spongiosis (arrows).

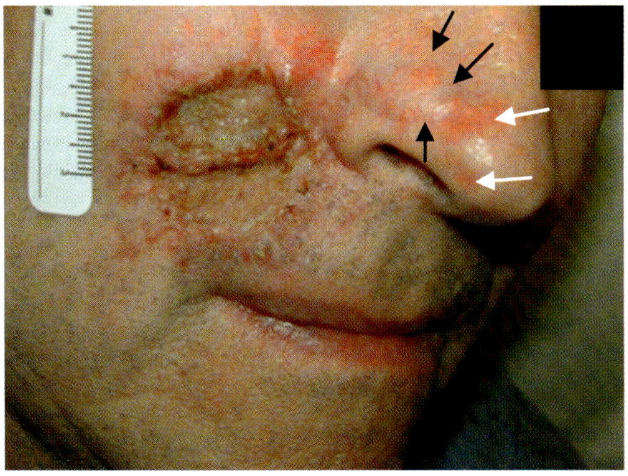

◀ **Figure 6.76** Case 2: a flesh-colored, slightly erythematous macule (white arrows) is seen on the right side of the nasal tip extending into a skin flap from previous surgery (black arrows). Visual examination revealed no areas of increased pigmentation, and the border of the lesion was difficult to discern.

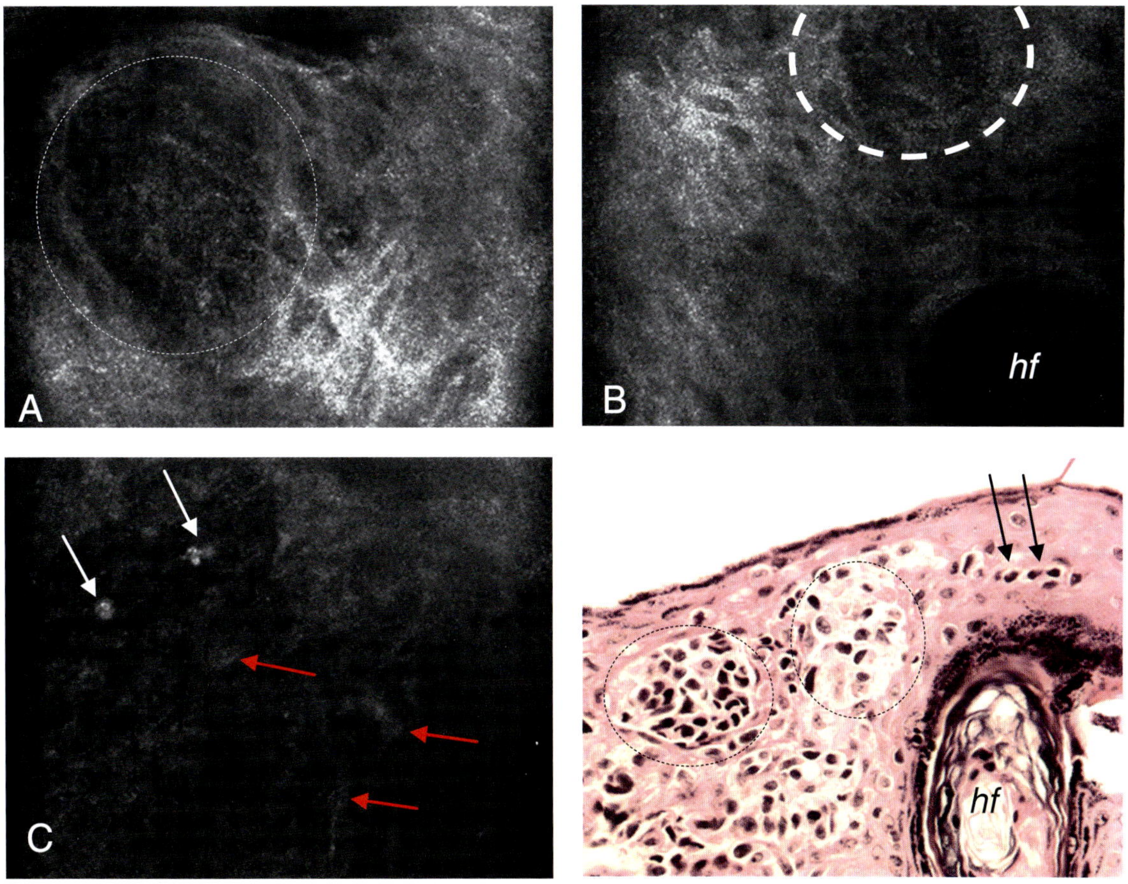

▲ **Figures 6.77–6.80** Case 2: representative RCM images (0.475 mm × 0.340 mm) from the area of interest reveals features suspicious for amelanotic melanoma. RCM (A) at the level of the stratum granulosum/upper stratum spinosum shows loss of the normal honeycomb pattern and a cluster of atypical nucleated cells with slightly refractile granular cytoplasms and dendritic processes (circle). RCM at the level of the stratum spinosum (B) shows similar findings and an adjacent hair follicle (hf). Another RCM image (C) from the upper stratum spinosum reveals loss of the normal honeycomb pattern and a large, ill-defined cluster of weakly refractile dendritic cells (red arrows) containing rare bright, round cells (white arrows). Histology (40×) from the RCM-guided biopsy shows atypical poorly melanized melanocytes singly (arrows) and in discohesive clusters (circles) at all levels of the epidermis, compatible with melanoma in situ.

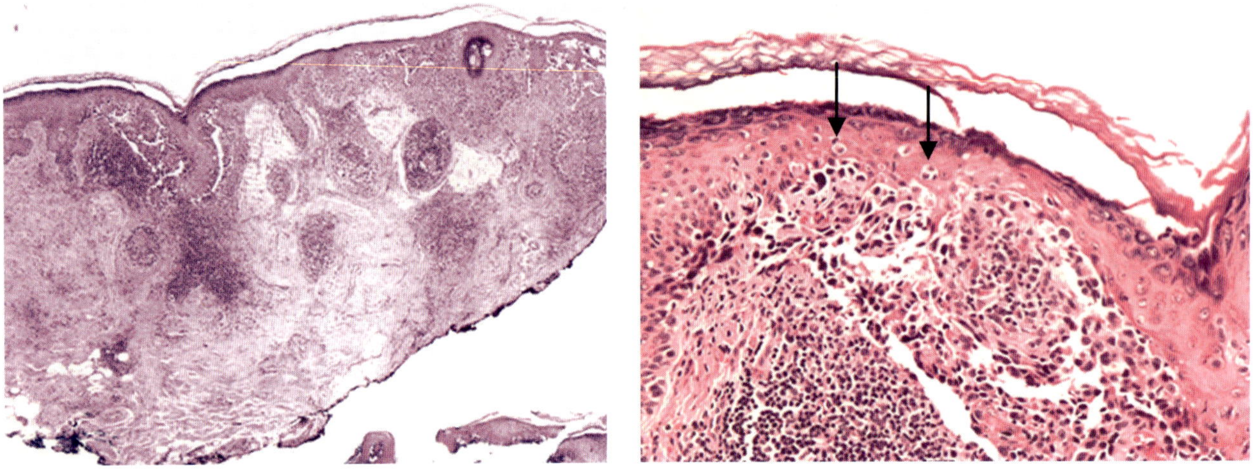

▲ **Figures 6.81, 6.82** Case 2: histology (4×, left) of the excision specimen confirmed the diagnosis of melanoma in situ, lentigo maligna type, with adnexal involvement. Histology (20×, right) reveals confluent, discohesive aggregates of poorly melanized, atypical melanocytes within the lower portion of the epidermis and pagetoid scatter of melanocytes (black arrows) at all levels of the epidermis. A prominent inflammatory response is seen in the dermis.

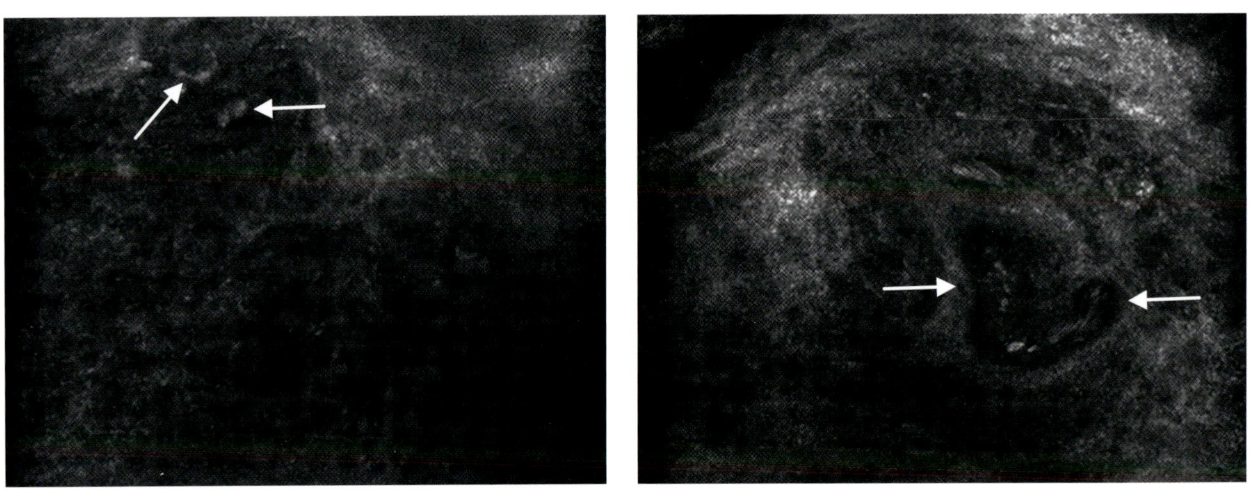

▲ **Figures 6.83, 6.84** Case 2: RCM images (0.475 mm × 0.340 mm) of the residual lesion before imiquimod therapy show loss of the normal honeycomb pattern, refractile round–oval and dendritic cells, and subtle, ill-defined cell aggregates (arrows) in the stratum spinosum (left) and a prominent, dilated blood vessel (arrows) in the dermis (right).

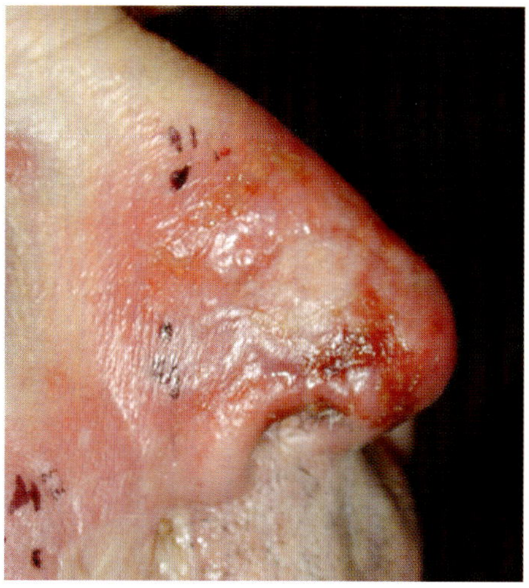

◀ **Figure 6.85** Case 2: clinical image obtained upon completion of 6 weeks of topical imiquimod therapy reveals significant erythema, edema, oozing, and serosanguinous crusting in treated areas.

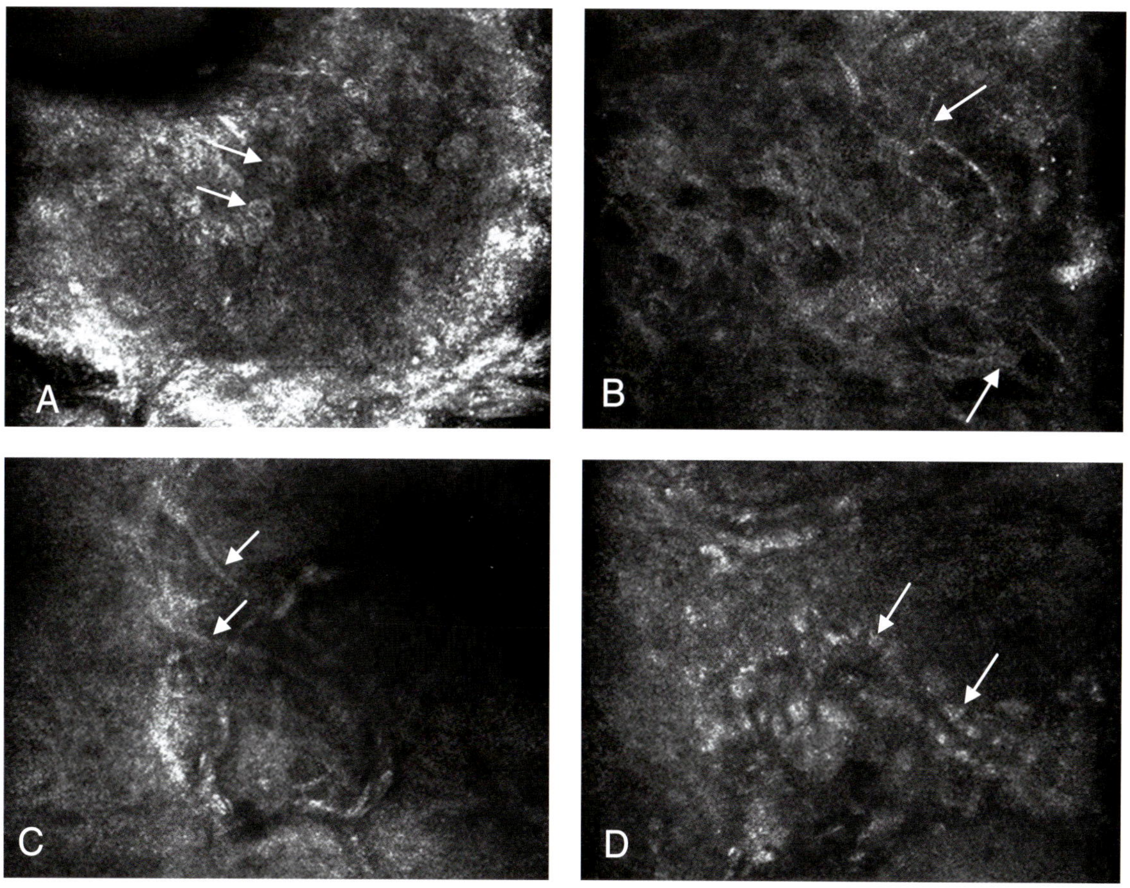

▲ **Figures 6.86–6.89** Case 2: RCM images (0.475 mm × 0.340 mm) were obtained upon completion of 6 weeks of imiquimod therapy. The stratum corneum (A) is altered, containing individual corneocytes and parakeratotic nuclei (white arrows). The granular layer (B) shows extensive disruption of the honeycomb pattern and refractile dendritic cells (arrows) with long, thin dendrites, which may correspond to Langerhans cells. Within the dermis, multiple elongated canalicular structures (arrows) consistent with blood vessels (C) and numerous bright round-to-oval cells (arrows) compatible with inflammatory cells (D) are seen.

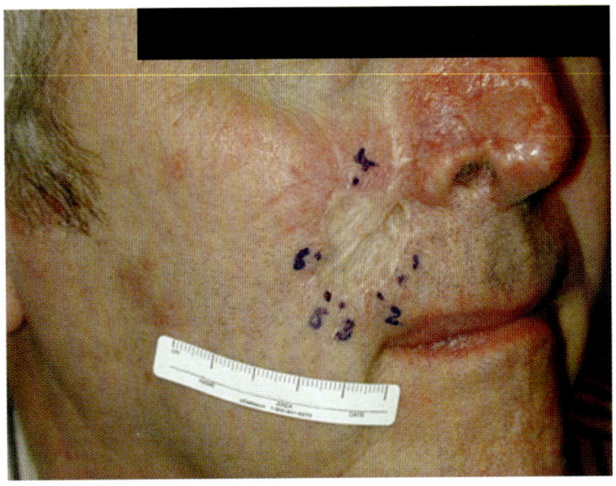

◀ **Figure 6.90** Case 2: digital photograph obtained 6 weeks after cessation of imiquimod treatment reveals slight residual erythema, but no oozing or crusting.

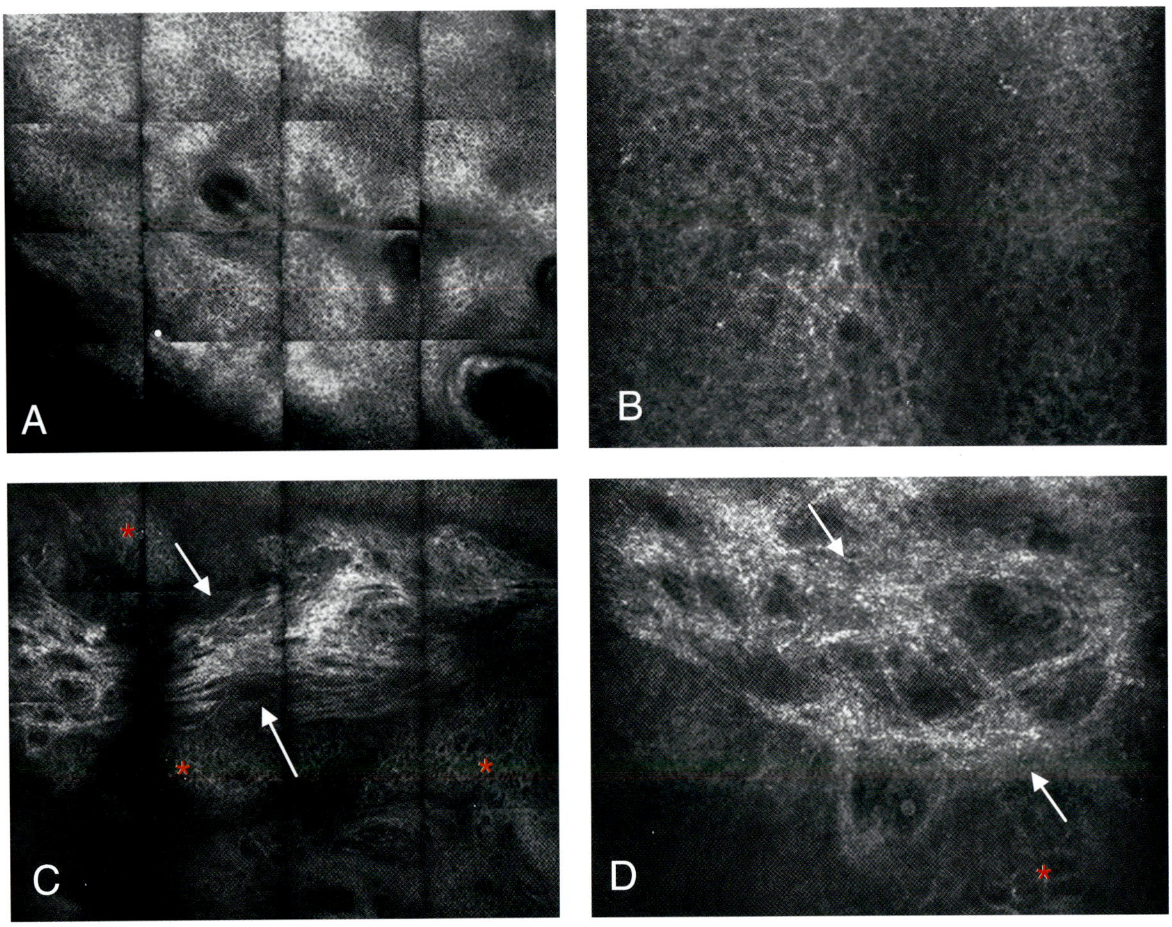

▲ **Figures 6.91–6.94** Case 2: the lesional area was evaluated by RCM 6 weeks after cessation of imiquimod therapy. RCM mosaic (A, 1.900 mm × 1.360 mm) and image (B, 0.475 mm × 0.340 mm) at the level of the stratum granulosum/upper stratum spinosum show restoration of the normal honeycomb pattern and a notable absence of atypical refractile cells, dendritic cells, and inflammatory cells. RCM mosaic (C, 1.900 mm × 1.360 mm) and image (D, 0.475 mm × 0.340 mm) at the level of the superficial dermis show zonated, highly refractile thickened collagen bundles arranged in parallel to one another (arrows), compatible with scar, and adjacent fine, moderately refractile collagen fibers arranged in a reticulated pattern (asterisks).

CHAPTER 6d

RCM-assisted in-vivo margin mapping

Sanjay K Mandal, Ashfaq A Marghoob, Cristiane Benvenuto-Andrade, Ruby Delgado, Salvador González, and Allan C Halpern

Ideal treatment for melanoma and non-melanoma skin cancers is complete excision of the tumor with histologically verified clear margins. However, despite careful macroscopic visual examination, it is often difficult, if not impossible, to clinically determine the precise histologic boundary between tumor and normal skin. This is particularly true for ill-defined non-pigmented basal cell carcinomas (BCCs), some lentigo maligna/lentigo maligna melanomas (LM/LMMs) and amelanotic melanomas. Imaging modalities such as dermoscopy, reflectance confocal microscopy (RCM), optical coherence tomography, and high-resolution ultrasound may enable clinicians to visualize tissue details with sufficient resolution to determine the lesion's borders. Amongst these modalities, RCM provides the highest resolution, approaching that of histology.[1]

The utility of RCM in assessing the lateral extent of some atypical melanocytic proliferations has been evaluated in several studies. Busam et al first described the utility of RCM for delineating the margins of amelanotic melanoma prior to surgical excision of the tumor.[2] This was subsequently confirmed in a study by Curiel-Lewandrowski et al.[3] They showed that RCM was able to assist in detecting residual or recurrent melanoma in patients with previously excised amelanotic melanomas. These preliminary reports suggest that RCM may be a useful adjunct to surgical therapy for some melanomas. In addition, RCM may prove useful for monitoring melanoma response to non-invasive therapies (e.g. the off-label use of topical imiquimod for lentigo maligna).

LM/LMMs are often clinically challenging. These lesions can progress to metastatic disease and, when excised with inadequate margins, have a high likelihood of recurrence. Unlike most melanomas, which have distinct clinical borders, LM/LMM characteristically arise on chronically sun-damaged skin in older individuals and often have poorly defined borders.[4] Even histologically, it is often difficult to delineate the margin of complex LM/LMM due to the presence of background solar damage with associated melanocytic atypia and solar lentigines.[5] The problem is compounded by the common occurrence of these lesions on the face, with the attendant cosmetic and functional implications of wider margins. Accordingly, the recommended 5 mm excision margin for in-situ melanomas may not be adequate or readily achievable for some LM cases.[6,7] Thus, accurate and precise presurgical margin mapping for melanoma has largely focused on this subset of the disease.

In clinical practice, the biopsy-proven LM/LMM lesion is initially evaluated by simple visual inspection and palpation. Wood's lamp examination and dermoscopy can be helpful for the detection of subclinical extension and the distinction between melanoma and neighboring solar lentigo.[8,9] As noted above, RCM may permit further refinement of the surgical margin by non-invasively sampling within and beyond the optimized clinical/Wood's lamp/dermoscopic border. In the preliminary studies that have been performed to date, multiple punch biopsies have demonstrated good correlation of RCM findings with histology at the margins of LM/LMM. A further advantage of RCM is that it permits interrogation of skin at a distance from the lesion, permitting comparison to the patient's background photodamage. In the cases outlined below, the lesions were 'mapped' with RCM, punch biopsies were performed of representative RCM positive and negative sites, and the adequacy of the final surgical excision was assessed via permanent histology utilizing both hemotoxylin and eosin (H&E) and immunohistochemically stained sections.[10]

CASE PRESENTATIONS

Case 1

A 79-year-old man presented for evaluation of an irregularly pigmented lesion on the scalp which developed adjacent to the scar of a previously excised melanoma. Clinical examination revealed a 20 mm × 20 mm irregularly shaped ill-defined brown patch adjacent to the previous excision scar (Figure 6.95). A biopsy from the pigmented patch revealed lentigo maligna melanoma, primarily in situ with focal microinvasion. It was difficult to clinically determine the border of the pigmented patch due to the presence of diffuse background lentigines.

Clinical, Wood's light, and dermoscopic examination were utilized to mark the presumed border of the LMM. Following this, RCM was utilized to image multiple foci within and outside the demarcated area. Some of the foci were selected based on clinical, Wood's lamp, and dermoscopic findings, while others were selected randomly (Figures 6.96–6.98). RCM images were correlated to histology from five pairs of corresponding punch biopsies (Figures 6.99–6.102). The final surgical excision margin was determined based on the confocal mapping (Figures 6.103, 6.104). The surgical margins were reported to be adequate and free of melanoma on permanent section histology. The patient remains free of melanoma recurrence 4 years post excision.

Case 2

A 90-year-old female presented with a 22 mm × 11 mm irregular and ill-defined pigmented patch on her right cheek (Figure 6.105). A biopsy from the center of the lesion revealed melanoma in situ. Due to the ill-defined border and the presence of background lentigines, delineation of the border of the melanoma on clinical inspection was difficult. Wood's lamp examination revealed two additional foci of pigmentation, which were not apparent on initial unaided visual inspection (Figure 6.105). The multistep in-vivo margin mapping procedure described above was used to help determine the border of this melanoma (Figures 6.105–6.107). Once the lesion's border was refined based on the confocal findings, five punch biopsies were obtained for histologic confirmation (Figure 6.108). RCM findings and corresponding punch biopsy histologic findings (Figures 6.109–6.120) helped guide the surgeon in determining the final surgical margin of excision (Figure 6.121). The lesion was subsequently excised (Figure 6.122) and the surgical margins were reported to be adequate and clear of melanoma on permanent histology sections. Currently, there is no evidence of local recurrence 8 months post excision.

Key steps for RCM-assisted in-vivo margin mapping

- Clinical inspection and palpation of the lesion
- Delineation of the lesion's border using Wood's lamp and dermoscopy
- Selection of foci for RCM examination inside and outside Wood's lamp and dermoscopy delineated border
- Refinement of the lesion's border based on RCM findings
- Histologic confirmation of RCM findings with paired punch biopsies
- Final refinement of the lesion's border based on histologic findings
- Mapping of definitive surgical margin
- Excision with appropriate margin of normal skin, confirmed by permanent histology using H&E and immunohistochemical stains

While there are a growing number of case reports of the use of RCM for margin mapping of LM/LMM, it is important to emphasize that this technique remains in the investigational stage of development. The reported cases have utilized fixed tissue rings, which has limited the area of skin examined. The recent advent of a handheld scanning device should, in theory, permit more rapid and exhaustive margin sampling. On the other hand, much additional research is needed to define the optimal parameters for the technique and validate its utility. Based on the promising preliminary data, it can be hoped that, with refinements, RCM will permit improved presurgical margin mapping not only for melanoma but also for other lesions such as large indistinct BCCs or extramammary Paget's disease.

REFERENCES

1. González S, Swindells K, Rajadhyaksha M et al. Changing paradigms in dermatology: confocal microscopy in clinical and surgical dermatology. Clin Dermatol 2003; 21:359–69.
2. Busam KJ, Hester K, Charles C et al. Detection of clinically amelanotic malignant melanoma and assessment of its margins by in vivo confocal scanning laser microscopy. Arch Dermatol 2001; 137:923–9.
3. Curiel-Lewandrowski C, Williams CM, Swindells KJ et al. Use of in vivo confocal microscopy in malignant melanoma: an aid in diagnosis and assessment of surgical and nonsurgical therapeutic approaches. Arch Dermatol 2004; 140:1127–32.
4. Chang AE, Karnell LH, Menck HR. The National Cancer Data Base report on cutaneous and noncutaneous melanoma: a summary of 84,836 cases from the past decade. The American College of Surgeons Commission on Cancer and the American Cancer Society. Cancer 1998; 83:1664–78.
5. Acker SM, Nicholson JH, Rust PF et al. Morphometric discrimination of melanoma in situ of sun-damaged skin from chronically sun-damaged skin. J Am Acad Dermatol 1998; 39:239–45.
6. Agarwal-Antal N, Bowen GM, Gerwels JW. Histologic evaluation of lentigo maligna with permanent sections: implications regarding current guidelines. J Am Acad Dermatol 2002; 47:743–8.
7. Wildemore JK, Schuchter L, Mick R et al. Locally recurrent malignant melanoma characteristics and outcomes: a single-institution study. Ann Plast Surg 2001; 46:488–94.
8. Paraskevas LR, Halpern AC, Marghoob AA. Utility of the Wood's light: five cases from a pigmented lesion clinic. Br J Dermatol 2005; 152:1039–44.
9. Robinson JK. Use of digital epiluminescence microscopy to help define the edge of lentigo maligna. Arch Dermatol 2004; 140:1095–100.
10. Chen CS, Elias M, Busam K et al. Multimodal in vivo optical imaging, including confocal microscopy, facilitates presurgical margin mapping for clinically complex lentigo maligna melanoma. Br J Dermatol 2005; 153:1031–6.

RCM-ASSISTED IN-VIVO MARGIN MAPPING

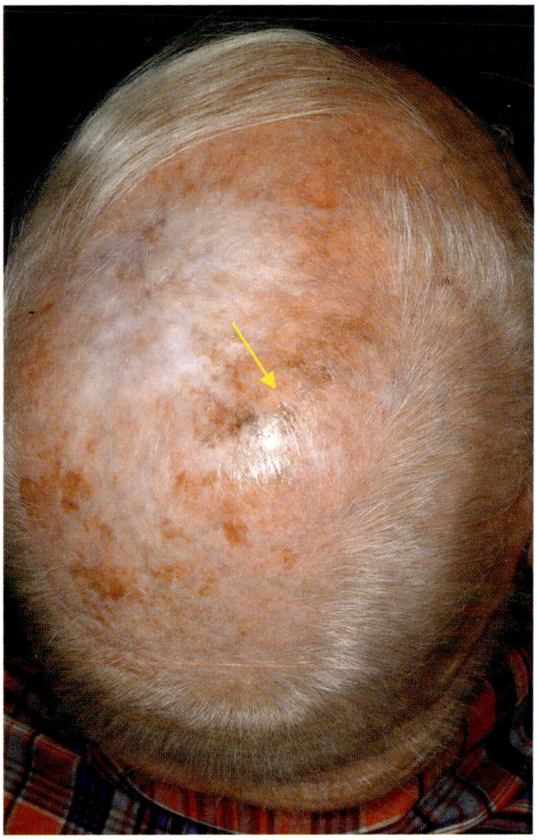

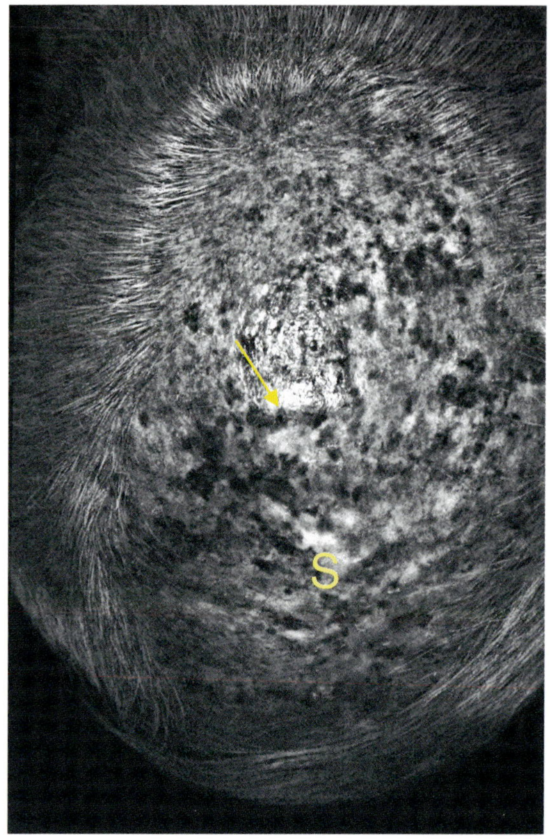

▲ **Figures 6.95, 6.96** Case 1: a 79-year-old white male presented with a pigmented patch which developed adjacent to a scar from a previously excised melanoma (arrow). Wood's lamp image of the scalp reveals the irregular pigmented area (arrow) next to the scar (S) in addition to multiple lentigines.

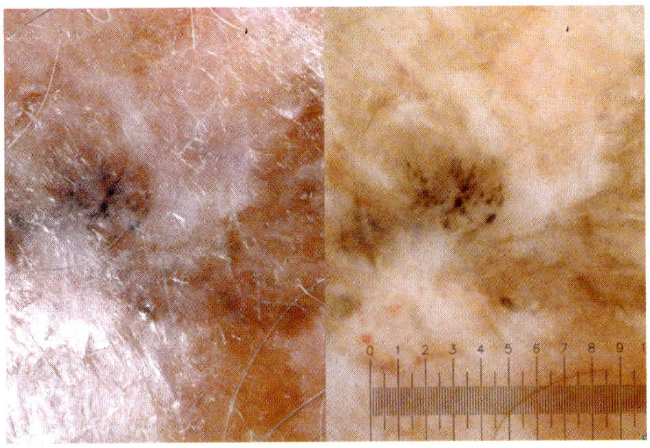

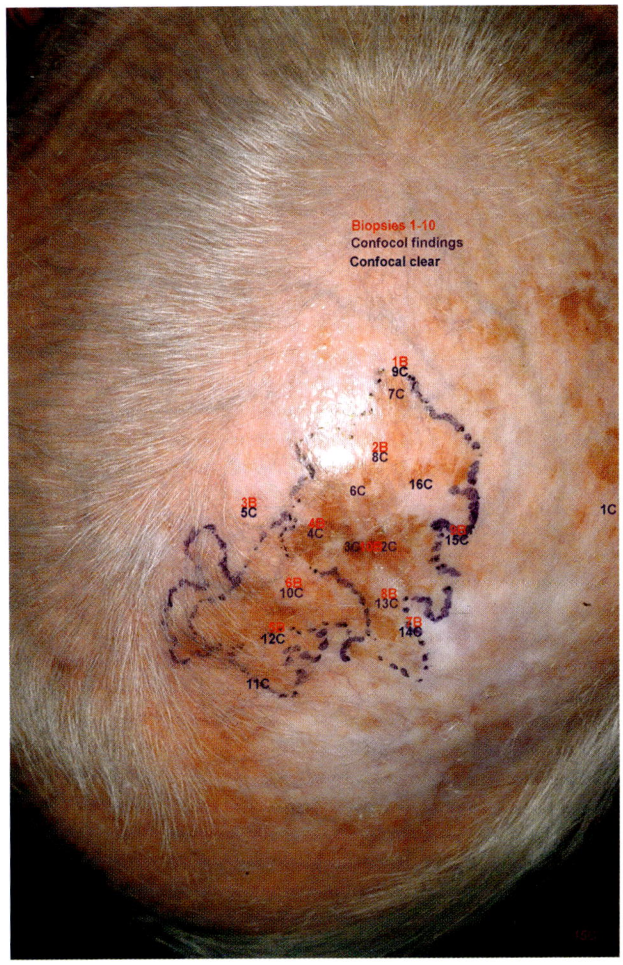

▶ **Figures 6.97, 6.98**

Case 1: close-up clinical and dermoscopic images of the pigmented area reveal an irregular, ill-defined pigmented lesion with a pigment network and irregular blue-gray dots arising at the edge of a scar. Based on Wood's lamp and dermoscopy findings, multiple foci were chosen for confocal examination. Foci suspicious for melanoma are marked in purple, foci revealing normal skin are marked in blue, and the corresponding biopsy sites are marked in red.

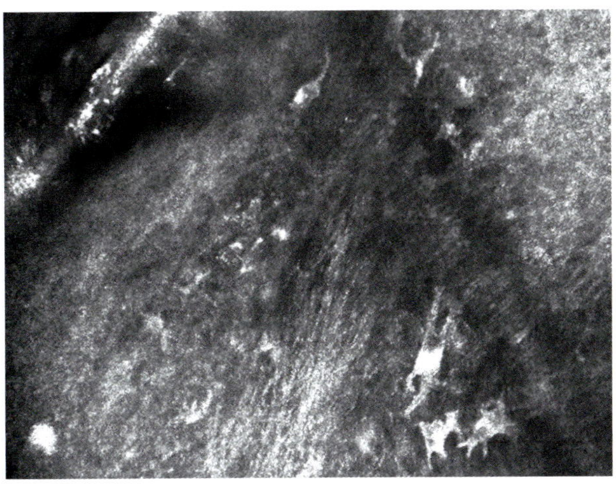

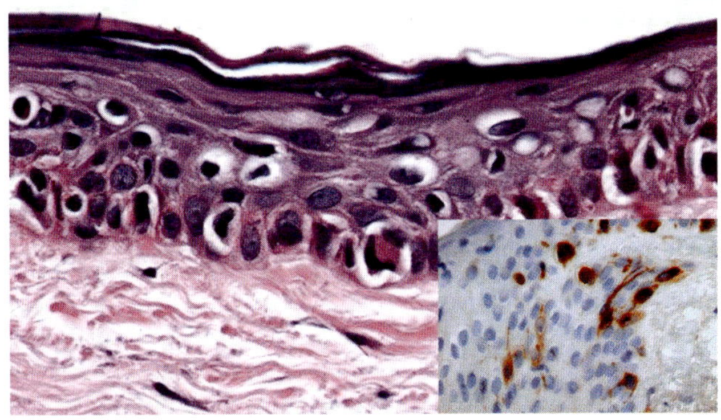

▲ **Figures 6.99, 6.100** Case 1, site 2B/8C: RCM (0.5 mm × 0.5 mm) at the level of the stratum spinosum reveals multiple bright dendritic cells and loss of the normal honeycomb pattern, suggestive of melanoma. Histopathology (40×) with corresponding Melan-A immunohistochemical stain (inset) show an increased number of atypical melanocytes, some of which are dendritic in shape.

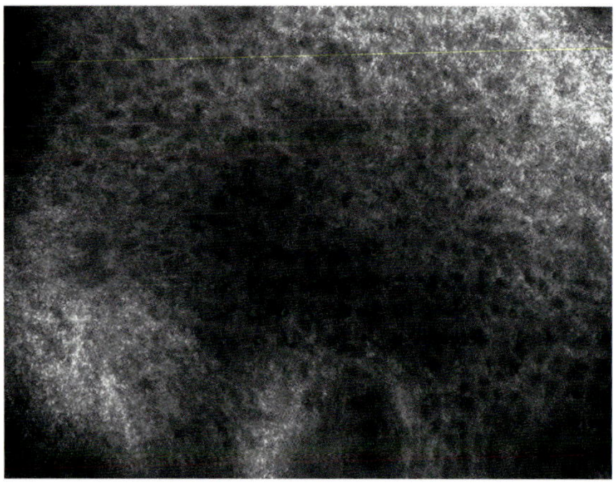

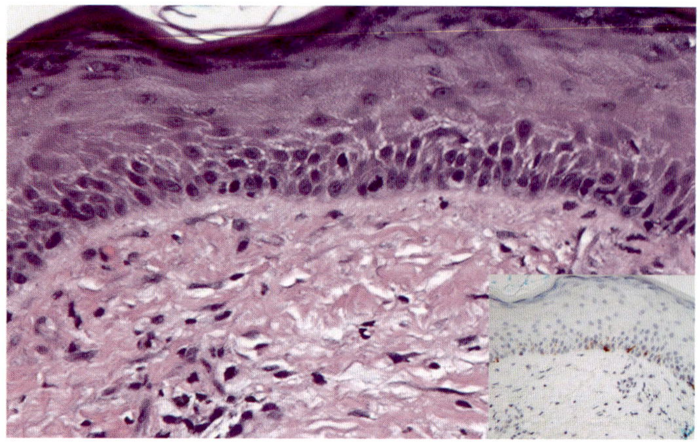

▲ **Figures 6.101, 6.102** Case 1, site 3B/5C: RCM (0.5 mm × 0.5 mm) at the level of the stratum granulosum/spinosum shows a normal honeycomb architecture. Histopathology (20×) with corresponding Melan-A immunohistochemical stain (inset) from a normal uninvolved area.

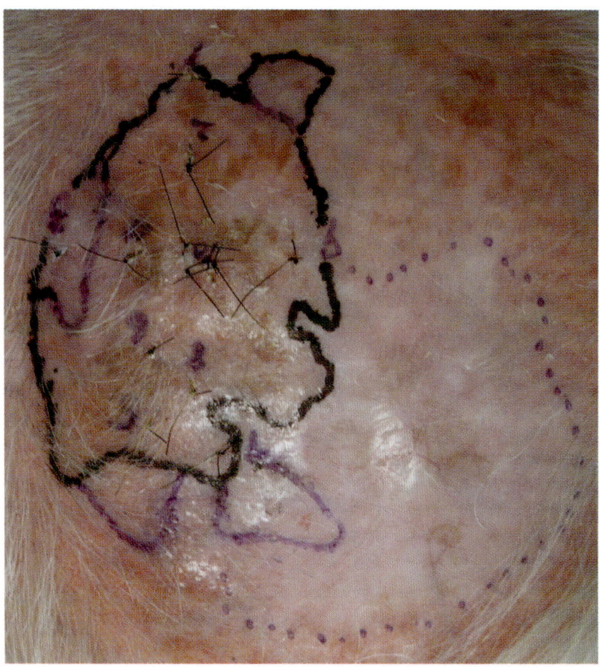

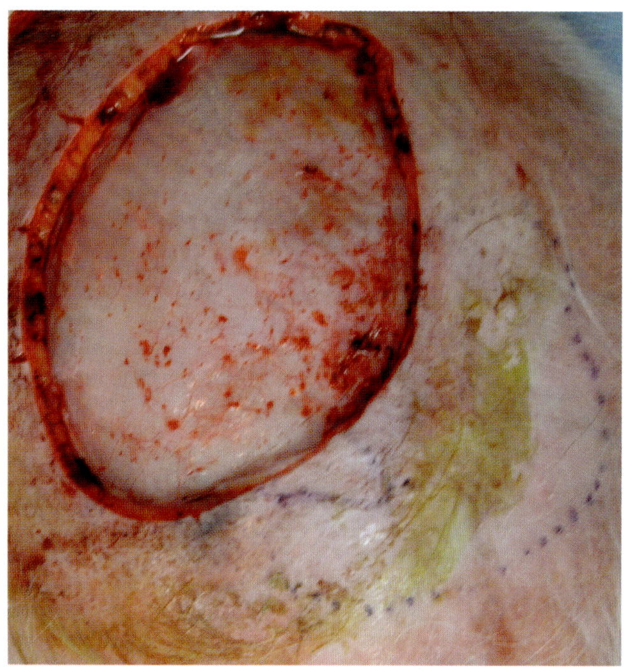

▲ **Figures 6.103, 6.104** Case 1: the final refined margin was based on the confocal findings and the results of the paired 4 mm punch biopsies, taken from within and outside the in-vivo RCM determined border for the purpose of histologic confirmation. The final excision margin was adequate and clear of melanoma.

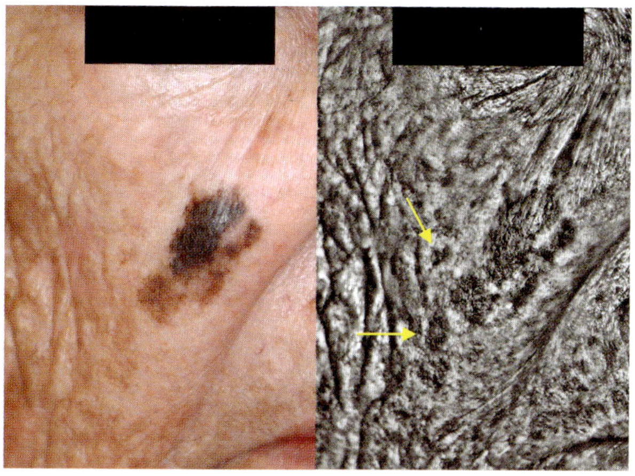

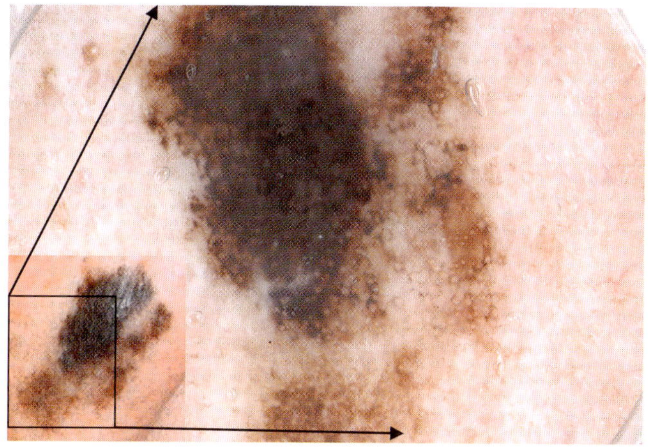

▲ **Figures 6.105, 6.106** Case 2: this irregular pigmented lesion on the cheek of a 90-year-old woman on Wood's light examination shows two additional areas of pigmentation (yellow arrows) beyond the clinically visualized lesional border. Dermoscopy revealed a central blotch, blueish veil with annular granular areas, and rhomboidal structures at the periphery.

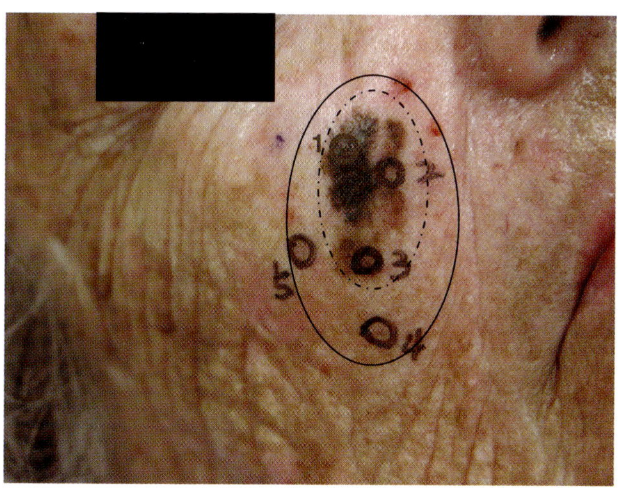

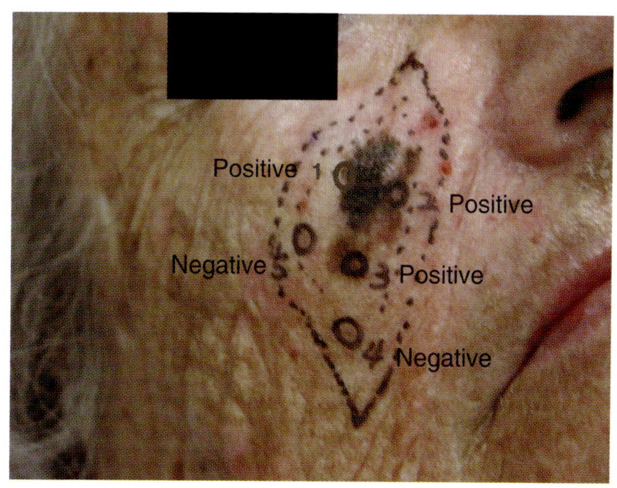

▲ **Figures 6.107, 6.108** Case 2: multiple foci were selected for confocal examination, as described in the text above. Left: the dotted oval line represents the border of the melanoma based upon clinical and dermoscopic examination and the solid oval line represents the refined border based upon the Wood's lamp examination. Right: the dotted outer-most inked line represents the refined margin based on confocal examination.

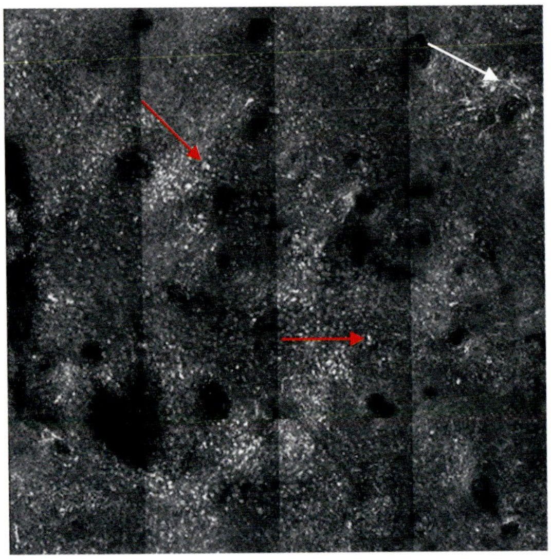

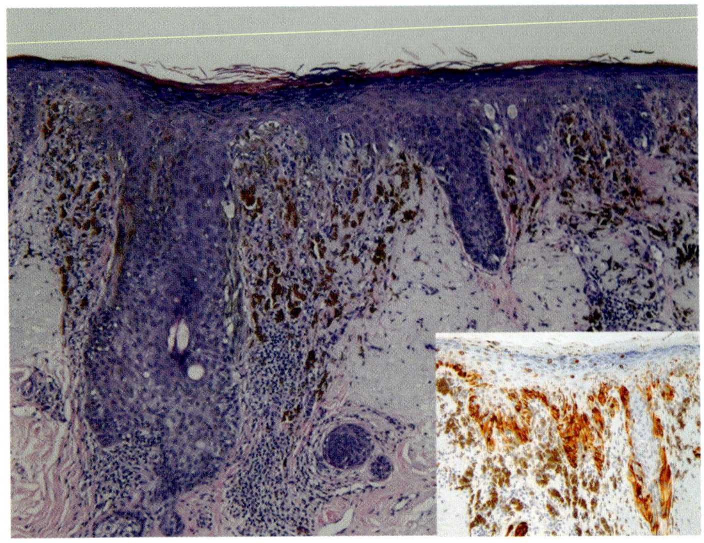

▲ **Figures 6.109, 6.110** Case 2, site 1: RCM mosaic (2 mm × 2 mm) at the level of the lower stratum spinosum/superficial stratum basalis reveals a cobblestone pattern, which is somewhat disrupted by refractile particles and elongated dendritic structures, many of which are located around hair follicles. A few atypical refractile nucleated polygonal (red arrows) and dendritic cells (white arrow) are seen. Corresponding histopathology (10×) shows focally invasive malignant melanoma. Melan-A immunohistochemical stain (10×, inset) highlights the full-thickness upward scatter of melanocytes as well as the extension down adnexal epithelium and focal dermal invasion.

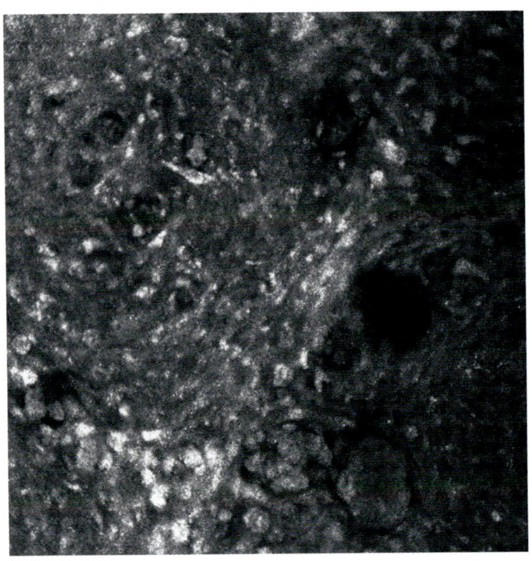

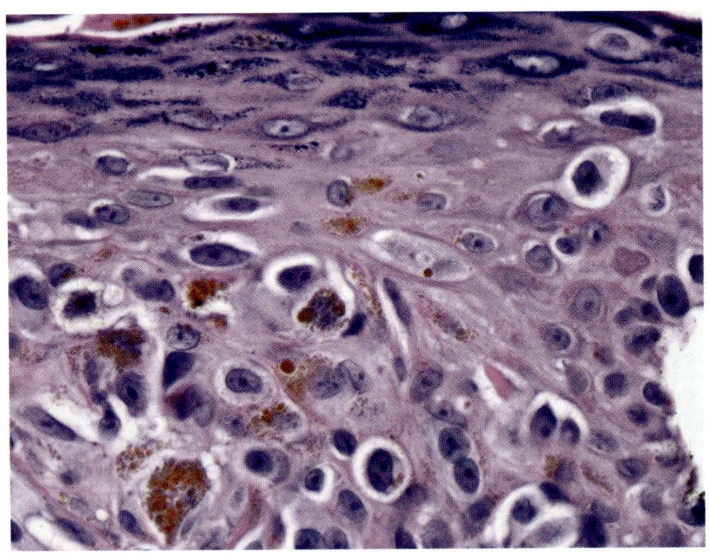

▲ **Figures 6.111, 6.112** Case 2, site 1: RCM (0.5 mm × 0.5 mm) reveals bright epithelioid and dendritic melanocytes at the suprabasal level, suggestive of melanoma. Histopathology (40×) shows the in-situ component of the melanoma, including atypical melanocytes within the stratum spinosum and granulosum. Some of the spinous keratinocytes are pigmented.

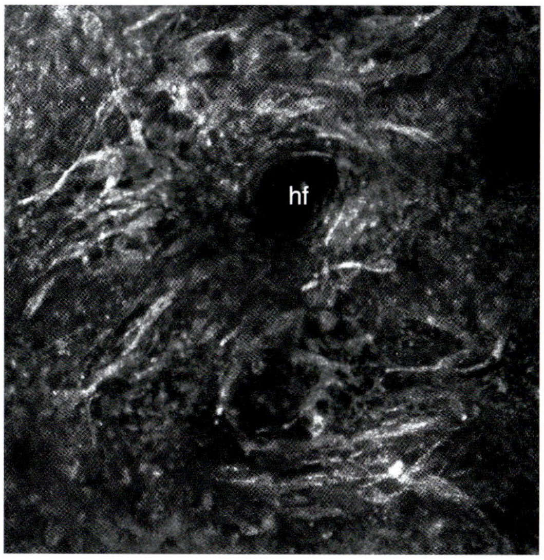

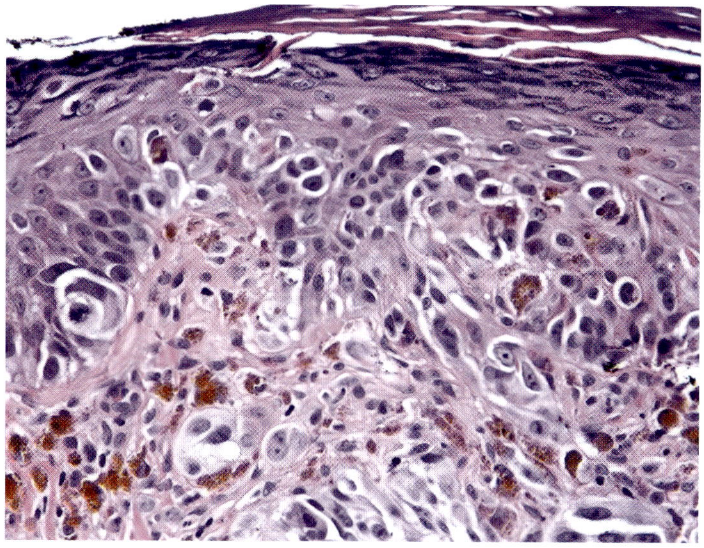

▲ **Figures 6.113, 6.114** Case 2, site 1: RCM (0.5 mm × 0.5 mm) at the level of the basal layer shows numerous atypical bright dendritic cells, dendritic structures, and refractile particles around a hair follicle (hf), compatible with melanoma. Histopathology (20×) shows in-situ and invasive melanoma.

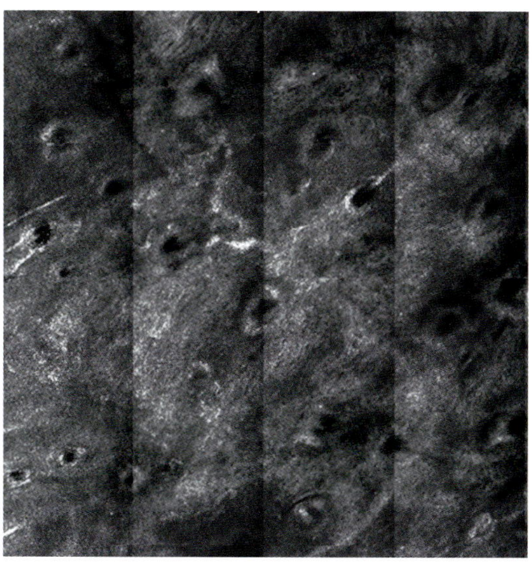

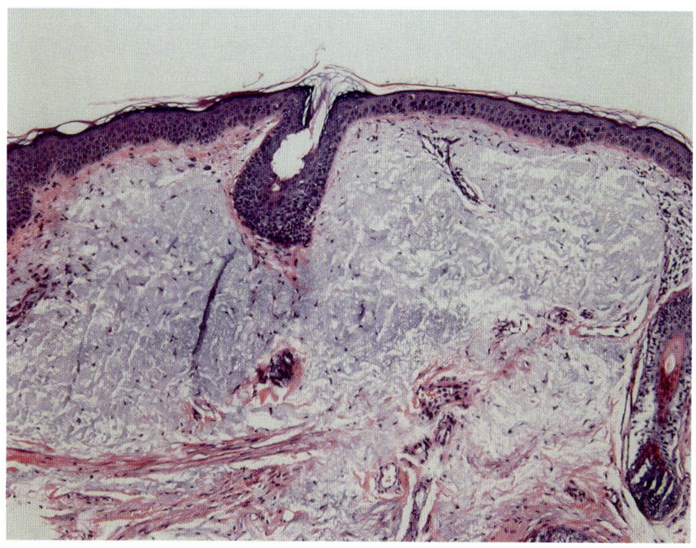

▲ **Figures 6.115, 6.116** Case 2, site 4: RCM mosaic (2 mm × 2 mm) obtained at the suprabasal level shows multiple hair follicles and normal epidermal architecture. Notably, there is no evidence of a melanocytic proliferation. Corresponding histopathology (10×) from the confocally negative (normal) area shows features of chronic actinic damage, but no melanocytic proliferation.

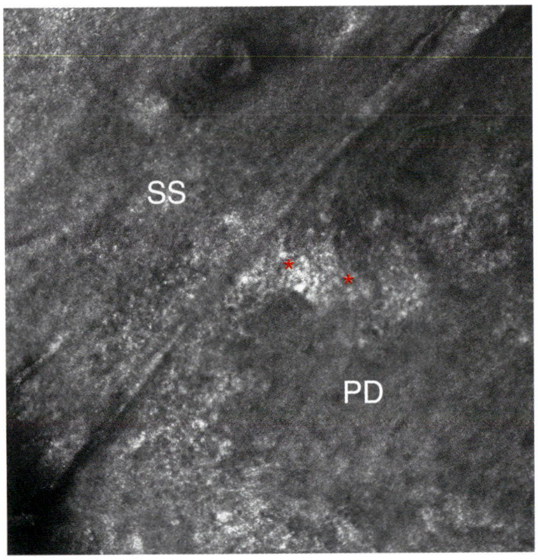

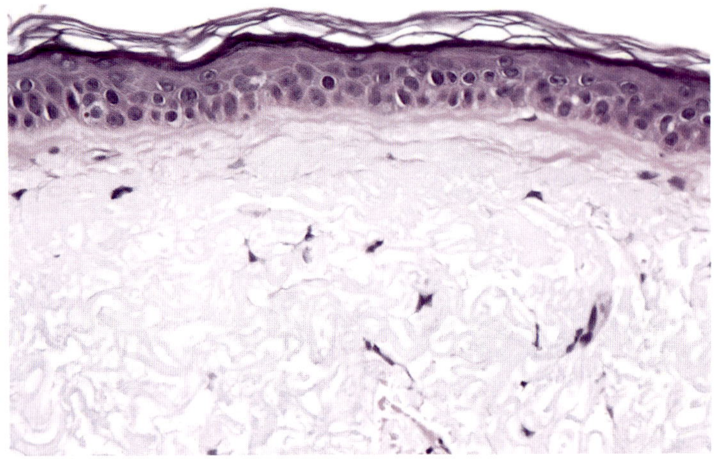

▲ **Figures 6.117, 6.118** Case 2, site 4: RCM image (0.5 mm × 0.5 mm) of DEJ in an area with flattened rete ridges allows for the simultaneous visualization of the lower stratum spinosum (SS), basal layer (asterisks), and papillary dermis (PD). Normal honeycomb pattern of the stratum spinosum, irregular pigmentation of the basal layer with slight variation in keratinocytic nuclear size, and amorphous spiral and lacy structures in the dermis are compatible with background actinic damage. Features of a melanocytic proliferation are notably absent. Histopathology (20×) shows irregular epidermal pigmentation, minimal keratinocytic atypia, and extensive solar elastosis of chronically sun-damaged skin.

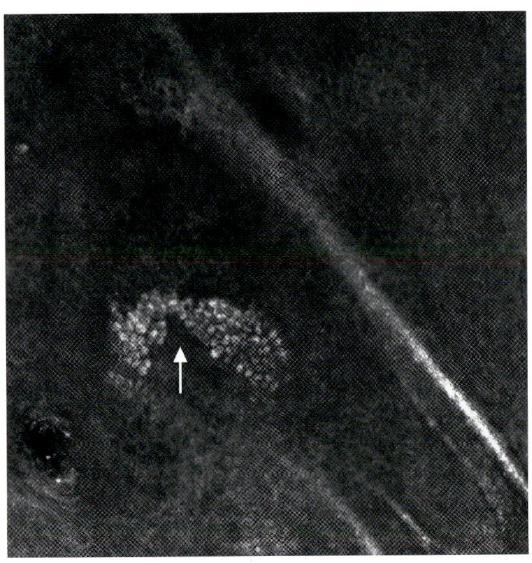

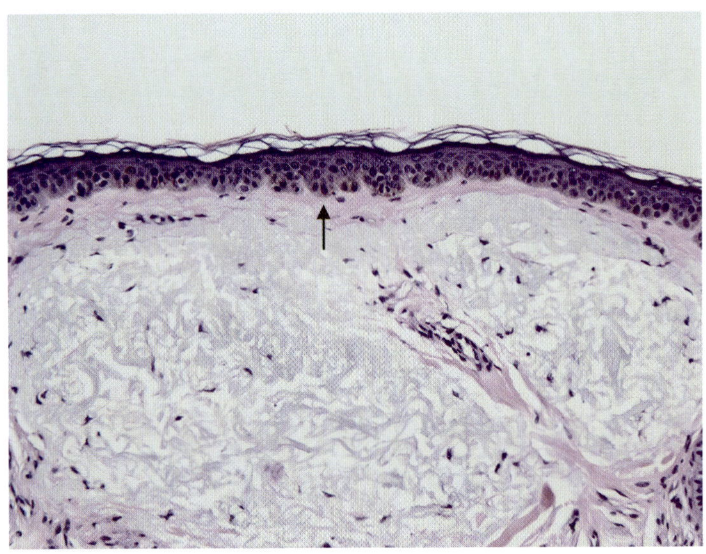

▲ **Figures 6.119, 6.120** Case 2, site 4: RCM (0.5 mm × 0.5 mm) at the level of the lower stratum spinosum reveals a normal honeycomb pattern interrupted by a small, well-demarcated area of bright cells in a carpet-like distribution showing a normal cobblestone pattern (white arrow), suggestive of lentigo. Corresponding histopathology (10×) shows focal presence of hyperpigmented rete ridges (black arrow), compatible with solar lentigo.

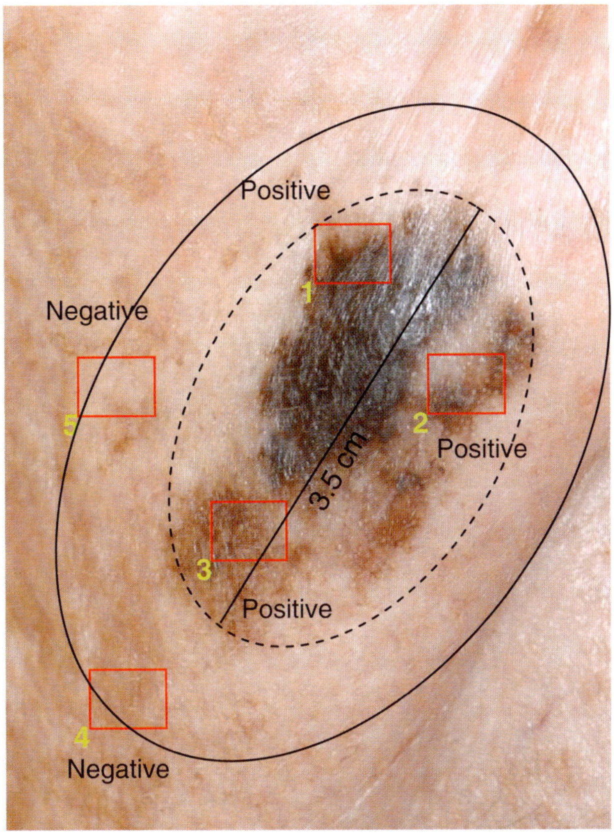

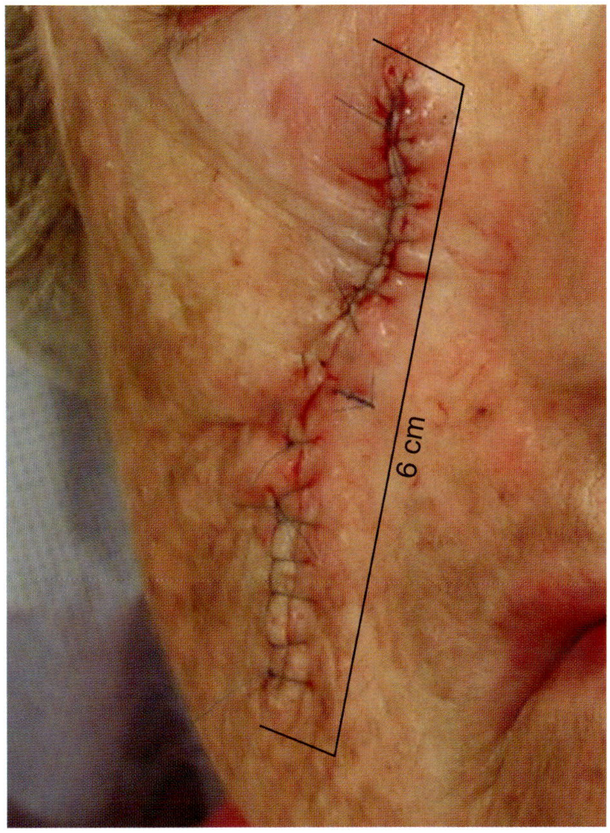

▲ **Figures 6.121, 6.122** Case 2: based on the confocal findings, which were confirmed histopathologically with punch biopsies marked 1 through 5 (red squares), the border of the lesion was redefined (dashed oval line) and the lesion's final greatest diameter was 3.5 cm. The lesion was surgically excised with a 1 cm margin of normal skin, resulting in the 6 cm long scar on the right. The excision specimen showed residual melanoma with clear and adequate margins on histopathology.

CHAPTER 6e

RCM-assisted ex-vivo margin assessment

Daniel S Gareau, Yogesh G Patel, Milind Rajadhyaksha, and Kishwer S Nehal

Potential clinical applications for reflectance confocal microscopy (RCM) include screening and diagnosis, image-guided biopsy, pre- and intraoperative mapping of tumor margins to guide surgery, and monitoring of treatment efficacy. These are applications in vivo. Other possible applications include surgical pathology ex vivo, such as detection of non-melanoma cancers in skin excisions during Mohs' surgery and detection of residual tumor in biopsies.

Mohs' micrographic surgery is a well-known procedure that uses frozen histology to guide precise excision of skin cancers. The classic indication for Mohs' surgery is non-melanoma skin cancer – i.e. basal cell carcinoma (BCC) and squamous cell carcinoma (SCC). BCCs and SCCs occur most commonly on the face, with consequent functional and cosmetic implications following treatment. Mohs' surgery has the highest cure rate as well as superior tissue conservation for primary and recurrent BCCs and SCCs, compared to any other treatment modality.[1]

The Mohs' procedure begins with excision of the tumor, followed by immediate preparation of frozen histologic sections. The surgeon examines the histologic sections for tumor in the peripheral and deep margins. If the margins are positive for tumor, another excision is performed and frozen histologic sections prepared. Excisions are performed and histologic sections prepared and examined in a repeated cycle until the last section is negative for cancer. Preparation and evaluation of frozen sections requires 20–45 minutes per excision. Furthermore, during the preparation, the patient has to wait under local anesthesia with an open wound. Typically, two and often several more excisions are required, such that the procedure typically lasts 2 hours or longer. Thus, the Mohs' procedure can be slow, tedious, and expensive. A non-invasive optical imaging modality, such as RCM, may enable rapid detection of BCCs and SCCs in fresh surgical skin excisions at the bedside during surgery and minimize the need for frozen histology. Confocal imaging may guide Mohs' surgery in real time and benefit both the patient and the surgeon.

Reflectance confocal microscopic detection of nuclei in BCC nests in Mohs' excisions is facilitated by the clinically well-known method of acetowhitening.[2,3] Topically treating (i.e. immersing or washing) a skin excision in 5% acetic acid for 30 seconds causes compaction of chromatin, which increases light backscatter, making nuclei appear bright on RCM (Figures 6.123, 6.124). Acetowhitening strongly enhances the brightness, contrast, and detectability of nuclei in BCC nests relative to the surrounding dermis (Figures 6.125, 6.126). The use of acetic acid as an exogenous contrast agent to 'optically stain' nuclei may be considered analogous to the staining with hematoxylin and eosin (H&E) of frozen sections.

Reflectance confocal microscopy typically provides a field-of-view of 0.5–0.2 mm, with a magnification of 40–100× and a resolution of 0.1–1.0 μm. However, Mohs' surgical excisions are much larger, typically 5–20 mm in size. The Mohs' surgeon usually examines the histology of the entire excision at low magnification, typically 2×, and with low resolution of 4 μm. To create such a large field-of-view on RCM, a two-dimensional sequence of images is captured and stitched together using software into a seamless composite mosaic. For example, with a 30× objective lens, up to 35 × 35 images may be stitched into a mosaic that displays a field-of-view of 15 mm × 15 mm.[4] This field-of-view is approximately equivalent to that seen with 2× magnification on light microscopy. With dense crowding of the acetowhitened nuclei, aggregates of nodular and micronodular BCC are easily distinguished from the darker dermis on ex-vivo RCM mosaics (Figure 6.127), which correspond well to frozen histology (Figure 6.128). RCM submosaics (Figure 6.129) allow for closer inspection at higher magnification of the morphologic features which define BCC, with comparable clarity to that of frozen histology (Figure 6.130). Unlike BCCs, however, SCCs may be subtle on ex-vivo RCM mosaics (Figure 6.131), requiring interrogation of submosaics at higher magnifications of 4–10× (Figure 6.132). The corresponding histology is also shown (Figure 6.133).

Presently, preparing an ex-vivo RCM mosaic requires 5–9 minutes, depending on the size of the surgical excision. Faster mosaicing within 3–5 minutes is anticipated with further advances in confocal and tissue mounting instrumentation. In addition to speed, other advantages include evaluation of *true* tumor margins directly in fresh surgical excisions (rather than trimmed margins from a frozen section block), more conservation of tissue, and absence of wrinkling and freezing artifacts.

The acetowhitening method with RCM uses only reflectance contrast and currently enables rapid detection of superficial, large nodular and small micronodular BCCs.[5] However, tiny nests or thin strands of infiltrative and sclerosing BCCs are not easily detected. These nests or strands consist of very few cells and therefore tend to remain obscured within the surrounding bright dermis. Preliminary results suggest that SCCs, too, may be difficult to detect using ex-vivo RCM with acetowhitening. This may be due to the strongly bright appearance of keratinized cytoplasm in SCCs such that the acetowhitened bright nuclei lack relative contrast and detectability. Consequently, similar to the use of two or more stains in histology, multiple optical stains or modes of contrast may be necessary. Several multimodal methods of contrast are being developed, using combinations of fluorescence and fluorescence anisotropy,[6,7] fluorescence and autofluorescence,[8,9] autofluorescence and second harmonics,[10] Raman scattering[11] and fluorescence spectroscopy,[12] and near-infrared reflectance spectroscopy.[13] Such multimodal methods may enable rapid detection of all BCCs, including infiltrative and sclerosing types, as well as SCCs with high sensitivity and specificity.

Beyond Mohs' surgery of skin cancers, such methods of ex-vivo confocal mosaicing with the use of contrast agents may enable rapid surgical pathology at the bedside, reducing the need for frozen histology in other settings. Examples include the evaluation of thyroid nodules and parathyroid glands in head and neck excisions, breast tissue from needle-core biopsies and lumpectomies, and biopsies from liver, bladder, and other tissues. Additionally, ex-vivo RCM may enable intraoperative evaluation of tissue that is difficult or impossible to section using frozen rather than formalin-fixation techniques, such as fatty tissue and bone, respectively.

Key features of RCM-assisted margin assessment

- Ex vivo RCM allows for detection of BCC and SCC in surgical excision margins without the need for frozen section histology.
- Pre-imaging tissue immersion in acetic acid enhances rapid detection of BCC.
- Ex vivo RCM evaluates true tumor margins (rather than trimmed) resulting in maximal conservation normal skin.
- Ex vivo RCM shows promise for future applications, such as confirmation of biopsy adequacy and intraoperative pathological consultation on tissue that is not amenable to frozen sectioning.

REFERENCES

1. Rowe DE, Carroll RJ, Day CL Jr. Long-term recurrence rates in previously untreated (primary) basal cell carcinoma: implications for patient follow-up. J Dermatol Surg Oncol 1989; 15:315–28.

2. Rajadhyaksha M, Menaker G, Flotte T et al. Confocal examination of nonmelanoma cancers in thick skin excisions to potentially guide Mohs micrographic surgery without frozen histopathology. J Invest Dermatol 2001; 117:1137–43.

3. Rajadhyaksha M, Menaker G, Dwyer PJ. Confocal cross-polarized imaging of skin cancers to potentially guide Mohs micrographic surgery. Optics Photonics News 2001; 12:30.

4. Patel YG, Nehal KS, Aranda I et al. Confocal reflectance mosaicing of basal cell carcinomas in Mohs surgical skin excisions. J Biomed Opt 2007; 12(3):034027.

5. Chung VQ, Dwyer PJ, Nehal KS et al. Use of ex vivo confocal scanning laser microscopy during Mohs surgery for nonmelanoma skin cancers. Dermatol Surg 2004; 30:1470–8.

6. Yaroslavsky AN, Barbosa J, Neel V et al. Combining multispectral polarized light imaging and confocal microscopy for localization of nonmelanoma skin cancer. J Biomed Opti 2005; 10:14011.

7. Yaroslavsky AN, Neel V, Anderson RR. Fluorescence polarization imaging for delineating nonmelanoma skin cancers. Opt Lett 2004; 29:2010–2.

8. Wennberg AM, Gudmundson F, Stenquist B et al. In vivo detection of basal cell carcinoma using imaging spectroscopy. Acta Derm Venereol 1999; 79:54–61.

9. Stenquist B, Ericson MB, Strandeberg C et al. Bispectral fluorescence imaging of aggressive basal cell carcinoma combined with histopathological mapping: a preliminary study indicating a possible adjunct to Mohs micrographic surgery. Br J Dermatol 2006; 154:305–9.

10. Lin SJ, Jee SH, Kuo CJ et al. Discrimination of basal cell carcinoma from normal dermal stroma by quantitative multiphoton imaging. Opt Lett 2006; 31:2756–8.

11. Nijssen A, Bakker Schut TC, Heule F et al. Discriminating basal cell carcinoma from its surrounding tissue by Raman spectroscopy. J Invest Dermatol 2002; 119:64–9.

12. Brancaleon L, Durkin AJ, Tu JH et al. In vivo fluorescence spectroscopy of nonmelanoma skin cancer. Photochem Photobiol 2001; 73:178–83.

13. McIntosh LM, Jackson M, Mantsch HH et al. Infrared spectra of basal cell carcinomas are distinct from non-tumor-bearing skin components. J Invest Dermatol 1999; 112:951–6.

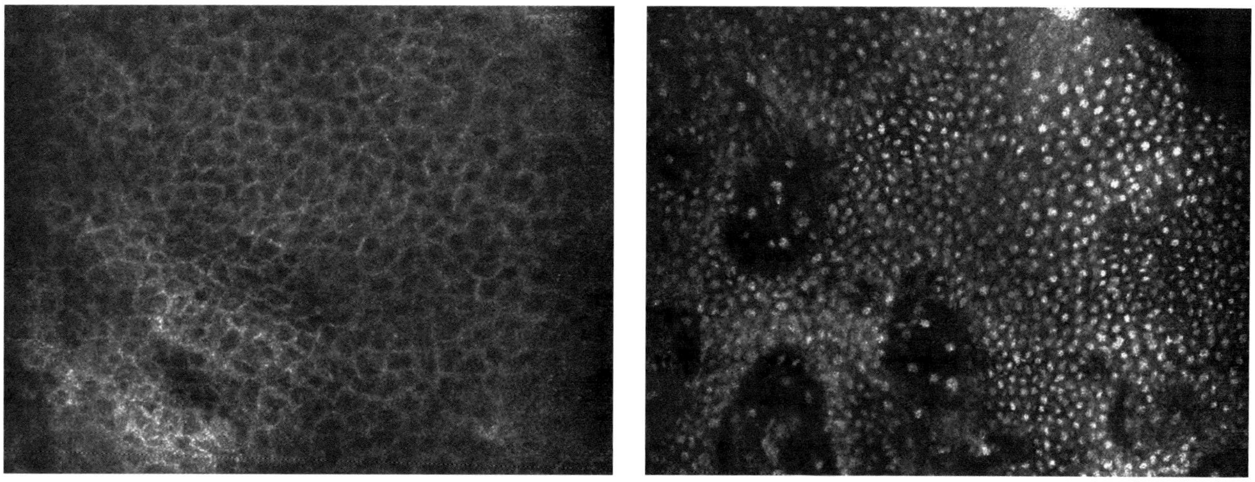

▲ **Figures 6.123, 6.124** RCM images (0.5 mm × 0.375 mm) of normal epidermis before (left) and after (right) acetowhitening. Chromatin compaction brightens nuclei, inverting nuclear contrast from dark to bright.

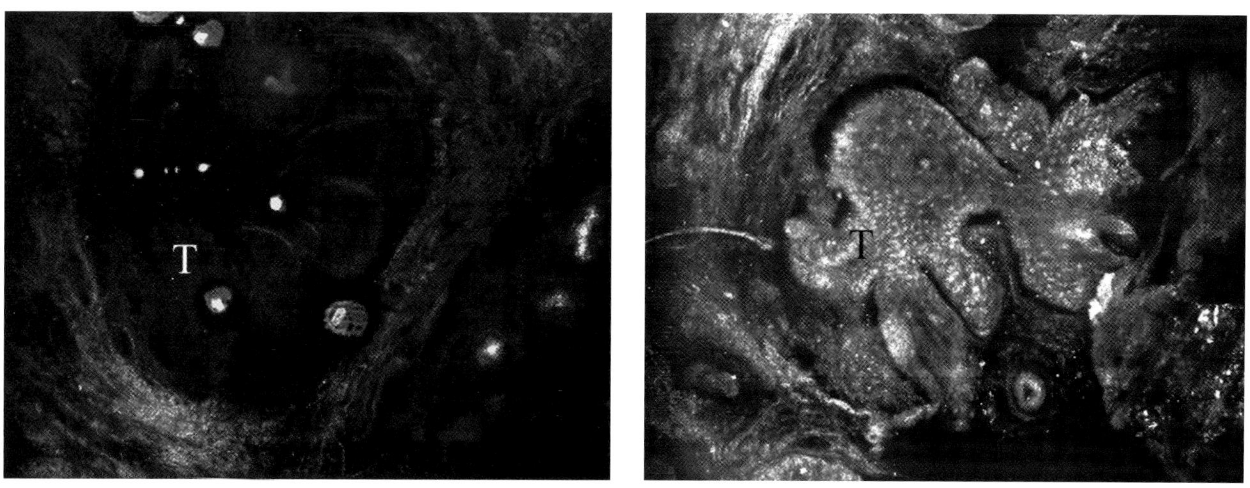

▲ **Figures 6.125, 6.126** RCM images (0.5 mm × 0.375 mm) of BCC tumor nest (T) before (left) and after (right) acetowhitening. After acetowhitening, the tumor has increased brightness and contrast with respect to the surrounding dermis.

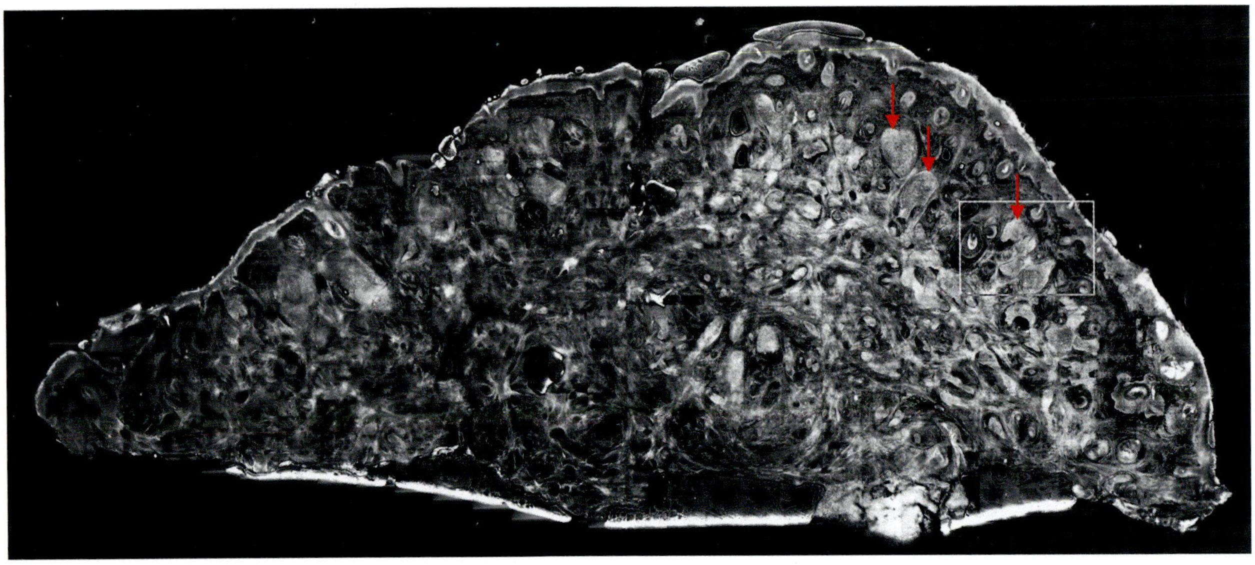

▲ **Figure 6.127** RCM mosaic (15 mm × 7 mm) of a Mohs' surgical skin excision, showing micronodular and nodular BCC at the approximate equivalence of 2× magnification. Nests of BCC (red arrows) are seen, along with normal skin landmarks, such as epidermis along the superior border, hair follicles, and dermis. The area in the white box corresponds to the submosaic shown in Figure 6.129.

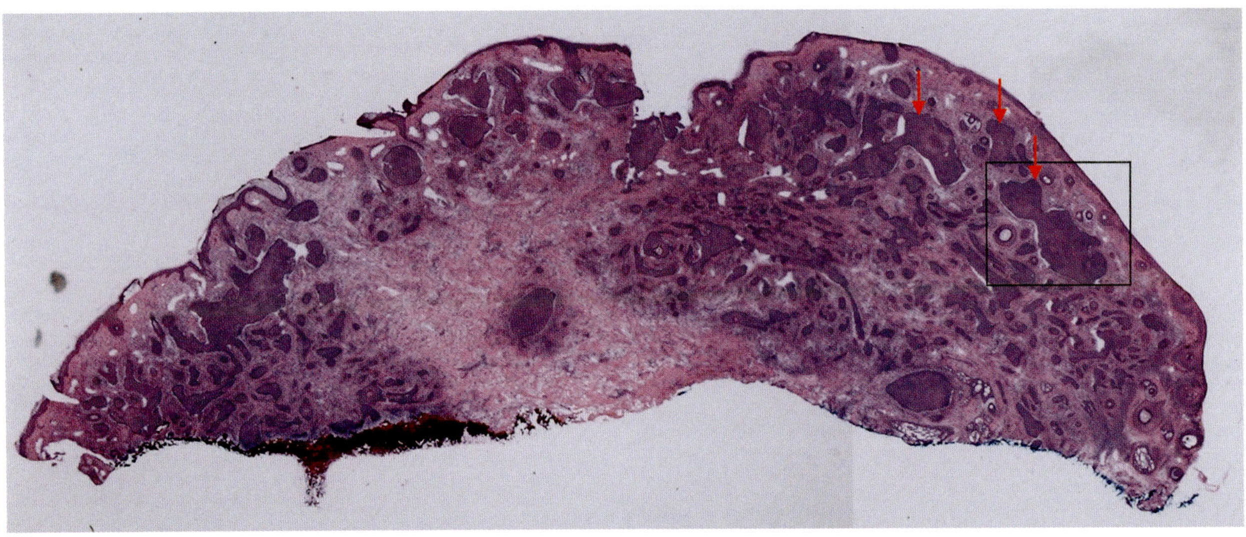

▲ **Figure 6.128** Frozen histology (2×) corresponding to Figure 6.127 shows variably sized nests of basaloid cells throughout much of the dermis. On low power, morphologic detail in mosaics compares closely to that seen on histology. The comparison is not exact, because the confocal microscopy was performed after 3–4 sections were prepared for routine Mohs' pathology. Hence, the RCM and histology sections shown represent different levels within the tissue, separated by approximately 20 µm. The area in the black box corresponds to the high-power image shown in Figure 6.130.

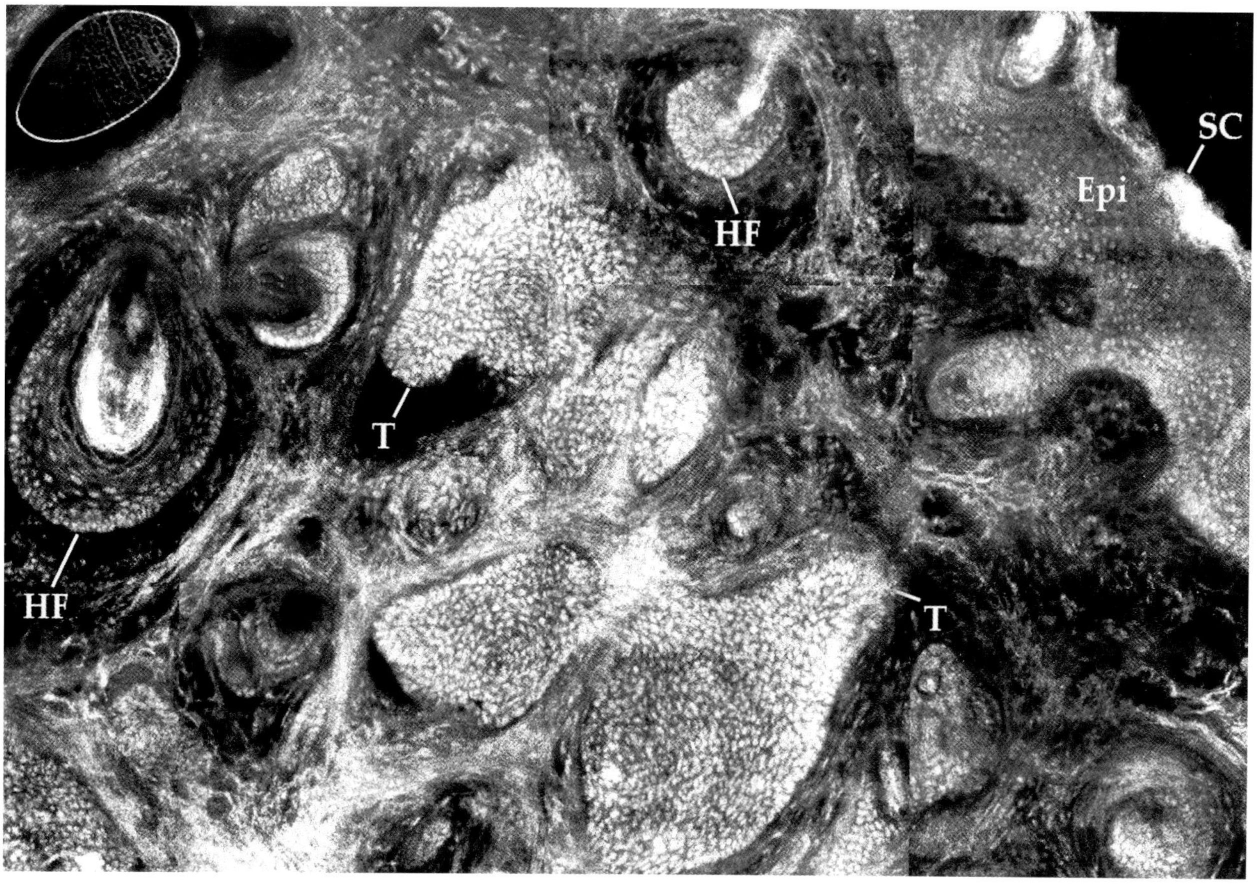

▲ **Figure 6.129** RCM submosaic (1.6 mm × 1.1 mm) from the mosaic in Figure 6.127 (box), showing a smaller area with higher magnification and higher resolution. With acetowhitening, key morphologic features of BCC (T), such as increased nuclear-to-cytoplasmic ratio (which causes the tumor nests to be very bright), elongated nuclei, polarization of nuclei, and peripheral palisading of nuclei, are easily appreciated. Normal structures, such as hair follicles (HF), epidermis (Epi), and epidermal differentiation to stratum corneum (SC), are also well visualized using this technique.

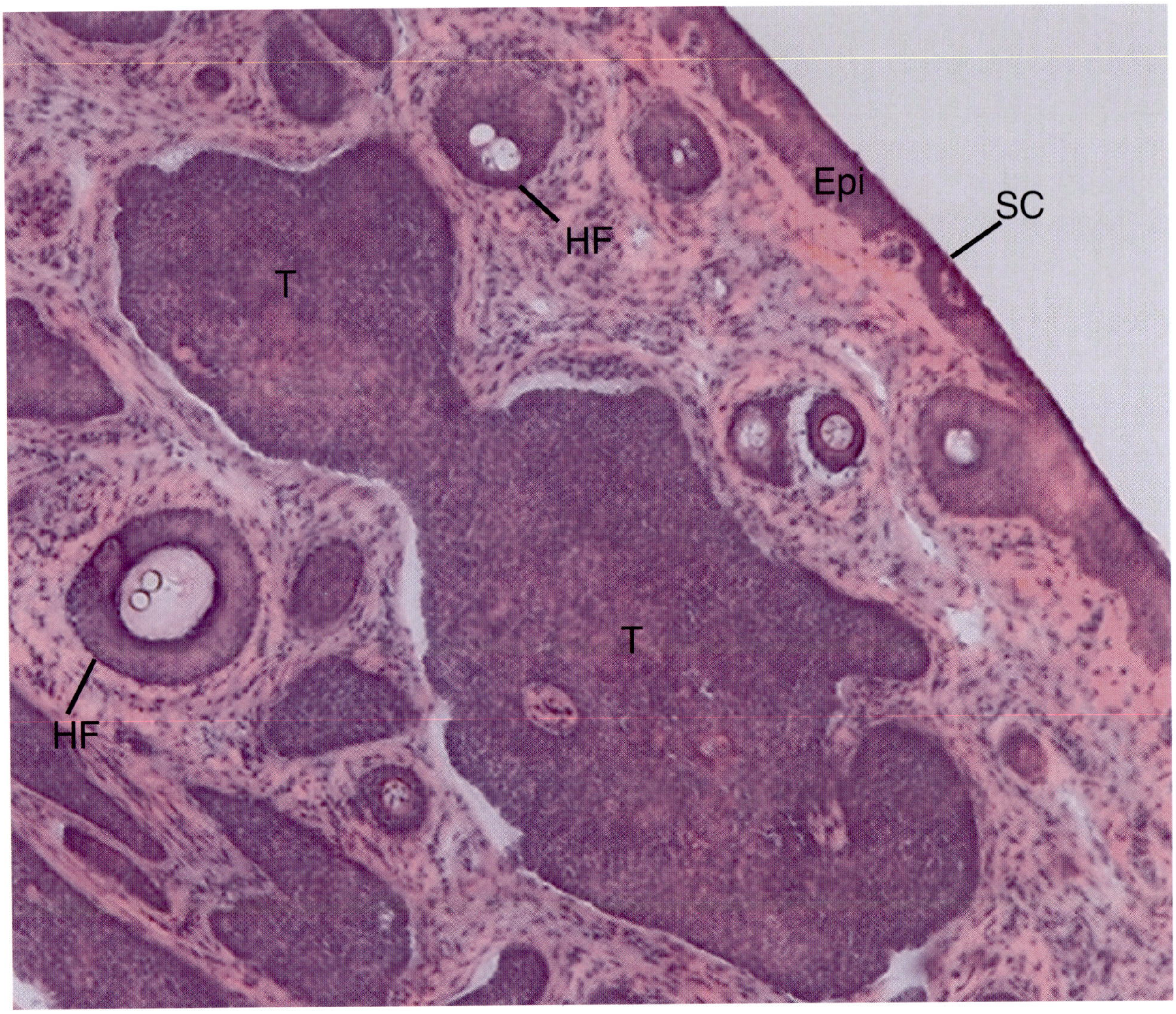

▲ **Figures 6.130** Frozen histology (10×) shows a detail of the low-power image in Figure 6.128 (box). On higher power, freeze artifact is more apparent. BCC can be detected when all features are present, but due to the artifact, less nuclear and cytoplasmic detail can be appreciated. If cut tangentially, without the hair shaft, hair follicles (HF) could be confused with tumor (T). Epidermal (Epi) differentiation to stratum corneum (SC) is less easily visualized in frozen section as compared to ex-vivo RCM (Figure 6.129).

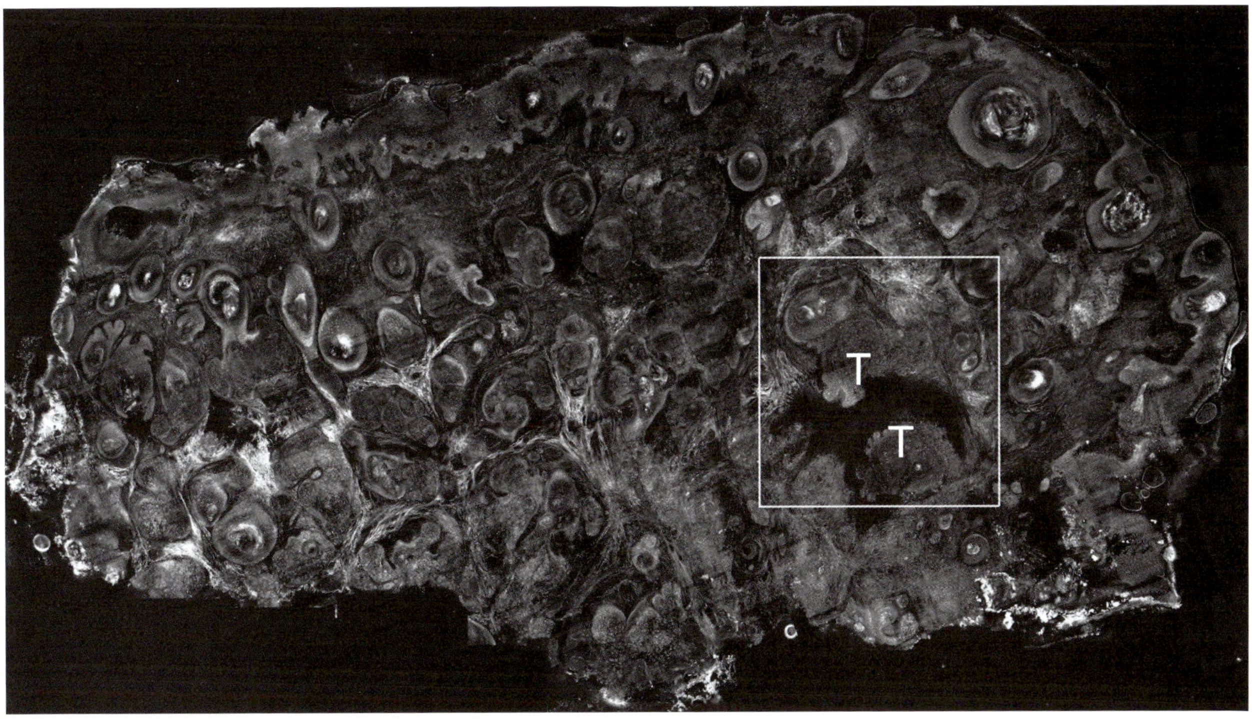

▲ **Figure 6.131** RCM mosaic (5.2 mm × 2.4 mm) of SCC. Note the tumor (T) is less easy to differentiate from surrounding structures as compared to BCC.

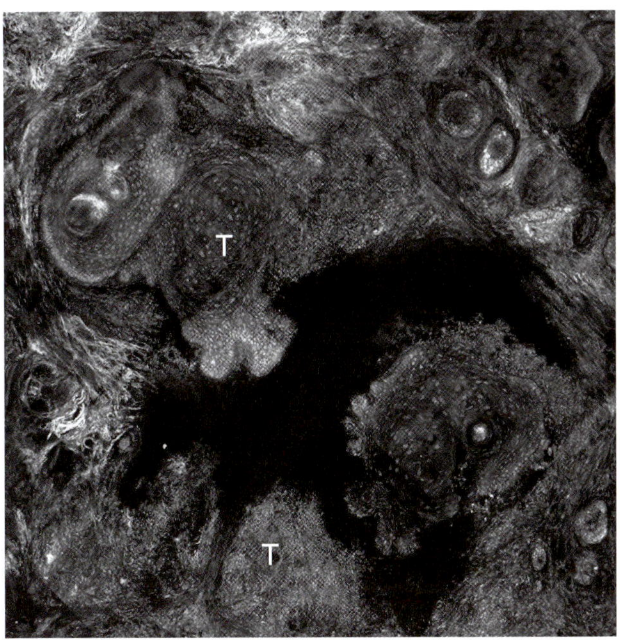

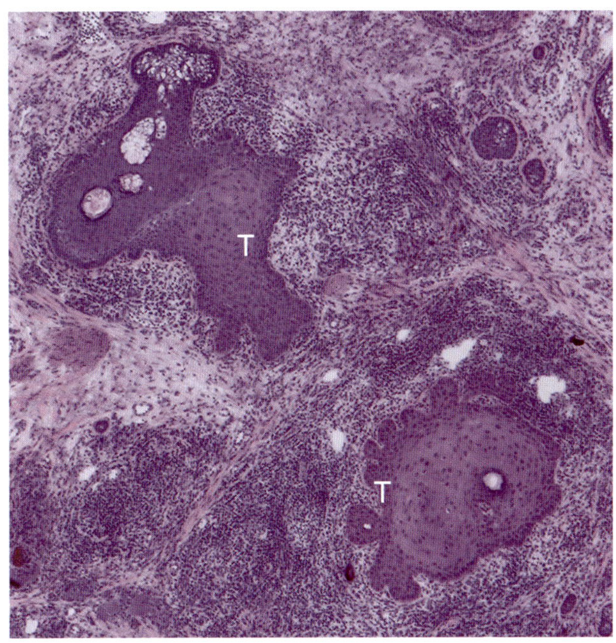

▲ **Figures 6.132, 6.133** RCM submosaic (1 mm × 1 mm) and frozen histology (10×) from boxed in area in Figure 6.131 show the SCC at higher magnification and resolution. Tumor (T) is seen extending along and budding from hair follicles. At this higher magnification, the cytologic atypia, which differentiates tumor from normal squamous epithelium, can be seen.

CHAPTER 7

Future perspectives

Salvador González, Melissa Gill, and Allan C Halpern

In this chapter, we briefly review the current state of reflectance confocal microscopy (RCM) as demonstrated pictorially in this atlas, discuss the current limitations of RCM skin imaging, and speculate on the future of RCM imaging in clinical practice.

CURRENT STATUS OF SKIN RCM IMAGING

As demonstrated throughout this atlas, RCM is an exciting new technology for in-vivo skin imaging. It is currently capable of providing quasi-histologic horizontal sections of the skin non-invasively and at the bedside in real time. In pigmented skin, the naturally occurring contrast provided by subcellular structures mainly melanosomes and melanin permits easy recognition of individual cells. Image quality is generally good and has become much more consistent over time. Most importantly, as depicted in the atlas, a growing body of knowledge has led to a rudimentary understanding of the correlation of in-vivo RCM images with histology and early clinical studies are demonstrating the utility of RCM to inform diagnosis and management of skin cancers.

There have also been significant strides made in clinical RCM instrumentation. The current generation of commercially available RCM instruments are about the size of small dental X-ray machines and can be readily applied to most anatomic sites. With the use of a tissue ring, small areas of the skin can be automatically imaged in a systemic fashion with resulting composite optical sections (mosaics) at various depths within the skin. A handheld device is available for real-time interrogation of larger areas of skin by simply gliding the instrument across the skin surface. Currently, commercially available systems typically utilize near-infrared laser light with resulting fairly consistent imaging down to the papillary dermis, but other light sources are available that have the potential to enhance resolution in the epidermis.

LIMITATIONS/CHALLENGES OF CLINICAL RCM

Although RCM is a very exciting and promising new technology, it has several inherent limitations and hurdles that need to be overcome to make it clinically useful. These limitations and challenges relate to the optical properties of the skin, the instrumentation, and the interpretation of the RCM images.

The optical properties of the skin present several challenges to RCM imaging. The stratum corneum and the dermal–epidermal junction (DEJ) both represent optical boundaries. The former can be addressed with an index-matched fluid interface and appropriate lens selection, although hyperkeratosis can still lead to image degradation. Similarly, contour irregularities of the skin surface can be addressed with varying imaging configurations. The DEJ, however, creates a greater challenge, which currently leads to reduced resolution in the dermis.

Superficial light scattering and absorption also compromise imaging beyond the epidermis. Further improvements in depth of imaging will probably entail optimization of the power and wavelength of light used as well as post-image processing (e.g. de-convoluting algorithms).

As noted above, RCM instrumentation for clinical imaging has improved dramatically in recent years. The large very expensive bench-top models commonly used in the laboratory have given way to new more compact and less-expensive machines suitable for bedside imaging. As with other early-generation medical imaging technologies, these instruments leave room for improvement. Ongoing adaptations of the technology hold significant promise for smaller, increasingly robust, and more versatile instruments. Software advances predicated on DICOM (Digital Imaging and Communications in Medicine) compatibility have permitted more intuitive and efficient image acquisition, archiving, and navigation analogous to radiologic PACS (picture archiving and communications system). The recent incorporation of macroscopic clinical and dermoscopic images into the system permits navigation of the microscopic images within a clinically relevant contextual framework. Further technical development is required to achieve these results without the restriction of the currently used adhesive tissue rings.

Image interpretation presents the last and perhaps greatest challenge to the diffusion of this technology into clinical practice. While acetic acid can be used to accentuate cellular detail in ex-vivo tissue and aluminum chloride in surgically exposed tissue, no extrinsic contrast agents have yet been developed for imaging intact skin. In the absence of selected contrast agents, many cellular elements demonstrate similar morphology on RCM (e.g. dendritic melanocytes and Langerhans cells). As demonstrated throughout the atlas, a new lexicon is evolving for the description of RCM skin morphology. Much additional work is needed to better define the RCM characteristics of normal skin at different anatomic sites and in different physiologic settings and to identify diagnostic RCM features for specific skin lesions. As in the case of routine histology, accurate RCM diagnosis will require consideration of the clinical and anatomic context, and RCM diagnosis will probably remain subjective and dependent on the expertise of the examiner.

FUTURE DIRECTIONS

Despite the aforementioned limitations, RCM imaging holds significant promise for the future. As demonstrated in this atlas, the high-resolution in-vivo and ex-vivo subsurface images provided by RCM have potential application for the diagnosis, surgical management, and assessment of response to non-invasive therapies for cutaneous neoplasms. With increasing interest in cosmetically sensitive, minimally invasive procedures and cosmetic dermatology, RCM may become an increasingly important tool. At present, even experienced dermatologists occasionally misdiagnose melanoma as lentigo and proceed with laser therapy, cryotherapy, or chemical bleaching without a confirmatory biopsy, delaying diagnosis and therapy. As more non-dermatologists begin performing these procedures, this error rate may increase. In the future, in-vivo RCM screening of lesions before empiric therapy may prevent some of these adverse outcomes. RCM imaging with sufficient resolution to resolve individual cells and scanning rates, permitting real-time assessment of blood flow, also holds significant potential for the evaluation of inflammatory skin conditions. This will probably best be achieved by combining RCM with complementary imaging modalities such as dermoscopy, high-frequency ultrasound, and optical coherence tomography.

Another exciting aspect of RCM is that it is inherently well suited to be used as a telemedicine application. As the images are acquired in digital format, images viewed at the bedside equal those viewed remotely. Furthermore, standardization and automation of image acquisition, combined with newly developed viewing software, allows remote readers to navigate through a lesion in the *x*, *y*, and *z* planes. Lesions could be interpreted live or remotely as a patient waits or stored for analysis at a later date. Difficult lesions could easily be shared instantaneously with colleagues anywhere in the world. If used in combination with available digital dermoscopy systems, RCM may improve care for patients in remote locations without ready access to dermatologic care. Likewise, ex-vivo RCM may offer intraoperative pathologic consultation to surgeons without access to frozen section pathology.

Most importantly, improvements in image processing (e.g. 3-D reconstruction) and diffusion of the technology into the hands of more investigators will probably lead to novel and heretofore unsuspected insights into RCM image interpretation for both clinical and research applications. These advances will be dramatically facilitated by the digital nature of the images which lend themselves to the establishment of large collaborative image databanks that can be made accessible to a broad scientific and clinical community. We look forward to seeing what the future will hold!

APPENDIX I

Glossary

Giovanni Pellacani, Marco Ardigo, Sara Bassoli, Caterina Longo, Stefania Seidenari, Allan C Halpern, Melissa Gill, and Salvador González

In this glossary, we have included histologic (H) and dermoscopic (D) terms used in the atlas to describe structures seen on reflectance confocal microscopy (RCM). Also, we have provided a preliminary set of definitions for RCM terms (R) used throughout the atlas. The latter terms borrow heavily on their histologic correlates. When relevant, we have included (in parenthesis) the lesions which commonly exhibit the defined feature.

Blood vessels (H): dark, tubular, oval or circular lumina containing variably refractile cells corresponding to white and red blood cells. Dynamic blood flow and leukocyte trafficking can be observed in real time or on video capture.

'Carpet-like' distribution (R): hyperrefractile small round cells with a similar architecture to the surrounding epidermis, giving the impression that a bright carpet has been placed on the epidermis (lentigo).

Cell cluster (R): clusters of refractile cells forming oval-to-roundish structures corresponding to melanocytic nests. These can be located anywhere in the epidermis or dermis, and can be seen in nevi or melanoma. Their distribution, quality, and context determine where they fall in the spectrum between benign and malignant.

According to their morphology, cell clusters are divided into different types:

- **Dense cell cluster** (R): compact aggregate with a sharp margin formed by cells with similar morphology and refractility (nevi > melanoma).
- **Dishomogeneous cell cluster** (R): aggregates formed by cells which vary in shape, size, and refractility (melanoma > nevi).
- **Loose (also called sparse) cell cluster** (R): irregularly aggregated and sparse cells, usually irregular in morphology and refractivity confined within a darker well-demarcated area (melanoma > nevi).
- **Cerebriform cell cluster** (R): confluent amorphous aggregates of low-reflecting cells exhibiting granular cytoplasm without evident nuclei and ill-defined borders with fine hyporeflective 'fissure'-like areas, creating a brain-like appearance (melanoma).

Cerebriform architecture of the epidermis (R): epidermal architecture characterized by (1) dark areas (resembling the sulci of the brain) containing variable amounts of refractile material which correspond to fissures on dermoscopy and keratin-filled surface invaginations on histology and (2) gray anastomosing ribbons (resembling the gyri of the brain) which correspond to ridges on dermoscopy and interwoven, acanthotic cords and tongues of basaloid cells on histology (seborrheic keratoses, lentigo, lentigo maligna).

Cobblestone pattern (R): small, polygonal bright cells separated by less refractile borders due to the presence of keratinocytic supranuclear melanin caps (basal layer of pigmented normal skin, some nevi, some melanomas, pigmented seborrheic keratosis, and lentigo).

Collagen, bundled (H, R): thicker, refractile bundles arranged in fascicles, seen in the reticular dermis.

Collagen, reticulated (H, R): fine refractile fibrils arranged in a reticulated web, seen in the papillary dermis.

Collarette structure (R): defined sharp lateral demarcation of the lesion seen at confocal mosaic images (clear cell acanthoma).

Cornoid lamellae (H): parakeratosis and disruption of stratum corneum at the site of cornoid lamella, better seen in superficial mosaics of RCM images (porokeratosis).

Crown vessels (D): vascular structures surrounding the sebaceous gland in the dermis, similar to the feature seen on dermoscopy (sebaceous hyperplasia).

Dermal papillary ring (R): rimming of dermal papillae by a monolayer of uniform refractile cells at the level of the DEJ due to the presence of physiologic melanin in basal keratinocytes.

Disarranged pattern (R): disarray of the normal honeycomb or cobblestone pattern of the epidermis (mycosis fungoides, basal cell carcinoma, actinic keratosis). This pattern may be associated with unevenly distributed bright granular particles and cells (melanocytic tumors).

Edged papilla (R): highly bright dermal papillary ring rimming dermal papilla at the level of the DEJ due to an increased number of melanocytes and pigmented keratinocytes (nevi > melanoma).

Elongated monomorphic nuclei (R): tight aggregates of cells with elongated, monomorphic dark nuclei and minimal cytoplasm (basal cell carcinoma).

Glomeruloid vessels (D, R): prominent vessels with glomeruloid-like features, following serpiginous lines, visible at the level of the upper dermis (clear cell acanthoma).

Honeycomb pattern (R): the normal appearance of stratum granulosum and spinosum composed of 15–35 μm polygonal cells with dark nuclei and bright and thin cytoplasm.

Horn cyst (H, R): round, black space filled with brightly refractile material visible within a tumor island and corresponding to a horn cyst on histology (trichoepithelioma).

Hyporefractile dermal papillary rings (R): decreased refractility of the epidermal basal layer as compared to non-lesional skin, probably due to leukocyte permeation of the basal layer (mycosis fungoides).

Junctional thickenings/expansion (R): enlargement of the rete ridges (interpapillary space) formed by aggregated cells. This feature corresponds to confluence of junctional melanocytic aggregates on histology (melanoma, nevi).

Keratin-filled cystic inclusions (D, H, R): well-defined, round, whorled collections of brightly refractile material surrounded by cords of keratinocytes corresponding to comedo-like openings and milia-like cysts on dermoscopy, and to horn pseudocysts on histology (seborrheic keratosis).

Keratinocytic atypia (H): enlarged, pleomorphic keratinocytic nuclei with haphazard orientation, contrasting with small, uniform, evenly spaced nuclei from normal skin (actinic keratosis, squamous cell carcinoma, basal cell carcinoma).

Non-edged papilla (R): dermal papilla without a demarcated rim of bright cells, but separated by a series of large reflecting cells, corresponding to a disarrangement of the rete ridges by a 'disorderly' proliferation of melanocytes not confined to the sides and tips of rete ridges (melanoma > nevi).

Nuclear peripheral palisading (H, R): a peripheral row of tumor cells containing elongated monomorphic nuclei arranged in parallel to one another and perpendicular to the edge of the tumor aggregate (basal cell carcinoma, trichoepithelioma).

Nuclear polarization (R): elongated monomorphic nuclei polarized along the same axis. This may be manifested as **nuclear peripheral palisading** or **nuclear streaming** (basal cell carcinoma).

Nuclear streaming (R): aggregates of cells with elongated monomorphic nuclei, all oriented along the same axis (basal cell carcinoma).

Onion skin-like stroma (H, R): fibrotic stroma that concentrically encases tumor islands in parallel bands creating an 'onion skin' appearance (trichoepithelioma).

'Pagetoid' cells (H, R): roundish or dendritic nucleated cells, often about twice the size of keratinocytes, with a dark nucleus and bright cytoplasm above the basal layer. Cell size, pleomorphism, cell density, and distribution throughout the lesion can be evaluated (melanoma > nevi).

Parakeratotic cells (H): hyperrefractile round-to-oval cellular structures located at the level of the stratum corneum, some with visible central dark nuclei (porokeratosis, actinic keratosis, squamous cell carcinoma).

Pautrier's microabscesses (H): well-defined, round, vesicle- and microvesicle-like dark spaces filled with weakly refractile round cells, which can be seen at all levels of the epidermis on RCM mosaics (mycosis fungoides).

Peritumoral cleft-like dark spaces (R): cleft-like non-reflective dark spaces present at the periphery of tumor aggregates (basal cell carcinoma).

Polymorphous, crowded, hyperrefractile dermal papillary rings (R): round, oval, annular-to-irregular polycyclic-shaped dermal papillae surrounded by a bright uniform monolayer of cells (lentigo).

Sheet-like cell distribution (H, R): cells seen at the transition from epidermis to dermis which are not aggregated in clusters but closely distributed in the same plane. Dermal papillae are not distinguishable due to loss of the normal rete ridge pattern. The cells are refractile, often monomorphic and roundish or spindled in shape (melanoma).

Swiss-cheese-like architecture (R): multiple black vascular lumina with variably refractile walls that are organized into lobules separated by stromal septa (angioma).

Tethering of dermal papillary rings (R): presence of sclerotic collagen bundles just below the DEJ which appear connected to highly bright dermal papillary rings and give the impression that they are pulling on the rete (dermatofibroma).

Trabeculae, cord-like structures, tumor islands (H): distinct aggregates of tightly packed cells, forming trabeculae or cord-like structures and nodules (epithelial tumors).

APPENDIX 2

Key RCM features: a quick reference

Basic principals of reflectance confocal microscopy

Table 1.1 Typical parameters of confocal microscopy compared to routine histology

Parameter	*Confocal*	*Histology*
Wavelength	Selectable, 400–1064 nm	Broadband white light, 400–700 nm
Maximum imaging depth	50–100 μm at 488 nm	–
	150–250 μm at 830 nm	
	300–400 μm at 1064 nm	
Section thickness	1–5 μm	5 μm
	Noninvasive, optical	Physical
Lateral resolution	0.1–1 μm	0.1–4 μm
Numerical aperture	0.7–1.4	0.1–1.4
Immersion media	Water or oil immersion	Air or oil immersion
Magnification	40–100×	1–100×
Field of view	0.5–0.2 mm	20–0.2 mm
Pinhole size	50–500 μm	–
Contrast mechanism	Endogenous reflective microstructures	Exogenous absorbing dyes
Contrast agents/stains	Melanin	Hematoxylin and eosin
	Keratin	Methylene blue
	Collagen	Toluidine blue

Normal skin

Table 2.1 Depth of normal skin structures on RCM

Structure	*Depth*	*Mean keratinocyte width*
Stratum corneum	0–15 μm	25–50 μm
Stratum granulosum	10–20 μm	25–35 μm
Stratum spinosum	20–100 μm	15–25 μm
Stratum basalis	40–130 μm	7–12 μm
Papillary dermis	50–150 μm	–
Reticular dermis	>150 μm	–

Table 2.2 Refractile structures in decreasing brightness

High refractility	Bright
Melanin-containing cells	
Melanocyte cytoplasm	
Melanophage cytoplasm	
Pigmented keratinocyte cytoplasm	
Keratin-containing structures	
Stratum corneum	
Infundibular epithelium	
Hair shaft	
Acrosyringium	
Activated Langerhans cell cytoplasm	
Granulocyte (WBC) cytoplasm	
Medium refractility	
Spinous keratinocyte cytoplasm	
Sebocyte cytoplasm	
Keratohyaline granules	
Nucleoli	
Collagen	
Low refractility	
Red blood cells	
Lymphocytes	
Skin folds (very low)	
Nuclei (very low)	
No refractility	
Air	
Serum	Dark

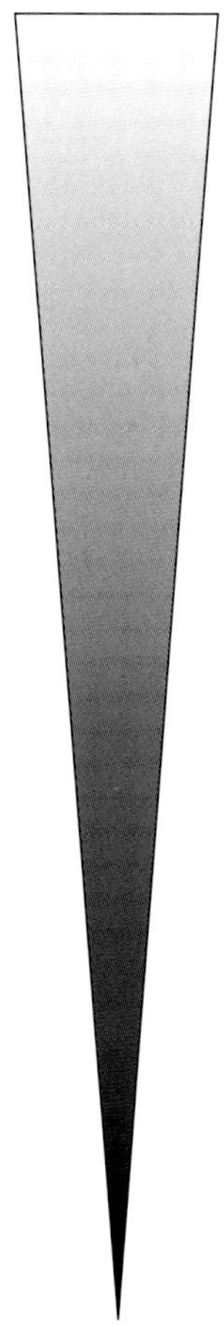

Key RCM features of normal skin

- Stratum corneum: highly refractile and granular
- Stratum granulosum: regular honeycomb pattern formed by polygonal cells with moderately refractile granular cytoplasm and dark central nuclei
- Stratum spinosum: regular honeycomb pattern formed by smaller polygonal cells with moderately refractile cytoplasm and dark central nuclei
- Stratum basalis (skin phototypes II–VI): bright supranuclear melanin caps form a regular cobblestone pattern
- Stratum basalis (skin phototype I): poorly pigmented basal cells are difficult to distinguish from surrounding cells
- Dermal–epidermal junction (skin phototypes II–VI): bright basal cells with dark basal nuclei form rings around dark central dermal papillae or bright dermal papillary rings
- Dermal–epidermal junction (skin phototype I): weakly refractile basal cells form rings around relatively brighter central dermal papillae or dark dermal papillary rings
- Dermis: moderately refractile collagen bundles and blood vessels with dark lumina containing bright granulocytes and weakly refractile erythrocytes

Seborrheic keratosis

Key RCM features of seborrheic keratosis

- Cerebriform architecture of the epidermis
- Keratin-filled cystic inclusions
- Plump, bright round or polygonal cells in the upper dermis (melanophages)
- Bright cobblestone pattern of stratum spinosum (pigmented SK)

Clear cell acanthoma

Key RCM features of clear cell acanthoma

- Sharp lateral circumscription
- Often surrounded by collarette of refractile scale
- Glomeruloid vessels expanding the dermal papillae

Porokeratosis

Key RCM features of disseminated superficial actinic porokeratosis

- Cornoid lamella at the periphery
- Sharp demarcation from surrounding skin
- Mild superficial disruption of the stratum corneum with focal parakeratosis
- Pleomorphism of the granular/spinous layer
- Architectural disarray of the epidermis

Squamous neoplasia

Key RCM features of actinic keratosis

- Superficial disruption of the stratum corneum with detached corneocytes and parakeratosis
- Pleomorphism of the epidermis
- Architectural disarray of the epidermis

Key RCM features of squamous cell carcinoma

- Superficial disruption of the stratum corneum
- Pleomorphic parakeratosis
- Severe atypical pleomorphism of the epidermis
- Severe architectural disarray of the epidermis
- Atypical aggregates of keratinocytes in the dermis (if light penetration possible)

Basal cell carcinoma

Key RCM features of BCC

- Elongated monomorphic nuclei
- Polarization of elongated nuclei along the same axis of orientation:
  - Streaming: polarization of nuclei in an entire aggregate of tumor cells
  - Peripheral palisading of nuclei: peripheral monolayer of tumor cells oriented parallel to each other and perpendicular to the stroma
- Prominent inflammatory cell infiltrate
- Increased vascularity
- Variable epidermal disarray (nucleated corneocytes, loss of the honeycomb pattern, and keratinocytic nuclear pleomorphism)

Key RCM features of nodular basal cell carcinoma

- Lobulated nodules, islands, or trabeculae of tightly packed refractile cells
- Peripheral palisading of elongated monomorphic nuclei
- Peritumoral cleft-like dark spaces
- Variably refractile stroma

Key RCM features of superficial basal cell carcinoma

- Intraepidermal or immediately subepidermal aggregates of cells with elongated monomorphic nuclei
- Streaming, or polarization of aggregated tumor cells along the same axis
- Peritumoral weakly refractile round cells
- Abundant, dilated peritumoral blood vessels with active leukocyte trafficking

Key RCM features of infiltrative basal cell carcinoma

- Dermal aggregates of cells with elongated monomorphic nuclei
- Streaming, or polarization of aggregated tumor cells along the same axis
- Jagged or poorly defined tumor aggregate borders
- Abundant, dilated peritumoral blood vessels with active leukocyte trafficking
- Peritumoral weakly refractile round cells
- Architectural disarray of the epidermis

Key RCM features of pigmented BCC

- Brightly refractile nucleated dendritic cells within tumor aggregates
- Brightly refractile dots and granular structures scattered among tumor cells
- Brightly refractile plump oval- to stellate-shaped cells in the tumoral stroma
- RCM features characteristic of the histologic architectural subtype of BCC

Lentigo

Key RCM features of lentigo

- Preserved honeycomb and cobblestone pattern of the epidermis
- Hyperrefractile dermal papillary rings composed of uniform, round cells
- Polymorphous, crowded dermal papillae
- Plump bright cells (melanophages) may be present in the dermis

Key RCM features of lentigo simplex

- Preserved honeycomb and cobblestone pattern of the epidermis
- Hyperrefractile dermal papillary rings composed of uniform, round cells
- Polymorphous, crowded dermal papillae with round, ovoid, or annular contours
- Plump bright cells (melanophages) may be present in the dermis

Key RCM features of solar lentigo

- Preserved honeycomb and cobblestone pattern of the epidermis
- Hyperrefractile dermal papillary rings composed of uniform, round cells
- Polymorphous, crowded dermal papillae with ovoid to annular or polycyclic contours
- or cerebriform architecture of the epidermis
- or well-demarcated hyperrefractile cobblestone pattern of the epidermis
- Plump bright cells (melanophages) may be present in the dermis

Key RCM features of ink spot lentigo

- Preserved honeycomb and cobblestone pattern of the epidermis
- Variable presence of brightly refractile particles/globules within the superficial epidermis
- Carpet-like distribution of uniform, small round bright cells in the lower epidermis, or a diffuse cobblestone pattern (if present, dermal papillary rings often blend into the stratum spinosum)
- Hyperrefractile dermal papillary rings composed of uniform, round cells
- Polymorphous, crowded dermal papillae with round, ovoid, annular, or polycyclic contours

Congenital and common acquired melanocytic nevi

Key RCM features of benign melanocytic nevi

- Well circumscribed and symmetrical
- Preservation of the normal honeycomb and cobblestone patterns of the epidermis
- Uniformly sized and shaped dermal papillary rings
- +/– Edged papillae
- Dense, homogeneous cell clusters, uniform in size and shape, and distributed evenly

Key RCM features of congenital melanocytic nevi

- Well circumscribed and symmetrical
- Preservation of the normal honeycomb and cobblestone patterns of the epidermis
- Uniformly sized and shaped dermal papillary rings
- +/– Edged papillae
- Dense or slightly loose, homogeneous cell clusters, uniform in size and shape, and distributed evenly
- Cell clusters or aggregates in a periadnexal and/or perivascular distribution

Key RCM features of common acquired melanocytic nevi

- Well circumscribed and symmetrical
- Preservation of the normal honeycomb and cobblestone patterns of the epidermis
- Uniformly sized and shaped dermal papillary rings
- +/– Edged papillae
- Dense, homogeneous cell clusters, uniform in size and shape, and distributed evenly
- **Lentiginous nevi:** expanded cobblestone pattern and edged papillae are typical

Dysplastic nevi

Key RCM features of dysplastic nevi

- Variable distortion of normal epidermal honeycomb and cobblestone patterns
- Slight-to-complex distortion of the DEJ architecture:
  - Variation in size and shape of dermal papillae
  - Altered contour of the rete ridges
- Junctional cell cluster disarray:
  - Variation in size, shape, and location of cell clusters
  - Enlarged, misshapen cell clusters
  - Presence of cell clusters in suprapapillary plates
- Variable cellular atypia
- Dense cell clusters predominate

Malignant melanoma

Table 4.1 RCM and histopathologic features of cutaneous melanomas

Histopathologic feature	*Correlating RCM feature*
Altered epidermal background	Disarranged Pattern: disruption of the normal honeycomb and cobblestone patterns of the epidermis
Pagetoid melanocytosis	'Pagetoid' cells: bright round or dendritic cells in the spinous or granular cell layer
Atypical melanocytes	Cellular atypia: large bright cells +/- coarse dendritic processes
Increased density of solitary units	Increased number of bright cells, some of them with dendritic or roundish morphology at the dermal-epidermal junction
Disordered growth pattern of melanocytes in rete ridges	Non-edged papillae: dermal papillae without a demarcated rim of bright cells, but separated by a series of large reflecting cells
Discohesive nests, internally pleomorphic nests, or confluently aggregated melanocytes	Cell clusters with loose, dishomogenous or cerebriform morphology
Sheets of melanocytes	Sheet-like distribution of cells

Table 4.2 Pitfalls in the diagnosis of melanoma using RCM

RCM feature	*Pitfall*
'Pagetoid' cells in spinous layer	May mistake Langerhans cells for dendritic melanocytes May be benign pagetoid melanocytes of Spitz nevus, acral or traumatized/irritated nevus
Pigmented nest	May be a 'pseudonest' composed of pigmented keratinocytes (clonal seborrheic keratosis)
Non-edged papillae	May be present in nevi (dysplastic or Spitz nevi)

Key RCM features of in-situ melanoma

- Bright roung or dendritic cells in the spinous or granular cell layer (**'pagetoid' cells**)
- Increased number of bright cells, some of them with dendritic or roundish morphology, at the dermal-epidermal junction
- **Junctional thickenings** or **cell clusters** that are **loose** or **dishomogenous**
- Large bright cells with variable dendritic processes, including coarse processes (**cellular atypia**)
- Dermal papillae without a demarcated rim of bright cells, but separated by a series of large reflecting cells (**non-edged papillae**)
- Disarray of the normal architecture of the superficial layers of the epidermis; i.e., loss of the honeycomb and cobblestone pattern (**disarranged pattern**)
- Lentigo maligna type may show rare or no 'pagetoid' cells, but often shows disruption of the normal epidermal architecture at all levels including the DEJ, prominent coarse branching dendrites and atypical bright nucleated cells at the DEJ as confluent single cells and clusters with extension down adnexal structures.

Key RCM features of invasive melanoma

- RCM features of in-situ melanoma
- Individual atypical nucleated and reflective cells in the dermis
- **Dermal cell clusters** with **loose, dishomogeneous** or **cerebriform** morphology
- Cells in a **sheet-like distribution**
- Superficial spreading melanoma with a nodular component typically shows 'Pagetoid' infiltration and a disarranged pattern; about half have non-edged papillae
- Purely nodular melanoma contains few 'pagetoid' cells, little to no alteration of the epidermal architecture and non-edged papillae are infrequent
- Lentigo maligna melanoma may show few 'pagetoid' cells, but the epidermal architecture is usually disrupted; the transition from the confluent proliferatin of atypical cells at the DEJ to those within the dermis may be difficult to discern due to effacement of rate ridges

Key RCM features of amelanotic melanoma

- RCM features characteristic of the histological architectural subtype of melanoma, but composed of melanocytes that are only slightly reflective

Blue nevus

Key RCM features of blue nevus

- Normal/unaltered epidermis
- Brightly refractile, dendritic cells between collagen bundles in the dermis
- Scattered plump bright cells (melanophages) in the dermis

Spitz nevus

Key RCM features of Spitz nevus

- 'Pagetoid' melanocytosis, predominantly constituted by small dendritic cells
- Rim of dense cell clusters at the periphery
- Dense cell clusters distributed throughout the lesion
- Non-edged papillae and atypical cells in the basal layer and dermal–epidermal junction
- Regular roundish edged papillae
- Increased vascularity
- Large confluent irregular dermal clusters of reflective polygonal cells

Trichoepithelioma

Key RCM features of trichoepithelioma

- Dermal basaloid tumor cell islands tightly wrapped in stroma
- Brightly refractile stroma arranged in parallel bundles
- Horn cysts within tumor islands

Sebaceous hyperplasia

Key RCM features of sebaceous hyperplasia

- Dilated central follicular infundibulum
- Enlarged morula-like clusters of round cells with bright speckled cytoplasms (sebaceous lobules)
- Crown vessels

Dermatofibroma

Key RCM features of dermatofibroma

- Normal honeycomb or cobblestone pattern of the epidermis
- Increased density of bright dermal papillary rings
- Thickened, refractile collagen bundles
- Variable tethering of dermal papillary rings by sclerotic collagen bundles

Angioma

Key RCM features of cherry hemangioma

- Normal epidermis
- Dilated vascular lumina separated by thin septa in the upper dermis
- Blood cells moving briskly through the vascular lumina

Key RCM features of angiokeratoma

- Thickened stratum corneum
- Large, ectatic vascular lumina just below the DEJ
- Blood cells packing vascular lumina

Mycosis fungoides

Key RCM features of patch-type mycosis fungoides

- Small weakly refractile round-to-oval cells within the spinous layer
- Hyporefractile dermal papillary rings

Key RCM features of plaque-type mycosis fungoides

- Small weakly refractile round-to-oval cells scattered within the spinous layer
- Intraepidermal vesicle-like dark spaces filled with small, weakly refractile, round-to-oval cells
- Hyporefractile dermal papillary rings

Key RCM features of tumor-type mycosis fungoides

- Variable presence of small, weakly refractile, round-to-oval cells within the spinous layer
- Variable presence of intraepidermal vesicle-like dark spaces filled with small, weakly refractile, round-to-oval cells
- Variable presence of hyporefractile dermal papillary rings
- Variable presence of small, weakly refractile, round-to-oval cells filling the papillary dermis

Adjunct to clinical diagnosis

Key points for the use of RCM as an adjunct to clinical diagnosis

- RCM examination can increase the clinician's suspicion that a clinically and dermoscopically equivocal lesion is indeed skin cancer (i.e. increased sensitivity)
- RCM examination can increase the clinician's confidence that a lesion that appears clinically and dermoscopically banal is indeed benign (i.e. increased specificity)
- RCM may provide complementary information on nondescript lesions, resulting in an increased diagnostic accuracy and also impacting management

RCM-guided biopsy site selection

Key RCM features of RCM-guided biopsy site selection

- RCM allows one to screen several lesions at the cellular level for features that may be diagnostic histologically, increasing the likelihood of achieving a diagnostic and representative biopsy.
- RCM enables one to examine the entirety of a single large lesion at the cellular level for features that may be diagnostic histologically, helping to ensure that a small biopsy is representative of the lesion as a whole.
- RCM-guided biopsy may achieve specific diagnoses with fewer biopsies and thus enable earlier diagnosis and treatment.

RCM-assisted assessment of treatment response

Key RCM features of RCM to monitor treatment response

- RCM allows for in vivo monitoring of cutaneous disease longitudinally over time.
- RCM can assist in the management of skin cancer with either large extent (i.e. actinic field cancerization), or where the full extent of the lesion cannot be delineated easily (i.e. amelanotic melanoma).
- Indications for the use dof RCM to monitor treatment response:
  - When non-invasive therapies adre a viable alternative to surgical or other invasive treatment.
  - When residual or recurrent disease is not amenable to surgical resection.

RCM-assisted in-vivo margin mapping

Key steps for RCM-assisted in-vivo margin mapping

- Clinical inspection and palpation of the lesion
- Delineation of the lesion's border using Wood's lamp and dermoscopy
- Selection of foci for RCM examination inside and outside Wood's lamp and dermoscopy delineated border
- Refinement of the lesion's border based on RCM findings
- Histologic confirmation of RCM findings with paired punch biopsies
- Final refinement of the lesion's border based on histologic findings
- Mapping of definitive surgical margin
- Excision with appropriate margin of normal skin, confirmed by permanent histology using H&E and immunohistochemical stains

RCM-assisted ex-vivo margin assessment

Key features of RCM-assisted margin assessment

- Ex vivo RCM allows for detection of BCC and SCC in surgical excision margins without the need for frozen section histology.
- Pre-imaging tissue immersion in acetic acid enhances rapid detection of BCC.
- Ex vivo RCM evaluates true tumor margins (rather than trimmed) resulting in maximal conservation normal skin.
- Ex vivo RCM shows promise for future applications, such as confirmation of biopsy adequacy and intraoperative pathological consultation on tissue that is not amenable to frozen sectioning.

Index

Page numbers in *italics* indicate figures or tables.